Experimental Models in Serotonin Transporter Research

The serotonin transporter is a key brain protein that modulates the reuptake of the neurotransmitter serotonin from synaptic spaces back into the presynaptic neuron. In this book, an international team of top experts introduce and explicate the role of serotonin and the serotonin transporter in both human and animal brains. They demonstrate the relevance of the transporter and the serotonergic system to substrates of neuropsychiatric disorders, and explain how this knowledge is translated into valid animal models that will help foster new discoveries in human neurobiology. Writing for graduate students and academic researchers, they provide a comprehensive coverage of a wide spectrum of data from animal experimentation to clinical psychiatry, creating the only book exclusively dedicated to this exciting new avenue of brain research.

ALLAN V. KALUEFF is Assistant Professor of Physiology in the Department of Physiology and Biophysics at the Georgetown University Medical Center, Washington DC, USA. His research has been recognized by numerous prestigious scientific awards, and has focused on the role of the serotonin transporter as a contributor to neuropsychiatric disorders in various animal models.

JUSTIN L. LAPORTE worked at the National Institute of Mental Health (Bethesda, USA) and employed behavioral pharmacology and molecular genetics approaches to elucidate the pathogenetic mechanisms of psychiatric disorders with a specific focus on the role of the serotonin transporter.

Experimental Models in Serotonin Transporter Research

ALLAN V. KALUEFF
Georgetown University Medical Center

JUSTIN L. LAPORTE
National Institute of Mental Health

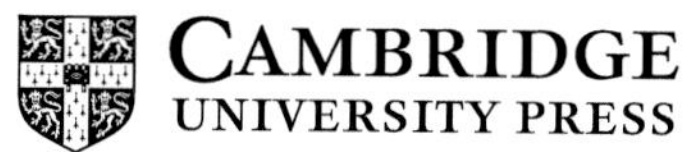

CAMBRIDGE
UNIVERSITY PRESS

University Printing House, Cambridge CB2 8BS, United Kingdom

One Liberty Plaza, 20th Floor, New York, NY 10006, USA

477 Williamstown Road, Port Melbourne, VIC 3207, Australia

314-321, 3rd Floor, Plot 3, Splendor Forum, Jasola District Centre, New Delhi - 110025, India

103 Penang Road, #05-06/07, Visioncrest Commercial, Singapore 238467

Cambridge University Press is part of the University of Cambridge.

It furthers the University's mission by disseminating knowledge in the pursuit of education, learning and research at the highest international levels of excellence.

www.cambridge.org
Information on this title: www.cambridge.org/9780521514873

First published 2010

A catalogue record for this publication is available from the British Library

Library of Congress Cataloging in Publication data
Experimental models in serotonin transporter research / [edited by] Allan V. Kalueff, Justin L. Laporte.
p. ; cm
Includes bibliographical references and index.
ISBN 978-0-521-51487-3 (hardback)
1. Serotonin. 2. Carrier proteins. 3. Serotoninergic mechanisms.
I. Kalueff, Allan V. II. LaPorte, Justin L. III. Title.
[DNLM: 1. Serotonin–metabolism. 2. Serotonin Plasma Membrane Transport Proteins–metabolism. 3. Disease Models, Animal. 4. Mental Disorders–drug therapy. 5. Models, Psychological. 6. Serotonin Uptake Inhibitors–pharmacology. QV 126 E976 2010]
QP364.7.E985 2010
612.8′042–dc22

2009015599

ISBN 978-0-521-51487-3 Hardback

Contents

The colour plates will be found between pages 84 and 85.

Contributors

Joëlle Adrien
INSERM and University Pierre and Marie Curie Paris

Chloé Alexandre
INSERM and University Pierre and Marie Curie Paris

Anne Milasincic Andrews
Pennsylvania State University

Lipa Cicin-Sain
Rudjer Boskovic Institute

Alexander Cools
UMC St. Radbout

Edwin Cuppen
Hubrecht Institute for Developmental Biology and Stem Cell Research

Bart Ellenbroek
University of Nijmegen

Tracey L. Gilman
Pennsylvania State University

F. Scott Hall
Molecular Neurobiology, NIDA, NIH

Khalisa N. Herman
NICHD, NIH

Judith Homberg
UMC St. Radboud

Branimir Jernej
Rudjer Boskovic Institute

Allan V. Kalueff
Georgetown University Medical Center

Justin L. LaPorte
NIMH, NIH

Clément Léna
Ecole Normale Supérieure and CNRS

Klaus Peter Lesch
University of Würzburg

Dennis L. Murphy
NIMH, NIH

Qian Li
University of Kansas

Beth A. Luellen
Pennsylvania State University

Jocelien Olivier
UMC St. Radbout

Maria T. G. Perona
NIDA, NIH

Antonio M. Persico
University "Campus Bio-Medico"

Daniela Popa
INSERM and University Pierre and Marie Curie Paris

Renee F. Ren-Patterson
NIMH, NIH

Etienne Sibille
University of Pittsburgh

Ichiro Sora
NIDA, NIH

Stephen J. Suomi
Laboratory for Comparative Ethology, NICHD, NIH

Adam Tripp
University of Pittsburgh

George R. Uhl
NIDA, NIH

James T. Winslow
NIMH, NIH

Preface: Focus on the serotonin transporter

The serotonin transporter (SERT) has gained research popularity due to its prominent role in normal and aberrant brain processes. This key brain protein reuptakes serotonin from the synaptic cleft into presynaptic neurons, thereby modulating serotonergic neurotransmission. An entire class of psychotropic drugs, the serotonin reuptake inhibitors (SRIs), is dedicated to the action of this single protein. The fact that selective SRIs are becoming the world's most prescribed psychotropic medication emphasizes the utmost importance of SERT research for clinical psychiatry. The growing body of knowledge on SERT's role in the brain also emphasizes the need for experimental models of SERT function. Collectively, this has stimulated the compilation of this book, the aim of which is to provide a comprehensive update spanning the breadth of SERT research from animal models to their clinical parallels.

Although the exact functional mechanisms of SERT are not yet fully elucidated, it is thought to contain 12 hydrophobic transmembrane domains and to bind Na^+, Cl^-, and serotonin simultaneously. This results in a conformational change in the molecule, forming a barrier against the exterior of the cell, and opens the protein inwardly to the cytoplasmic membrane. The serotonin then disassociates from SERT, and the transporter returns to its original conformation receptive to extracellular serotonin once again. This process is the main mechanism of serotonin modulation in the brain, and the dysregulation of this system can affect brain and behavior markedly.

Genetic studies have also implicated SERT in many psychiatric disorders, including anxiety, major depression, cognitive dysfunctions, bipolar disorder, autism, and obsessive compulsive disorder. As will be discussed further in the book, genetic heterogeneity, phenotypic diversity, and gene $\times$ environment interactions contribute to the complexity of clinical and animal phenotypes. For example, a strong correlation between the SERT genetic variants and stressful life events indicates that SERT plays a key role in stress responses, which makes modeling these clinically relevant scenarios an important goal in neurobehavioral research.

Since human geneticists have identified the SERT gene, neurogeneticists have identified different polymorphisms, and their behavioral and neurobiological effects. Human SERT gene is 37.8 kb, and is located on chromosome 17q11.2. There are several known polymorphisms of the gene, some of which are exclusive to humans and non-human primates. Two major variants of the SERT promoter region, a "long" (L) allele and a "short" (S) allele, differentially modulate the activity of the SERT promoter region, and therefore the activity of the protein. Numerous studies have consistently confirmed that the S allelic variant results in lower expression and diminished function of SERT, which leads to altered responses to SRI treatment. In contrast, the individuals with the LL genotype were more sensitive to SRI antidepressants in different groups of patients with depression. Thus, the implementation of different genetic methods has begun to shed light on SERT's role in developing better treatments for psychiatric disorders.

The chapters collected in this book aim to reflect all these developments. Since altered serotonergic functioning is the neurochemical basis for many psychotropic drugs, the first two chapters summarize molecular synaptic adaptive responses to chronic antidepressant treatment. They will focus on alterations in SERT expression, extracellular and intracellular serotonin levels, and serotonergic innervation. The chapters will next contrast these data with studies on constitutive loss of SERT gene expression, and discuss whether presynaptic neuroadaptive responses are sufficient to explain the paradoxical increases in trait anxiety that accompany constitutive reductions in SERT expression in animals.

Since serotonin plays a critical role in brain development, chapter 3 will review the current knowledge of SERT's influence during the developmental stages. This chapter will concentrate on the trophic effects of serotonin cell development in mammals, and cover the role of SERT in brain development, neural plasticity, synaptogenesis, and cell proliferation. The available rodent experimental models will be discussed, as well as the clinical and translational implications for human neurodevelopment.

Continuing with the rodent models, there is also a chapter on behavioral and genomic correlates of targeted genetic manipulations in the mouse, with a focus on SERT and its role in emotional disorders. The chapter will also address the limitations and advantages of knock-down, knock-out, and over-expressing SERT for modeling aspects of anxiety-like and depression-related behaviors in rodents with regards to gender, genetic risk factors, and environmental modifiers.

Along this line, chapter 5 will more specifically focus on depression-like behaviors in mice in relation to SERT. The chapter will detail many rodent models of depression, and will discuss how they are created through genetic and epigenetic manipulations involving SERT. Special attention will be given to the biological and behavioral manifestations of SERT alterations, particularly examining the role of early-life serotonin in depression. The authors put forth an interesting developmental hypothesis of SERT dysfunction and examine its utility for translational research.

The book's next chapter will review a unique SERT knock-out rat model, covering experimental approaches in a slew of different paradigms, ranging from pharmacological phenotypes to social behaviors. Important comparisons will be made in a separate, but related, contribution on rats with high and low activity of platelet SERT phenotypes. Selective breeding for extreme values of platelet serotonin levels produced two sublines of rats with constitutional hyper and hypo-serotonemia. The chapter will discuss the changes in serotonin homeostasis in relation to the neurochemical, pharmacological, and behavioral phenotypes in these rats.

Addressing a more specific behavioral domain, chapter 8 will discuss how psychiatric disorders affect the reward system and related phenotypes. This chapter will specifically focus on the role of serotonin and SERT in mouse drug reward paradigms, also discussing the interaction between the serotonergic and dopaminergic systems in this domain. The chapter will also explain how SERT genetic variation may contribute to individual differences in response to drugs of abuse, as part of the polygenic and heterogeneous genetic basis of addiction.

While the previous chapters have focused on the genetic manipulations with SERT in animals, this can also be combined with other mutations: for example, with brain-derived neurotrophic factor (BDNF) gene. Several clinical reports have shown that SERT and BDNF genes may interact and co-determine psychiatric phenotypes. Chapter 9 will cover the relationship of SERT and BDNF, paralleling clinical data and experimental models such as SERT and SERT × BDNF knock-out mice. Emphasis will be put on SERT and BDNF genetic polymorphisms and their biomolecular effect on protein expression and neuronal survival, as well as the role of these interactions in the development of neuropsychiatric disorders.

Usefully complementing the rodent models, a chapter on SERT in non-human primates will make another step towards creating cross-species bridges between animal and human data. As clinical data link polymorphisms in the SERT gene with environmental risk factors of depression, anxiety, antisocial and borderline personality disorders, as well as substance abuse, investigations with the rhesus monkey reveal similar gene–environment interactions. This chapter will review the history of primate models in SERT research, and highlight the interaction between early experience and the resulting changes in behavior that are found in conjunction with alterations in serotonergic functioning.

The book's final chapter provides a logical recap that focuses on the application of basic research to the clinical field. The author addresses the topic of innate SERT variability from numerous experimental perspectives, emphasizing how the formerly distinct realms of social and biological sciences are now merging into a discipline of biosocial science. The chapter will address these new developments in relation to SERT research, and how they utilize techniques such as neuroimaging to ascertain the neurobiological substrates of the genetic variations, thereby providing new perspectives and hypotheses for clarifying the epigenetic mechanisms of brain disorders.

Overall, the collected chapters provide an excellent scholarly summary of neuroscientific investigations of SERT. The book caters to an international audience of basic and clinical neuroscientists who would like to gain knowledge in this rapidly developing field. Similarly, while providing an important update to professional researchers in the disciplines of psychology, biology, and neuroscience, the text will also remain accessible to students studying different topics of biological psychiatry.

Finally, the valuable contribution of the National Alliance for Research on Schizophrenia and Depression (NARSAD) – the world's leading charity dedicated to mental health research – must be acknowledged. NARSAD has an established history of promoting education and research on neuropsychiatric disorders, and the YI Award from this organization has been pivotal to the creation of this book. We take this opportunity to thank NARSAD for their important work, and hope that this multidisciplinary book on SERT will become yet another contribution to advancing translational neuroscience and biological psychiatry.

A.V. Kalueff and J.L. LaPorte
Washington DC

BETH A. LUELLEN, TRACY L. GILMAN AND
ANNE MILASINCIC ANDREWS

1

Presynaptic adaptive responses to constitutive versus adult pharmacologic inhibition of serotonin uptake

ABSTRACT

Many antidepressants are believed to relieve depressed mood and excessive anxiety by inhibiting the reuptake of serotonin so as to cause increases in extracellular serotonin. This homeostatic alteration is thought to underlie further adaptive processes – which have not been fully clarified – that together constitute the cellular mechanisms of current antidepressant therapy. Here, we review the literature on presynaptic adaptive responses to chronic antidepressant treatment, focusing on alterations in serotonin transporter (SERT) expression, extracellular and intracellular serotonin levels, and serotonergic innervation. We contrast this with studies on constitutive loss of SERT gene expression. A partial genetic reduction in SERT expression results in modest increases in extracellular serotonin, while the total absence of SERT is associated with substantial increases in extracellular serotonin, decreases in intracellular serotonin, and a reduction in serotonin immunopositive cell bodies and axons in the dorsal raphe and hippocampus, respectively. Adaptive changes in SERT protein levels and extracellular and intracellular serotonin concentrations following many different regimens of chronic antidepressant administration were found to be more variable, often falling in between those resulting from partial and complete genetic ablation of SERT. This might reflect incomplete pharmacologic inhibition of SERT and the wide variety of drug administration paradigms utilized. The microdialysis literature, in particular, suggests that it is difficult to conclude that chronic antidepressant

Experimental Models in Serotonin Transporter Research, eds. A. V. Kalueff and J. L. LaPorte.
Published by Cambridge University Press.

treatment reliably causes elevated extracellular serotonin. However, with the exception of immunocytochemical studies, which were few and reported opposing findings, presynaptic adaptations occurring in response to antidepressants were qualitatively similar to those resulting from constitutive reductions in SERT. Thus, these particular presynaptic neuroadaptive responses by themselves are not sufficient to explain paradoxical increases in trait anxiety that accompany constitutive reductions in SERT expression in mice, rats, and humans.

INTRODUCTION

Long-term reduction in the recapture of serotonin (5-HT) from the extracellular space by the serotonin transporter (SERT) is a powerful adaptive force and the mechanisms of many antidepressants are believed to involve chronic SERT inhibition. However, changes in emotionally related behavior in response to reduced uptake occurring over different periods of life are dichotomous. Pharmacologic inhibition of SERT decreases anxiety and depressive symptoms in the subset of adult patients who respond to commonly prescribed antidepressants. By contrast, constitutive reductions in SERT expression occurring throughout development are correlated with increased anxiety-related behavior in mice (Holmes *et al.*, 2003a, 2003b) and heightened personality traits associated with negative emotionality in humans (Greenberg *et al.*, 2000; Lesch *et al.*, 1996; Schinka *et al.*, 2004; Sen *et al.*, 2004).

In this chapter, we examine the impact of genetically driven SERT deficiency on the neurochemistry of the presynaptic serotonergic system in rodent models. We compare this scenario to the relatively larger and more complex picture of presynaptic serotonergic responses to chronic antidepressant administration in adult animals. We focus on adaptations in the expression of SERT itself, effects on extracellular and intracellular serotonin levels, and changes in serotonergic neuronal architecture. Along with numerous studies published by many different authors, we integrate the results of our own studies on serotonin neurochemistry in SERT-deficient mice and present new data on the effects of reduced SERT expression on serotonergic innervation of the adult hippocampus. Our goal in analyzing and comparing these two bodies of literature is to determine whether differences in the effects of constitutive versus adult pharmacologic uptake inhibition on presynaptic neurochemistry provide a basis for understanding divergent phenotypic outcomes.

SEROTONIN TRANSPORTER EXPRESSION

Three different groups of investigators have produced mice with constitutive decreases in SERT expression (Bengel *et al.*, 1998; Lira *et al.*, 2003; Zhao *et al.*, 2006). SERT-deficient mice have been used to study the effects of reduced serotonin uptake on pre- and postsynaptic function with the goal of increasing information about the role of serotonin in modulating a number of important behaviors. Targeted disruption of exon 2, which contains the SERT gene start codon, results in a gene dose-dependent loss of full-length SERT mRNA (Bengel *et al.*, 1998). A truncated SERT message continues to be transcribed, which is translated into a non-functional and abnormally trafficked protein (Ravary *et al.*, 2001). In our initial study, SERT binding sites were assessed by quantitative autoradiography using [^{125}I]RTI-55, a cocaine analog with high affinity for SERT (Andrews *et al.*, 1996; Bengel *et al.*, 1997), in mice on a mixed 129 × CD-1 background (Bengel *et al.*, 1998). A 50% reduction in SERT density occurred in SERT+/− mice across a wide range of brain regions, while the complete absence of SERT was observed in null mutant mice (Figure 1.1; Bengel *et al.*, 1998; Perez *et al.*, 2006). A 50% decrease and a complete lack in SERT binding have also been reported in the CA3 region of the hippocampus of SERT+/− and SERT−/− mice, respectively, using the radiolabeled antidepressant [^{3}H]cyanoimipramine (Montanez *et al.*, 2003). These mice were produced from the same founders as mice initially reported by Bengel and coworkers, but they had been bred onto a C57BL/6J background. Sora and coworkers reported on SERT labeled by [^{3}H]paroxetine in SERT-deficient mice in the C57BL/6J background that had been cross-bred with mice deficient in the dopamine transporter (DAT; Sora *et al.*, 2001). Here, DAT+/+ × SERT+/− mice showed a ~50% decrease in SERT binding and SERT was not detected in DAT+/+ × SERT−/− mice. In mice generated independently using a similar gene inactivation strategy but bred onto a 129S6/SvEv background, autoradiography of brain sections with [^{125}I]DAM (5-iodo-2−[[2-2-[dimethylamino)methyl]phenyl]thio]benzyl alcohol) showed undetectable levels of SERT in SERT−/− mice compared to wildtype littermates (Lira *et al.*, 2003). Zhao *et al.* used a different gene targeting strategy to produce mice with a disruption of the C-terminus of the SERT gene in a 129S5 × C57BL/6J hybrid background (2006). Homozygous mutant mice also showed a complete loss of SERT analyzed by saturation binding with [^{3}H]citalopram in brain tissue homogenates (Zhao *et al.*, 2006).

The selectivity of two additional SERT ligands, AFM ([^{3}H]2-[2-(dimethylaminomethylphenylthio)]-5-fluoromethylphenylamine) and

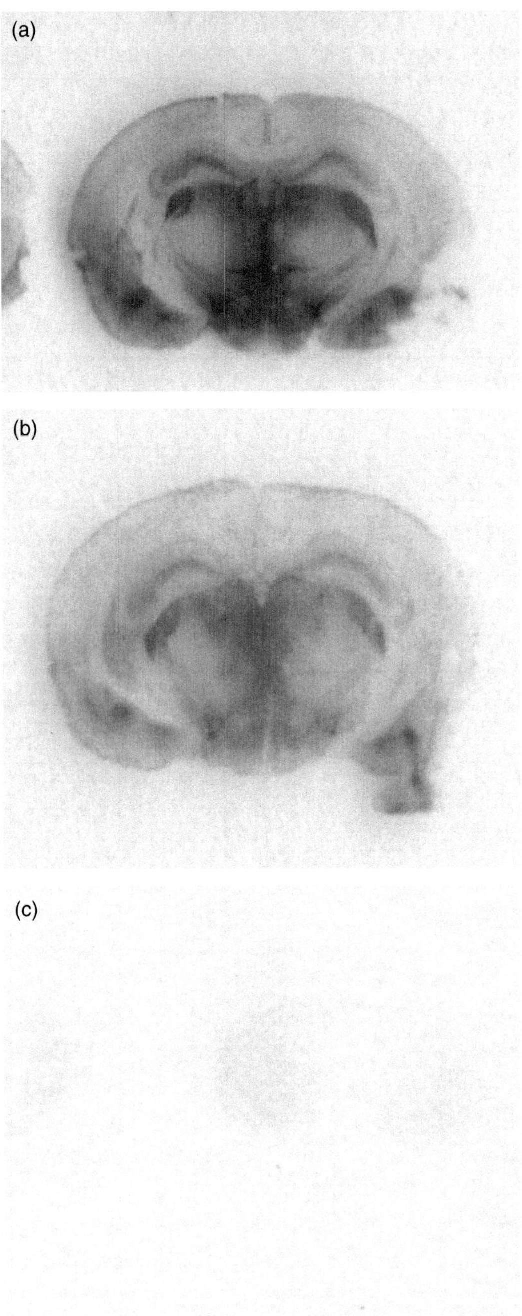

Figure 1.1 Serotonin transporter autoradiography in mice with constitutive Reductions in SERT. The cocaine analog [^{125}I]RTI-55 was used

DASB ([^{3}H]3-amino-4-[2-(dimethylaminomethylphenylthio)]benzonitrile), recently developed for positron emission tomography (PET) imaging, has been investigated by autoradiography in mice lacking one or both copies of the SERT gene (Li *et al.*, 2004). High densities of [^{3}H]AFM and [^{3}H]DASB binding were observed in the hippocampus, thalamus, raphe nuclei, and locus coeruleus of SERT+/+ mice. SERT+/− mice exhibited reduced binding to ~50% of that detected in wildtype mice. As anticipated, no binding was observed for either ligand in any of the brain regions analyzed in SERT−/− mice (Li *et al.*, 2004). Thus, there is agreement among published studies that intact serotonin transporter protein labeled by many different radioligands is reduced in a gene dose-dependent manner in SERT-deficient mice generated by alternate strategies in a variety of genetic backgrounds.

Many studies have been conducted that have assessed the effects of long-term pharmacologic inhibition of serotonin reuptake on SERT protein levels. Here, the majority of studies conclude that a reduction in SERT occurs after chronic administration of selective serotonin reuptake inhibitors (SSRIs) to mice (Hirano *et al.*, 2005; Mirza *et al.*, 2007) or rats (Benmansour *et al.*, 1999, 2002; Brunello *et al.*, 1987; Gould *et al.*, 2006, 2007; Horschitz *et al.*, 2001; Kovachich *et al.*, 1992; Pineyro *et al.*, 1994; Rossi *et al.*, 2008; Watanabe *et al.*, 1993). In these studies, SERT protein levels or binding sites have been evaluated by Western blot and immunochemistry or quantitative autoradiography, respectively. Decreases in SERT are reportedly widespread, occurring in subregions of the hippocampus (CA2, CA3 and dentate gyrus), the basolateral and central nuclei of the amygdala, (fronto)parietal cortex, perirhinal cortex, striatum, thalamus, and midbrain (Benmansour *et al.*, 1999, 2002; Gould *et al.*, 2006, 2007; Hirano *et al.*, 2005; Kovachich *et al.*, 1992; Mirza *et al.*, 2007; Pineyro *et al.*, 1994; Rossi *et al.*, 2008; Watanabe *et al.*, 1993). From these data, it appears that reductions in SERT occur in

Caption for Figure 1.1 (cont.)
to label serotonin transporter (SERT) binding sites in wildtype mice (a), mice lacking one intact copy of the SERT gene (b), and mice lacking both intact SERT gene copies (c). Representative coronal sections are shown at the level of the rostral hippocampus. Densitometric analyses (Bengel *et al.*, 1998; Perez and Andrews, 2005) have shown that SERT binding is reduced by ~50% in all brain regions in SERT+/− mice compared to SERT+/+ mice, and is not detected in any brain region in SERT−/− mice.

projection networks originating from both the dorsal and median raphe nuclei.

However, not all reports show decreased SERT levels in response to chronic SSRI administration. An early study by Hrdina and Vu (1993) reported that chronic treatment of rats with fluoxetine resulted in an increase in SERT labeling in cortical areas and the CA1 region of hippocampus, and a smaller increase in the superior colliculus. Some of these are the same regions where others have reported reductions in SERT protein levels. A number of studies have reported no change in SERT following long-term administration of the SSRI citalopram to rats (Cheetham *et al.*, 1993; Gobbi *et al.*, 1997; Gould *et al.*, 2006; Graham *et al.*, 1987; Kovachich *et al.*, 1992), with the exception of one study where a decrease in SERT levels following citalopram was observed (Brunello *et al.*, 1987). Interestingly, two of these same studies also noted reductions in SERT following chronic treatment with a different SSRI, sertraline (Gould *et al.*, 2006; Kovachich *et al.*, 1992). Interestingly, tianeptine, which is reported to be a serotonin reuptake enhancer, was also found to decrease SERT binding in cortex and hippocampus (Watanabe *et al.*, 1993).

In addition to in vivo experiments, the regulation of SERT by antidepressant treatment has been investigated in in vitro systems (Iceta *et al.*, 2007; Lau *et al.*, 2008). Iceta and coworkers studied an enterocyte-like cell line that natively expresses human SERT (2007). Their results showed that four consecutive days of treatment with fluoxetine reduced plasma membrane SERT without altering total SERT protein or mRNA levels. Similarly, in a recent study by Lau *et al.* (2008), citalopram treatment of human SERT-transfected HEK293 kidney cells resulted in the time-dependent translocation of SERT to intracellular compartments. Following treatment of murine stem cell-derived serotonergic neurons ($1C11^{5HT}$ cells) with citalopram, SERT was similarly internalized, in addition to being relocated from neurite extensions to cell bodies, without affecting cell morphology or neurite outgrowth (Lau *et al.*, 2008). Citalopram-free medium initiated the movement of SERT from the soma back to neurites and the same SERT reappeared on the cell surface, as evidenced by co-treatment with a protein synthesis inhibitor. In addition to providing new information about the mechanisms by which antidepressants modulate SERT, the results of these studies raise the possibility that earlier discrepancies regarding the effects of chronic antidepressant treatment on SERT expression may be due to methodological issues involving the labeling of SERT localized to different subcellular compartments. A number of intracellular signaling mechanisms have been reported to regulate SERT surface expression, including protein kinase C (Qian *et al.*, 1997; Ramamoorthy *et al.*, 1998). Substrates and antagonists of SERT, such as serotonin and antidepressants, respectively, mediate PKC-dependent SERT phosphorylation and the redistribution of cell-surface SERT (Blakely *et al.*, 2005; Ramamoorthy and Blakely, 1999). Therefore, additional experiments will be needed to differentiate SERT localized to different subcellular compartments and to address how changes in specific populations of SERT occur in response to chronic antidepressant treatment, particularly in vivo.

A number of additional factors come into play when interpreting data from studies on antidepressant-induced regulation of SERT. These include the possibility that specific SSRIs (or tricyclic antidepressants) have different effects, as evidenced in studies performed by two different groups (Gould *et al.*, 2006; Kovachich *et al.*, 1992). In addition, the route of administration is a consideration. For instance, Hrdina and Vu (1993) and Gobbi *et al.* (1997) both administered fluoxetine to rats for 21 days; however, the drug was given intraperitoneally and perorally, respectively. Differences in routes of administration might underlie some of the conflicting data resulting from these two studies. An additional issue involves whether drug levels in preclinical studies reach steady-state human therapeutic serum concentrations. In rodents, the half-lives of many antidepressants are significantly shorter than in humans (Fredricson Overo, 1982; Hiemke and Hartter, 2000; Melzacka *et al.*, 1984). The use of osmotic minipumps circumvents problems associated with metabolism, and many investigators have incorporated the use of these devices for this reason (Benmansour *et al.*, 1999, 2002; Gould *et al.*, 2006, 2007; Hirano *et al.*, 2005; Koed and Linnet, 1997; Lesch *et al.*, 1993; Neumaier *et al.*, 1996; Pineyro *et al.*, 1994). Interestingly, the majority of studies that did not utilize osmotic minipumps reported increases (Hrdina and Vu, 1993) or no change (Cheetham *et al.*, 1993; Gobbi *et al.*, 1997; Graham *et al.*, 1987; Spurlock *et al.*, 1994; Swan *et al.*, 1997) in SERT protein levels following chronic SSRI treatment with the exception of two studies (Kovachich *et al.*, 1992; Mirza *et al.*, 2007), as opposed to consistent decreases in SERT protein or binding reported in studies employing minipump administration.

The time between the cessation of drug treatment and the measurement of SERT, otherwise known as the washout period, may also influence results. Moreover, it will be important to understand whether the effects of chronic antidepressant treatment cause global changes in SERT expression, similar to those occurring in genetic models, or whether specific brain regions are modulated differently by pharmacologic inhibition of SERT. In summary, it seems that consensus has not been reached regarding the most appropriate methods for administering antidepressants, so as to determine more clearly how long-lasting inhibition of serotonin reuptake modulates serotonin transporter protein levels and dynamic regulation of subcellular SERT distribution in the brain.

At the level of transcription, reports on the regulation of SERT following long-term administration of antidepressants are inconsistent. A number of groups have reported no change in SERT mRNA levels after chronic administration of SSRIs to rats (Benmansour *et al.*, 1999; Koed and Linnet, 1997; Spurlock *et al.*, 1994; Swan *et al.*, 1997), or treatment of cells expressing human SERT (Iceta *et al.*, 2007), or murine stem cell-derived serotonergic neuron cells (Lau *et al.*, 2008). By contrast, Benmansour and colleagues found that 21 days of treatment with 10 mg/kg paroxetine via osmotic minipumps in rats had no effect on SERT mRNA levels in the median raphe; however, it resulted in a trend toward an increase in SERT mRNA in the dorsal raphe nucleus as quantified by in situ hybridization histochemistry (Benmansour *et al.*, 1999). In a later study, this group found that sertraline administration (7.5 mg/kg for 10 days) increased SERT mRNA levels by approximately 30% in the dorsal raphe, but these levels returned to baseline after 21 days of treatment (Benmansour *et al.*, 2002). Together, these two studies suggest that chronic antidepressant treatment regulates SERT transcription in the dorsal raphe nucleus, one of the main nuclei containing the serotonergic cell bodies that project to many areas of the forebrain. They also imply that changes in SERT mRNA may be transient, possibly explaining why no changes in SERT mRNA levels have been reported in other studies where intermediate time points were not investigated. Neumaier and coworkers also observed temporally related changes in SERT mRNA levels; however, in this study, chronic fluoxetine treatment (3 mg/kg/day) in rats via osmotic minipumps resulted in decreased SERT mRNA in the dorsal raphe after 7 days of treatment, with mRNA returning to control levels after 21 days of fluoxetine as determined by in situ hybridization (Neumaier *et al.*, 1996). Although Benmansour *et al.* and Neumaier *et al.* reported that the subchronic effects of antidepressant treatment on SERT mRNA levels changed in opposite directions, both studies point to the possibility of time-dependent alterations in SERT mRNA occurring after the initiation of antidepressant administration. In another study by Lesch and colleagues, a decrease in SERT mRNA levels (~30%) in the rat midbrain raphe complex was observed by Northern blot following treatment with fluoxetine (2.5 mg/kg) via osmotic minipump for 21 days (Lesch *et al.*, 1993). These results conflict with the other studies described above. Thus, regulation of SERT at the transcriptional level by chronic inhibition of serotonin reuptake is not fully understood. Here, inconsistencies in the results of the studies discussed are not due to a lack of steady-state drug levels since osmotic minipumps were used to deliver drugs in all cases.

Tricyclic antidepressants have also been investigated with regard to the role they play in the regulation of SERT mRNA, and the data are similarly lacking in agreement. For example, following chronic treatment of rats with imipramine, SERT mRNA levels were reported to increase (Lopez *et al.*, 1994), to decrease (Lesch *et al.*, 1993), or not to change (Burnet *et al.*, 1994; Koed and Linnet, 1997; Spurlock *et al.*, 1994) compared to levels in animals treated with vehicle. Chronic treatment with the atypical antidepressant tianeptine resulted in decreased SERT mRNA (Kuroda *et al.*, 1994). The use of in situ hybridization versus Northern blotting cannot be correlated with upregulation, downregulation, or a lack of effect on SERT mRNA, suggesting that these disparities do not arise from methodological issues. The studies discussed here are by no means exhaustive with regard to reports on the regulation of SERT mRNA by long-term antidepressant administration. However, they highlight some of the discrepancies in this area and indicate that there is much to learn before we understand how pharmacologic inhibition of 5-HT reuptake regulates SERT at the level of transcription, in addition to protein levels and membrane trafficking.

EXTRACELLULAR SEROTONIN LEVELS

Antidepressants including SSRIs, mixed serotonin and norepinephrine reuptake inhibitors (SNRIs), and tricyclic antidepressants are thought to act by blocking the reuptake of serotonin and/or norepinephrine at their respective transporters. This inhibition is hypothesized to increase extracellular neurotransmitter levels, which results in the alleviation of anxiety and depressive symptoms in some patients by additional adaptive mechanisms that have yet to be fully elucidated. Studies in mice constitutively lacking both copies of the SERT gene support the idea that the loss of serotonin reuptake results in elevated extracellular levels of 5-HT. Compared to wildtype mice, dialysate 5-HT levels were increased in SERT−/− mice in frontal cortex, striatum (Mathews *et al.*, 2004; Shen *et al.*, 2004; Trigo *et al.*, 2007), and ventral hippocampus (Whittington and Virag, 2006) as determined by in vivo microdialysis. Rats constitutively lacking SERT have also been reported to possess significantly increased amounts of dialysate 5-HT levels in the ventral hippocampus (Homberg *et al.*, 2007). Conversely, mice overexpressing SERT exhibit decreased extracellular 5-HT (Jennings *et al.*, 2006). Thus, constitutive absence of functional SERT protein results in augmented extracellular 5-HT levels in adult animals, while increased expression of SERT appears to diminish levels of extracellular 5-HT. On the contrary, chronic administration of antidepressants and, in particular, those purported to block the action of SERT have not resulted consistently in similar findings.

Many microdialysis studies have been carried out in rats to investigate the effects of chronic antidepressant treatment on dialysate 5-HT levels, with only one study having been conducted in mice (Gardier *et al.*, 2003). Table 1.1, which is organized by brain region, summarizes this literature and reveals the substantial disagreement that exists with regard to the effects of chronic antidepressants on dialysate 5-HT levels. For example, in the hippocampus, four studies reported increases (Gundlah *et al.*, 1997; Hajos-Korcsok *et al.*, 2000; Kreiss and Lucki, 1995; Wegener *et al.*, 2003), while the majority of studies carried out in this brain region found no change in basal dialysate 5-HT following long-term antidepressant administration (Bosker *et al.*, 1995a, 1995b; Gardier *et al.*, 2003; Hjorth and Auerbach, 1999; Invernizzi *et al.*, 1995; Keck *et al.*, 2005; Tachibana *et al.*, 2006). The most striking discrepancies are observed in studies using SSRIs, including citalopram (Gundlah *et al.*, 1997; Hjorth and Auerbach, 1994, 1999; Invernizzi *et al.*, 1995; Wegener *et al.*, 2003), fluoxetine (Kreiss and Lucki, 1995), fluvoxamine (Bosker *et al.*, 1995a, 1995b; Tachibana *et al.*, 2006), and paroxetine (Gardier *et al.*, 2003; Hajos-Korcsok *et al.*, 2000; Keck *et al.*, 2005). Chronic administration of tricyclic antidepressants (Gur *et al.*, 1999b; Hajos-Korcsok *et al.*, 2000; Newman *et al.*, 2000) and SNRIs (Gur *et al.*, 1999a, 2002a; Tachibana *et al.*, 2006) more consistently show no increase in hippocampal dialysate 5-HT levels.

In the hippocampus, discrepancies cannot be explained by the specific subregions investigated. For example, no changes in 5-HT levels after all classes of antidepressants have been observed in both the dorsal (Bosker *et al.*, 1995a, 1995b; Hjorth and Auerbach, 1994, 1999; Invernizzi *et al.*, 1995; Keck *et al.*, 2005; Tachibana *et al.*, 2006) and the ventral hippocampus (Gardier *et al.*, 2003; Gur *et al.*, 1999a, 1999b, 2002a; Newman *et al.*, 2000). Washout times are also not likely to be responsible for the discrepancies. The majority of hippocampal studies

Table 1.1. *Effects of different antidepressant drugs on dialysate 5-HT levels.*

Class	Drug	Dose (mg/kg/day)	ROA[1]	Days	Dialysate 5-HT[2]	Reference
Hippocampus						
SSRI	Citalopram	5 × 2	sc	14	nc	Hjorth and Auerbach (1994)
		10 × 2	sc	14	↑	Gundlah *et al.* (1997)
		10 × 2	sc	14	nc	Hjorth and Auerbach (1999)
		10 × 2	sc	14	nc	Invernizzi *et al.* (1995)
		20	minipump	21	↑	Wegener *et al.* (2003)
	Fluoxetine	15	ip	14	↑	Kreiss and Lucki (1995)
	Fluvoxamine	6.7	minipump	23	nc	Bosker *et al.* (1995b)
		30	oral	14	nc	Tachibana *et al.* (2006)
		30	oral	14	nc	Bosker *et al.* (1995a)
	Paroxetine	1	minipump	14	nc[a]	Gardier *et al.* (2003)
		5	oral	70	nc	Keck *et al.* (2005)
		5	sc	14	↑, nc[b]	Hajos-Korcsok *et al.* (2000)
TCA	Clomipramine	10	ip	28	nc	Gur *et al.* (1999b)
		10	minipump	28	nc	Newman *et al.* (2000)
	Desipramine	10	sc	14	nc	Hajos-Korcsok *et al.* (2000)
		15	ip	14	nc	Kreiss and Lucki (1995)
SNRI	Milnacipran	30	oral	14	nc	Tachibana *et al.* (2006)
	Venlafaxine	5	ip	28	nc	Gur *et al.* (1999a)
		5	minipump	28	nc	Gur *et al.* (2002a)

Table 1.1. (cont.)

Class	Drug	Dose (mg/kg/day)	ROA[1]	Days	Dialysate 5-HT[2]	Reference
Frontal cortex						
SSRI	Citalopram	5 × 2	sc	14	nc	Hjorth and Auerbach (1999)
		10	ip	14	↑	Golembiowska and Dziubina (2000)
		10 × 2	sc	14	nc	Gundlah *et al.* (1997)
		10 × 2	sc	14	nc	Hjorth and Auerbach (1999)
		20	minipump	13	↑	Ceglia *et al.* (2004)
		20	ip	14	↑, nc[c]	Arborelius *et al.* (1996)
	Fluoxetine	3	minipump	14	↑	Amargos-Bosch *et al.* (2005)
		3	minipump	14	↑, nc[d]	Hervas *et al.* (2001)
		5	ip	7	nc	Lifschytz *et al.* (2004)
		5	ip	12	↑	Newman *et al.* (2004)
		10	ip	11–12	↑	Gartside *et al.* (2003)
		10	ip	14	nc	Dawson *et al.* (2000)
		10	ip	14	nc	Dawson *et al.* (2002)
		10	ip	14	↑	Invernizzi *et al.* (1996)
		10	ip	14	↑, nc[e]	Johnson *et al.* (2007)
		10	oral	21	↑	Mitchell *et al.* (2001)
	Fluvoxamine	1	minipump	7	↑	Bel and Artigas (1993)
	Paroxetine	0.5 × 2	ip	14	nc	Malagie *et al.* (2000)
		1	minipump	14	nc[a]	Gardier *et al.* (2003)
		10	ip	14	↑	Owen and Whitton (2006)
		10	ip	21	↑	Owen and Whitton (2005)

TCA	Clomipramine	10	ip	14	↑	Owen and Whitton (2006)
		10	ip	21	↑	Owen and Whitton (2005)
		10	ip	28	↑	Gur *et al.* (1999b)
	Imipramine	4	minipump	14	↑	Bel and Artigas (1996)
		10	minipump	28	nc	Gur *et al.* (2002b)
SNRI	Duloxetine	6.25	oral	14	nc	Kihara and Ikeda (1995)
	Venlafaxine	5	ip	28	nc	Gur *et al.* (1999a)
		10	minipump	14	↑	Wikell *et al.* (2002)
NRI	Reboxetine	10	ip	14	↑	Owen and Whitton (2006)
		10	ip	21	↑	Owen and Whitton (2005)
		10	minipump	14	nc	Page and Lucki (2002)
		10 (13)[f]	minipump	14	nc	Invernizzi *et al.* (2001)
MAO	Tranylcypromine	0.5	minipump	14	↑	Ferrer and Artigas (1994)
Other	Tianeptine	5 × 2	ip	14	nc	Malagie *et al.* (2000)
	$LiCO_3$	0.2%[g]	oral	7	nc	Kitaichi *et al.* (2005)
Hypothalamus						
SSRI	Citalopram	50	oral	21	↑, nc[h]	Moret and Briley (1996)
	Fluoxetine	5	ip	7	nc	Lifschytz *et al.* (2004)
		5	ip	12	nc	Newman *et al.* (2004)
		10	ip	14	↑	Rutter *et al.* (1994)
	Paroxetine	10	ip	21	nc	Sayer *et al.* (1999)
TCA	Clomipramine	10	minipump	28	↑	Newman *et al.* (2000)
	Desipramine	10	ip	21	nc	Sayer *et al.* (1999)
	Imipramine	10	minipump	28	nc	Gur *et al.* (2004)

Table 1.1. (cont.)

Class	Drug	Dose (mg/kg/day)	ROA[1]	Days	Dialysate 5-HT[2]	Reference
SNRI	Venlafaxine	5	minipump	28	nc	Gur *et al.* (2002a)
Striatum						
SSRI	Fluoxetine	10	ip	14	↑	Rossi *et al.* (2008)
		15	ip	14	↑	Kreiss and Lucki (1995)
	Sertraline	10	minipump	21	nc	Rossi *et al.* (2008)
TCA	Desipramine	15	ip	14	↑	Kreiss and Lucki (1995)
NRI	Reboxetine	15	ip	14	nc	Sacchetti *et al.* (1999)
Raphe nuclei						
SSRI	Fluvoxamine	1	minipump	7	nc	Bel and Artigas (1993)
		30	oral	14	nc	Bosker *et al.* (1995a)
	Paroxetine	0.5×2	ip	14	↑	Malagie *et al.* (2000)
TCA	Imipramine	4	minipump	14	nc	Bel and Artigas (1996)
MAO	Tranylcypromine	0.5	minipump	14	↑	Ferrer and Artigas (1994)
SSRE	Tianeptine	5×2	ip	14	nc	Malagie *et al.* (2000)
Amygdala						
SSRI	Citalopram	~20	minipump	14	nc	Bosker *et al.* (2001)

Notes:
[1]Route of administration.
[2](↑) Increase in dialysate 5-HT was reported; (nc) no change in dialysate 5-HT was reported.

[a]Study conducted in mice (129/Sv) using zero net flux as opposed to basal dialysate studies in rats.

[b]Increase only when drug was given 2 × daily not when given 1 × daily.

[c]Increase was observed 10–12 h but not 18–20 h after the end of treatment.

[d]Increase was observed without a 48 h washout but not with a 48 h washout.

[e]Increase in two experiments in study; change only approached significance in a third experiment.

[f]Stated dose was 10 mg/kg/day but other information provided in the paper indicated a dose equal to 13 mg/kg/day.

[g]Rats were given chow containing 0.2% $LiCO_3$.

[h]Increase was observed without a 24 h washout but not with a 24 h washout.

listed in Table 1.1 reported a minimum of 22 h for drug washout, with a few exceptions where drugs were either not washed out prior to microdialysis (Bosker *et al.*, 1995b; Wegener *et al.*, 2003), or the washout period was not specified (Keck *et al.*, 2005; Tachibana *et al.*, 2006). Because only four studies have reported increases in extracellular hippocampal 5-HT, it is difficult to determine whether a correlation can be made between these studies and the routes of administration employed. For example, while oral administration of drugs consistently failed to increase hippocampal 5-HT levels, those studies that did report elevations utilized both subcutaneous and intraperitoneal injections, as well as osmotic minipumps. A wide variety of drugs have been studied, but dose–response relationships have not been investigated specifically, perhaps with the exception of citalopram. Even with this drug, there does not appear to be a trend across studies towards a dose–effect relationship in the hippocampus (Gundlah *et al.*, 1997; Hjorth and Auerbach, 1994, 1999; Invernizzi *et al.*, 1995; Wegener *et al.*, 2003).

Papers reporting on dialysate levels of 5-HT in the frontal cortex after chronic antidepressant treatment are more numerous but similarly divided in their observations. Some groups reported no change in 5-HT levels after chronic citalopram (Gundlah *et al.*, 1997; Hjorth and Auerbach, 1994, 1999), while others found that SSRIs, such as citalopram (Arborelius *et al.*, 1996; Ceglia *et al.*, 2004; Golembiowska and Dziubina, 2000) or fluvoxamine (Bel and Artigas, 1993), cause increases in dialysate 5-HT in frontal cortex. Administration of paroxetine has been shown to cause no change (Gardier *et al.*, 2003; Malagie *et al.*, 2000) or to elevate (Owen and Whitton, 2005, 2006) frontal cortex concentrations of dialysate 5-HT. In this brain region, there is evidence that a dose–response effect may account for different responses to paroxetine, with increases observed only at higher drug doses. However, additional studies will be necessary to confirm this. Contradictory results pertaining to the frontal cortex have also been published regarding fluoxetine, as it reportedly increases (Amargos-Bosch *et al.*, 2005; Gartside *et al.*, 2003; Hervas *et al.*, 2001; Invernizzi *et al.*, 1996; Mitchell *et al.*, 2001; Newman *et al.*, 2004) or does not influence (Dawson *et al.*, 2000, 2002; Hervas *et al.*, 2001; Lifschytz *et al.*, 2004) cortical levels of 5-HT in dialysates.

Closer inspection of the data reveals a number of perplexing inconsistencies in microdialysis studies on the effects of chronic antidepressant treatment on dialysate 5-HT in frontal cortex. For example, in comparing the results reported by Dawson and coworkers (2000, 2002), who studied the same dose of fluoxetine, using the same route of administration and rat strain as Gartside *et al.* (2003) and Invernizzi and coworkers (1996), only the latter two studies reported increases in cortical 5-HT levels. Another study found that after using the same dose and route of administration of fluoxetine for the same duration to the same rat strain as Amargos-Bosch *et al.* (2005), 5-HT levels were only increased if a 48-h drug washout period was omitted (Hervas *et al.*, 2001). These two examples highlight how discrepant results can occur in separate laboratories even when similar experimental protocols are utilized. A recent and particularly pertinent example by Johnson and coworkers (2007) highlights similar issues. Two experiments in this study showed significant increases in basal dialysate 5-HT levels in the frontal cortex after chronic fluoxetine administration, while a third, using the same treatment regimen, did not reach significance (Johnson *et al.*, 2007).

Therefore, we cannot definitively conclude from the microdialysis literature that chronic fluoxetine increases extracellular levels of 5-HT in frontal cortex. Furthermore, even though a range of doses has been used in different studies on fluoxetine, changes in cortical levels of 5-HT were not correlated with dose. Although it may be tempting to conclude that washout periods have an effect on neurotransmitter levels, as suggested by the work of Hervas and colleagues (2001), both increases (Johnson *et al.*, 2007; Mitchell *et al.*, 2001; Newman *et al.*, 2004) and a lack of change (Dawson *et al.*, 2000, 2002; Johnson *et al.*, 2007; Lifschytz *et al.*, 2004) have been observed after washout periods of at least 24 h.

Conflicting observations regarding 5-HT levels in frontal cortex are not restricted to SSRIs. In rats, chronic clomipramine administration was reported to result in increased dialysate levels of 5-HT in frontal cortex (Gur *et al.*, 1999b; Owen and Whitton, 2005, 2006), whereas administration of a different tricyclic antidepressant, imipramine, has (Bel and Artigas, 1996) or has not (Gur *et al.*, 2002b) produced similar results. Treatment with duloxetine, an SNRI, resulted in increased frontal cortex levels of 5-HT (Kihara and Ikeda, 1995); however, a different SNRI, venlafaxine, reportedly had no effect (Gur *et al.*, 1999a) or elevated (Wikell *et al.*, 2002) frontal cortex 5-HT in the extracellular space. Similarly, chronic exposure to the norepinephrine reuptake inhibitor (NRI) reboxetine has both failed to elicit changes (Invernizzi *et al.*, 2001; Page and Lucki, 2002) and to induce increases (Owen and Whitton, 2005, 2006) in frontal cortex 5-HT dialysate levels. Studies using chronic regimens of atypical antidepressant drugs are similarly inconsistent. The monoamine oxidase inhibitor (MAOI) tranylcypromine increased dialysate 5-HT in frontal cortex (Ferrer and Artigas,

1994), while tianeptine (Malagie *et al.*, 2000) or $LiCO_3$ (Kitaichi *et al.*, 2005) failed to increase dialysate 5-HT levels in this brain region.

Thus, reports on dialysate 5-HT levels in the frontal cortex following chronic administration of antidepressants are not consistent. With the possible exception of paroxetine, there does not appear to be a correlation between dose and the effects on cortical 5-HT. Although drugs given subcutaneously did not increase dialysate 5-HT, the majority of studies utilizing intraperitoneal injections or osmotic minipumps observed elevated 5-HT. Oral drug administration resulted in conflicting results with respect to changes in dialysate 5-HT in frontal cortex. Too few studies have examined the influence of SNRIs, MAOIs, or other classes of antidepressants (aside from SSRIs) on 5-HT levels in the cortex to draw conclusions regarding the effects of these drugs. Notably, frontal cortex was the brain region most often studied, yet the body of literature on this brain region is also the most divided.

Investigation of 5-HT levels in the hypothalamus in rats after chronic SSRI treatment has similarly resulted in contradictory outcomes. Several groups have reported no changes in basal levels of 5-HT (Lifschytz *et al.*, 2004; Moret and Briley, 1996; Newman *et al.*, 2004; Sayer *et al.*, 1999), although two groups have observed elevations in hypothalamic 5-HT (Moret and Briley, 1996; Rutter *et al.*, 1994). Furthermore, treatment with the tricyclic antidepressants imipramine (Gur *et al.*, 2004) or desipramine (Sayer *et al.*, 1999) did not change 5-HT levels in hypothalamus, while clomipramine was reported to increase dialysate 5-HT (Newman *et al.*, 2000). Only one SNRI, venlafaxine, has been studied and it was found to have no effect on dialysate hypothalamic 5-HT (Gur *et al.*, 2002a). With the exception of the study by Moret and Briley (1996), all of the papers pertaining to hypothalamus utilized a minimum of 24 h for drug washout. Based on these relatively few studies and the discrepant results in the hypothalamus, it is difficult to distinguish trends with regard to route of administration.

Only a handful of studies have examined dialysate levels of 5-HT in other brain regions including striatum, raphe nuclei, and amygdala in response to chronic antidepressant treatment. In striatum, levels of dialysate 5-HT were increased after fluoxetine (Kreiss and Lucki, 1995; Rossi *et al.*, 2008), but did not change following sertraline treatment (Rossi *et al.*, 2008). Similarly, while desipramine significantly increased striatal 5-HT (Kreiss and Lucki, 1995), the NRI reboxetine did not (Sacchetti *et al.*, 1999). Dialysate 5-HT levels in the raphe nuclei did not change after chronic fluvoxamine (Bel and Artigas, 1993; Bosker *et al.*, 1995a) or imipramine (Bel and Artigas, 1996), but were reported to rise following paroxetine (Malagie *et al.*, 2000). Likewise, the MAOI tranylcypromine increased dialysate 5-HT in the raphe nuclei (Ferrer and Artigas, 1994), but the atypical antidepressant tiantepine failed to elevate 5-HT in this brain region (Malagie *et al.*, 2000). A lone study to examine dialysate 5-HT in the central nucleus of the amygdala observed no changes after chronic citalopram (Bosker *et al.*, 2001).

It is more often than not accepted that chronic antidepressant treatment and, in particular, long-term administration of SSRIs results in elevated levels of extracellular serotonin in brain regions important for the modulation of emotional behavior, such as the frontal cortex, hippocampus, and hypothalamus. The analysis presented above demonstrates, however, that we are not yet in a position to draw this conclusion without ignoring almost half of the studies that indicate otherwise. Moreover, consideration of specific drugs, classes of drugs, and washout periods do not account for discrepant conclusions. Although a slight trend for subcutaneous injection and oral administration of drugs to fail to elicit changes in dialysate 5-HT across brain regions is noted, results from studies employing osmotic minipumps and intraperitoneal injections were evenly divided with regard to alterations in 5-HT levels. Future studies would need to compare routes of administration of antidepressants to conclude what influence this has on dialysate 5-HT levels determined by microdialysis.

One possible factor contributing to these variable outcomes involves issues surrounding in vivo recovery of 5-HT and the effect that reduced transport has on this factor. There are a number of quantitative microdialysis methods that have been developed (Kehr, 1993; Lonnroth *et al.*, 1987; Parsons and Justice, 1994) and utilized (Chefer *et al.*, 2006; Olson Cosford *et al.*, 1996) that attempt to account for the fact that recovery of neurotransmitters across microdialysis membranes is less than 100%. Furthermore, changes in the reuptake of neurotransmitters from the extracellular space, such as that occurring in response to antidepressant administration, are hypothesized to alter neurotransmitter concentration gradients in the tissue and, therefore, the flux (concentration per unit area per unit time) of neurotransmitter crossing the dialysis membrane.

We have used the method of zero net flux to correct for changes in the in vivo recovery of 5-HT theorized to occur as a result of reduced uptake in SERT-deficient mice (Mathews *et al.*, 2004). This method is based on the principle that when two solutions, such as the extracellular fluid in the brain and the artificial cerebrospinal fluid perfused into a microdialysis probe, are in contact across a semi-permeable membrane, no net diffusion will occur between the two when they contain equal concentrations of the target analyte (e.g. 5-HT). Thus, by perfusing different concentrations of 5-HT into the dialysis probe and determining how the concentrations of 5-HT in the dialysates change, extracellular neurotransmitter concentrations can be estimated that are corrected for in vivo probe recovery. In practice, different discrete concentrations of 5-HT perfused into the microdialysis probe (C_{in}) are related to the measured concentrations of 5-HT in the dialysate (C_{out}). The differences between the two are calculated ($C_{in} - C_{out}$) and plotted on the y-axis against C_{in} on the x-axis. Linear regression yields the concentration where no net diffusion occurs, which is the point where the regression line crosses the x-axis. The slope of the regression line is the extraction fraction (E_d), which estimates in vivo probe recovery. Using this method, we have been able to detect as little as 1–2-fold increases in extracellular 5-HT in frontal cortex and striatum in SERT+/− mice compared to SERT+/+ mice that are not evident in basal dialysate 5-HT levels uncorrected for in vivo recovery (Mathews *et al.*, 2004).

Zero net flux has only been employed in one study on the effects of chronic antidepressant treatment on extraneuronal 5-HT (Gardier *et al.*, 2003). Here, mice were administered 1 mg/kg/day paroxetine for 14 days by osmotic minipump. The authors reported no differences in extracellular 5-HT levels corrected for in vivo recovery in the hippocampus or frontal cortex. This dose of paroxetine has been shown to result in mouse plasma drug levels comparable to therapeutic levels observed in human patients (Hirano *et al.*, 2005). It also significantly decreases SERT binding sites within both the cerebral cortex and the hippocampus of mice as measured by autoradiography (Hirano *et al.*, 2005). The only difference between these two studies that might explain the lack of change in extracellular 5-HT levels was that Hirano *et al.* administered paroxetine by osmotic minipump for 21 days (2005), as opposed to a shorter 14-day regimen used by Gardier *et al.* (2003). Future studies using a longer duration administration might be useful for determining whether alterations in extracellular 5-HT occur in response to this dose of paroxetine.

As a whole, the antidepressant microdialysis literature suggests that additional work will need to be done to ascertain more fully the effects of long-term inhibition of reuptake on extracellular 5-HT levels. Additionally, it may be beneficial to use quantitative microdialysis, as well as other in vivo neurochemical methods such as voltammetry methods (Stuart *et al.*, 2004; Wightman, 2006), to determine changes in extracellular 5-HT levels following chronic administration of SSRIs and other antidepressants, as well as alterations occurring in response to constitutive deletions in SERT. Direct comparisons will allow assessment of the extent to which extracellular 5-HT is elevated in response to pharmacologic inhibition of SERT versus intermediate and complete SERT gene inactivation. We found no differences in extracellular levels of striatal dopamine in SERT-deficient mice (Mathews *et al.*, 2004); however, future studies might also benefit from investigating extracellular norepinephrine levels in SERT-deficient mice. Chronic administration of desipramine, which acts primarily as an inhibitor at the norepinephrine transporter, was reported to increase dialysate 5-HT in the striatum (Kreiss and Lucki, 1995). Thus, interactions between the norepinephrine and the 5-HT neurotransmitter systems may occur and underlie some of the complex mechanisms involved in the efficacy of antidepressants from different classes (Szabo *et al.*, 1999).

BRAIN TISSUE SEROTONIN LEVELS

The consequences of reducing 5-HT reuptake into presynaptic neurons via loss of SERT expression versus long-term pharmacologic inhibition of SERT have also been explored by determining concentrations of 5-HT in brain tissue. Barring a few exceptions, the data are in agreement that both genetic and pharmacologic reductions in SERT activity result in decreased 5-HT tissue levels. However, there is disagreement concerning the extent to which 5-HT is reduced following pharmacologic inhibition of 5-HT reuptake. Tissue 5-HT levels, which mainly reflect the combination of vesicular and cytoplasmic intracellular neurotransmitter pools, have been determined in a number of different studies on SERT-deficient mice. We originally reported that inactivation of one copy of the SERT gene has no effect on total tissue 5-HT content in frontal cortex, hippocampus, striatum, brain stem, and hypothalamus (Bengel *et al.*, 1998; Numis *et al.*, 2004) (Figure 1.2). By contrast, complete loss of SERT expression leads to 60–80% decreases in 5-HT in these brain regions. Fabre and colleagues (2000) reported similar magnitude reductions in 5-HT levels in cerebral cortex, hippocampus, striatum, and brain stem in SERT−/− mice. A recent study by Kim and coworkers (2005) confirmed no differences between brain tissue 5-HT levels in SERT+/+ and SERT+/− mice, but reported a slightly larger range of decreases in tissue 5-HT in SERT−/− mice to 40–70% of the levels measured in SERT+/+ mice. Tissue 5-HT levels have also been determined in BDNF+/+ × SERT−/− mice (BDNF, brain-derived neurotrophic factor; Ren-Patterson *et al.*, 2006). Here, 5-HT was decreased by

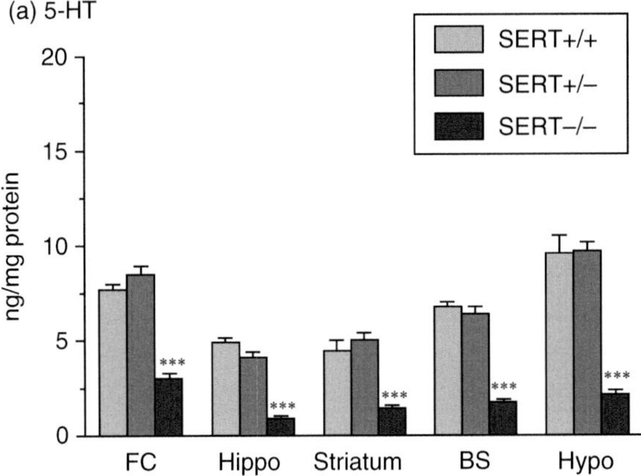

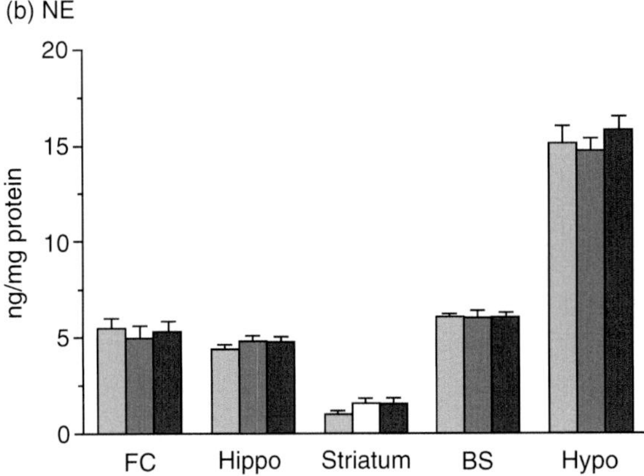

Figure 1.2 Tissue serotonin (a) and norepinephrine (b) concentrations in SERT-deficient mice determined by high performance liquid chromatography with electrochemical detection. FC, frontal cortex; Hippo, hippocampus; BS, brain stem; Hypo, hypothalamus. Probabilities are identified as $^{***}p<0.001$ for differences from SERT+/+ mice.

60–80% in hippocampus, hypothalamus, and brain stem and 50–65% in the striatum compared to BDNF+/+ × SERT+/+ mice bearing normal expression levels of both genes. In contrast to the association between reduced SERT expression and decreased tissue 5-HT levels, a recent paper by Jennings and colleagues reported that transgenic mice over-expressing the human serotonin transporter also show decreases in tissue 5-HT on the order of 15–35% in cortex, midbrain, brain stem, hippocampus, and hypothalamus compared to wildtype mice (Jennings *et al.*, 2006). Thus, both genetic deletion of SERT as well as increased expression of SERT may lead to reduced intracellular 5-HT, although the mechanisms that underlie changes in these two model systems may not be the same.

Statistically significant reductions in the major metabolite of 5-HT, 5-hydroxyindoleacetic acid (5-HIAA), have also been found in SERT−/− but not SERT+/− mice. In the same brain regions, 5-HIAA levels are generally reduced to a lesser extent compared to 5-HT in response to genetic deletion of SERT, whereby reductions in 5-HIAA ranged from 30 to 50% in SERT−/− mice (Bengel *et al.*, 1998; Fabre *et al.*, 2000; Kim *et al.*, 2005) and 10–50% in BDNF+/+ × SERT−/− mice (Ren-Patterson *et al.*, 2006). Tissue 5-HIAA levels in mice over-expressing SERT were not significantly different from those in wildtype mice (Jennings *et al.*, 2006). Tissue norepinephrine (NE) levels have also been measured in SERT-deficient mice (Numis *et al.*, 2004; Tjurmina *et al.*, 2002). Here, no differences in NE levels were observed in frontal cortex, hippocampus, hypothalamus, striatum, and brain stem in SERT+/− or SERT−/− mice (Figure 1.2; Numis *et al.*, 2004). Moreover, plasma and adrenal gland NE levels in SERT+/− and SERT−/− mice were also unaltered compared to levels in SERT+/+ mice (Tjurmina *et al.*, 2002).

Data regarding the effects of chronic antidepressant treatment on brain 5-HT levels are more variable. In an early study, mice receiving intraperitoneal fluoxetine injections for 14 days failed to show changes in whole brain 5-HT levels (Hwang *et al.*, 1980). However, this study also reported that the same fluoxetine regimen reduced 5-HIAA levels by 50% compared to control animals. Also, long-term treatment of rats with the SSRIs paroxetine or sertraline via osmotic minipump for 21 days has been reported to have no effect on tissue levels of 5-HT or 5-HIAA in the hippocampus, even when accompanied by a reduction in SERT binding by 80–90% (Benmansour *et al.*, 1999). In contrast, a number of other studies carried out in rats came to the alternate conclusion that chronic treatment with SSRIs results in decreased tissue 5-HT levels (Caccia *et al.*, 1992; Durand *et al.*, 1999; Hrdina, 1987; Nakayama *et al.*, 2003). Caccia *et al.* and Hrdina each reported that a 21-day regimen of fluoxetine given by intraperitoneal injections is associated with 5-HT levels in cortex that are decreased by 45% and 30%, respectively. Serotonin levels were also investigated in the hippocampus of rats treated for 21 days with the SSRIs fluoxetine or sertraline. Here, tissue 5-HT levels were decreased by 30–40% (Caccia *et al.*, 1992; Nakayama *et al.*, 2003). Moreover, Durand and coworkers reported a decrease in hypothalamic 5-HT and 5-HIAA levels in two different strains of rats receiving intraperitoneal fluoxetine for 21 days (Durand *et al.*, 1999). In cortex, hippocampus, and striatum, 5-HIAA levels were reportedly reduced by 10–35% in response to chronic administration of SSRIs (Hrdina, 1987; Nakayama *et al.*, 2003), whereas Caccia and colleagues observed larger decreases (50–60%) in 5-HIAA levels in cortex and hippocampus (Caccia *et al.*, 1992).

Therefore, the majority of studies suggest that chronic SSRI treatments result in reductions in intracellular 5-HT levels, which is similar to the effects of complete genetic loss of SERT. Decreases in 5-HIAA levels also occur regardless of whether reuptake is inhibited pharmacologically or genetically. Across the board, decreases in brain tissue 5-HT levels appear to be slightly higher and to occur more consistently in SERT−/− mice than in rodents receiving repeated antidepressant treatment. As suggested by the data on adaptive changes in SERT protein and extracellular 5-HT levels, variability in the effects of antidepressants on intracellular 5-HT levels may reflect incomplete inhibition of SERT, as a result of different drug doses and routes of administration. As such, the magnitude of adaptation may fall somewhere between that occurring in response to partial versus complete genetic ablation of SERT.

SEROTONIN SYSTEM ARCHITECTURE

In addition to investigating the aspects of presynaptic adaptation discussed above, we have begun to examine the effects of constitutive reductions in SERT expression on serotonergic innervation of the forebrain. We have hypothesized that the decreases in total tissue 5-HT levels in SERT−/− mice described above (Figure 1.2) reflect a reduced vesicular pool of intracellular 5-HT that arises from the loss of reuptake of 5-HT by SERT (Bengel *et al.*, 1998; Kim *et al.*, 2005). However, other studies have shown that constitutive loss of SERT has the ability to alter the architecture of the brain, including the serotonin system, during development (Altamura *et al.*, 2007; Lira *et al.*, 2003; Persico *et al.*, 2003; Salichon *et al.*, 2001). Thus, we reasoned that lower tissue 5-HT levels might also be accounted for by decreased serotonergic axonal innervation of the forebrain.

Using immunocytochemistry, we have labeled 5-HT-containing axons with a polyclonal antibody against 5-HT (ImmunoStar, Inc., Hudson, WI) and quantified axon numbers in subregions of the hippocampus with respect to genotype in SERT-deficient mice. Specifically, serotonergic neuronal innervation and morphology were examined in 3–4-month-old female SERT-deficient mice in a mixed CD1 × 129S6/SvEv background (n=6 SERT+/+, n=5 SERT+/− and n=5 SERT−/−). Axon quantification was performed using a Zeiss bright field microscope and Zeiss KS400 software (Carl Zeiss, Inc., Thornwood, NY) as described previously (Donovan *et al.*, 2002; Luellen *et al.*, 2006, 2007; Mamounas *et al.*, 1995). Dark field photomicrographs were selected to best represent the mean axon numbers determined by digital imaging for each treatment group. The brain regions of interest (ROIs) included the stratum radiatum layer of CA1, CA2, and CA3, the molecular layer of dentate gyrus (DG) and the granular layer of dentate gyrus (GrDG) of hippocampus. These regions were selected for study based on their innervation by the serotonin system and their involvement in the modulation of mood and anxiety-related behavior (Murphy *et al.*, 2004).

Analysis of variance revealed overall significant differences with respect to genotype in CA2 [$F(2,40)=14.8$; $p<0.001$], CA3 [$F(2,38)=3.4$; $p<0.05$], DG [$F(2,38)=3.5$; $p<0.05$], and GrDG [$F(2,38)=7.0$; $p<0.01$] regions of the hippocampus. Compared to SERT+/+ mice, mice with a 50% reduction in SERT expression showed no significant changes in 5-HT axon numbers in any of the hippocampal subregions studied, with the exception of a trend toward a significant increase in fibers in DG ($p=0.06$) (Figure 1.3A, 3B and 3D). By contrast, 35–70% decreases in axon numbers were observed in CA2 ($p<0.001$), CA3 ($p<0.05$) and GrDG ($p<0.01$) regions of hippocampus in mice completely lacking SERT (Figure 1.3A, 3C and 3D). Thus, the loss of serotonin reuptake occurring throughout development has the ability to alter serotonergic innervation in the adult hippocampus. Furthermore, decreased tissue levels of 5-HT in the hippocampus of SERT−/− mice might be due, in part, to decreased serotonergic axonal innervation, in addition to reflecting the effects of the absence of recycled 5-HT.

Reduced 5-HT axon numbers observed at 3–4 months of age in the hippocampus of SERT−/− versus SERT+/+ mice might result from elevated extracellular serotonin levels present during early developmental periods. However, direct assessment of extracellular 5-HT in mice during prenatal or early postnatal periods is not yet technically feasible. Nevertheless, findings from other studies lend support to the hypothesis that increased 5-HT during critical periods alters the development of the serotonin system and its postsynaptic targets. For example, mice administered a monoamine oxidase-A (MAO-A) inhibitor from embryonic day 15 to postnatal day 7 or mice lacking the MAO-A gene altogether show abnormal thalamocortical barrel field formation in the somatosensory cortex (Cases *et al.*, 1996; Rebsam *et al.*, 2002; Vitalis *et al.*, 1998). High 5-HT levels appear to be causal, since early

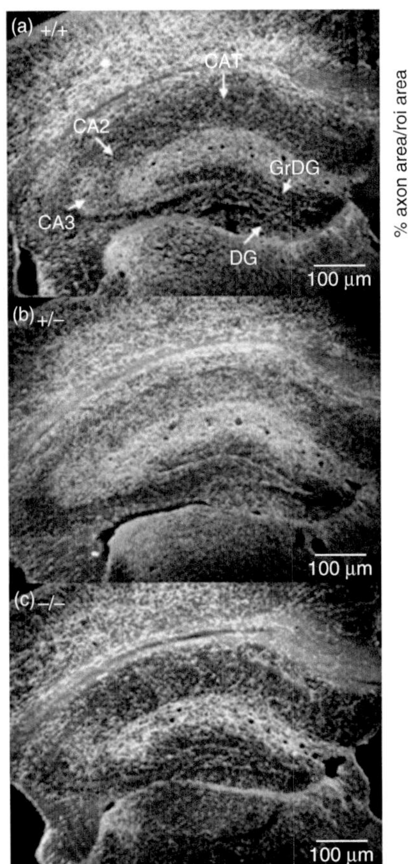

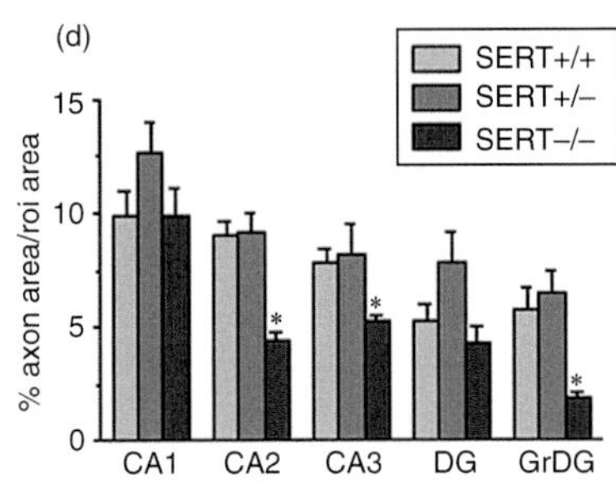

Figure 1.3 Representative darkfield photomicrographs and quantification of 5-HT axons in the hippocampus of 3–4-month-old SERT+/+, SERT+/–, and SERT–/– mice visualized by immunocytochemistry and measured by digitized axon analysis. Serotonin axon innervation is significantly decreased in the CA2 and CA3 subregions and the granular layer of dentate gyrus (GrDG) of the hippocampus in SERT–/– mice (c) compared to SERT+/+ mice (a,d). In d, the data are reported as mean percent axon area/region of interest area ± SEM. DG, dentate gyrus. Probabilities are identified as $^{*}p<0.05$ for differences from SERT+/+ mice.

intervention with the tryptophan hydroxylase inhibitor *p*-chlorophenylalanine (*p*CPA) to block 5-HT synthesis in MAO-A-deficient mice restores normal barrel formation (Cases *et al.*, 1996). Furthermore, mice lacking genes for both MAO-A and 5-HT1B receptors possess normal barrel patterns, suggesting that excess stimulation of 5-HT1B receptors by high extracellular 5-HT levels underlies the disruption of barrel formation

(Salichon *et al.*, 2001). Mice lacking SERT demonstrate similarly disrupted barrel patterns (Persico *et al.*, 2001; Salichon *et al.*, 2001). Additionally, SERT gene deletion has been reported to be associated with reduced numbers of serotonin immunopositive cell bodies in the dorsal raphe (Lira *et al.*, 2003).

In both the Lira study and the data presented above, antiserotonin antibodies were used to visualize serotonergic neurons and their projections. The possibility exists that decreases in stained structures detected might reflect decreased tissue 5-HT levels (Bengel *et al.*, 1998; Kim *et al.*, 2005). However, 5-HT-immunopositive staining is associated with amplification occurring at the levels of secondary antibody binding and conversion of substrate to product by horseradish peroxidase-conjugated secondary antibodies (Mamounas and Molliver, 1988; Mamounas *et al.*, 1991). All immunopositive structures with staining above a minimal threshold are detected and treated similarly in the digital imaging and quantification routines, regardless of the staining intensity. In this way, a reduced immunocytochemical signal is not necessarily expected when neurotransmitter levels are decreased. A more detailed discussion of this method, including additional information on interpreting immunocytochemical data, can be found in Luellen *et al.* (2006).

Similar to the other aspects of presynaptic serotonergic system structure and function discussed, there is disagreement in the literature as to the effects of chronic pharmacological inhibition of SERT on serotonergic innervation, although much less work has been done in this area. Recently, Williams and coworkers reported a threefold *reduction* in the density of 5-HT fibers in the inferior colliculus that was accompanied by modest reductions in 5-HT axon numbers in frontal and visual cortices in adult male mice chronically treated with imipramine or citalopram for 4 weeks (Williams *et al.*, 2005). No differences in 5-HT axon densities were observed in the pons, superior colliculus, motor cortex, or cerebellum in antidepressant-treated versus vehicle-treated mice. Quantitative analysis of the hippocampus was not carried out in this study.

By contrast, Zhou *et al.* demonstrated an *increase* in serotonergic innervation of the fronto-parietal neocortex (especially layers IV and V), primary olfactory (piriform) cortex, and subcortical limbic structures, including the ventral pallidum and nucleus accumbens shell, in 4–6-month-old male rats given either fluoxetine or tianeptine but not desipramine for 4 weeks (Zhou *et al.*, 2006). Effects in the hippocampus were not reported in this study either. No changes in tryptophan hydroxylase type-2 mRNA (TPH-2, the rate-limiting enzyme for 5-HT biosynthesis) or SERT mRNA levels were found in the raphe nuclei in fluoxetine-treated rats as determined by RT-PCR. The authors suggest that the increase in 5-HT- or SERT-immunopositive axons was not due to increased synthesis or uptake of 5-HT. Anterograde tracing of raphe axons with biotinylated dextran amine (BDA) revealed increased axonal branching in the piriform cortex in fluoxetine-treated animals (Zhou *et al.*, 2006). It is interesting to note that the atypical antidepressant tianeptine, which has been described as a serotonin reuptake enhancer, had similar effects to the SSRI fluoxetine in this study. These authors speculated that in both cases serotonin-specific effects on BDNF to promote sprouting in forebrain regions (Mamounas *et al.*, 2000) might be at work. In a separate study, it was postulated that upregulation of SERT expression in the frontal cortex, determined by [^{3}H]paroxetine binding in male rats receiving chronic fluoxetine treatments, might reflect increased 5-HT axonal growth and synaptogenesis in this region, possibly caused by 5-HT itself and/or the neurotrophic peptide, S100β (Wegerer *et al.*, 1999). The latter two arguments support the theory that increased plasticity is a key facet of antidepressant efficacy (Castren, 2004).

One difference between the study by Williams *et al.* and those carried out by Zhou *et al.* and Wegerer *et al.* is that mice were investigated in the former while rats were studied in the latter (Wegerer *et al.*, 1999; Williams *et al.*, 2005; Zhou *et al.*, 2006). It is possible that responses of mice versus rats to chronic antidepressant treatment might be different and contribute to the opposing changes in 5-HT innervation patterns observed in these studies. All of these studies utilized male animals in their experiments. It will be of interest to investigate the effects of chronic antidepressant administration on 5-HT innervation in female mice and rats in future studies to ascertain potential gender-related effects.

An important difference between studies on chronic antidepressant treatment compared to those focused on constitutive decreases in SERT expression is that reduced 5-HT reuptake occurs during critical prenatal and/or postnatal developmental periods in the latter. Similar to SERT-deficient mice and rats, increases in depressive behavior and altered reactivity to novel environments have been reported to occur following perinatal exposure of rats (Andersen *et al.*, 2002; Hansen *et al.*, 1997; Hilakivi and Hilakivi, 1987; Mirmiran *et al.*, 1981; Velazquez-Moctezuma and Diaz Ruiz, 1992; Vogel *et al.*, 1990), or postnatal exposure of mice to antidepressants (Ansorge *et al.*, 2004; Lisboa *et al.*, 2007;

Popa *et al.*, 2008). In mice, this effect does not appear to be associated with chronic inhibition of norepinephrine (Ansorge *et al.*, 2008) during the early postnatal period. Changes in mice treated during adulthood with fluoxetine (Ansorge *et al.*, 2008) or escitalopram (Popa *et al.*, 2008) do not produce similar effects and chronic administration of fluoxetine during adulthood reversed heightened depressive-like behaviors produced by postnatal treatment with escitalopram in mice (Popa *et al.*, 2008). Thus, inhibition of 5-HT uptake during a well-defined developmental window appears to recapitulate some, although not all, of the aspects of the phenotype associated with constitutive SERT deletion. Additionally, expression of 5-HT1A receptors during perinatal development is necessary to establish normal anxiety-like behavior in adult mice (Gross *et al.*, 2002). Together, these and other studies imply that alterations in serotonin neurotransmission during key periods of development induce life-long changes in neurochemistry, neuroanatomy, and behavior that may be different from those produced by chronic treatment in adulthood with antidepressants.

CONCLUSIONS

Although constitutive loss of one functional copy of the SERT gene leads to a 50% reduction in 5-HT reuptake in SERT+/− mice (Perez and Andrews, 2005; Perez *et al.*, 2006) that is accompanied by a 1–2-fold increase in extracellular 5-HT levels (Mathews *et al.*, 2004), the presynaptic serotonergic system appears capable of maintaining normal intracellular 5-HT levels (Bengel *et al.*, 1998; Numis *et al.*, 2004) and hippocampal serotonergic innervation. By contrast, complete constitutive loss of SERT is associated with dramatic changes in presynaptic homeostasis as reflected by increases in extracellular 5-HT on the order of 6–10-fold when corrected for in vivo recovery (Mathews *et al.*, 2004), and decreases in intracellular 5-HT levels ranging from 40 to 80% (Bengel *et al.*, 1998; Fabre *et al.*, 2000; Kim *et al.*, 2005). The latter may result from both a loss of recaptured 5-HT that is normally taken back up by SERT, as well as a decrease in the number of serotonergic axons, although additional work will need to be done to determine whether changes in innervation occur in other regions of the forebrain in SERT−/− mice. In SERT−/− mice, an increase in in vivo 5-HT synthesis rates that are not due to changes in TPH-2 levels also occurs (Kim *et al.*, 2005). Reuptake of 5-HT by alternate transporters under conditions of complete constitutive loss of SERT may also take place in some brain regions (Schmitt *et al.*, 2003; Zhou *et al.*, 2002), which, in addition to increased synthesis, may partly contribute to the homeostatic maintenance of tissue 5-HT levels in SERT−/− mice.

In humans, Lesch and Murphy have identified a 43-base pair insertion/deletion (indel) polymorphism (originally thought to be a 44 bp indel) in the promoter region of the human serotonin transporter gene (Heils *et al.*, 1996; Wendland *et al.*, 2006). Men and women expressing one or two copies of the short form of the 5-HTTLPR gene variant score higher on measures of anxiety-related personality traits (Greenberg *et al.*, 2000; Lesch *et al.*, 1996). This important discovery has spawned numerous studies aimed at replicating and extending these results. Two recent meta-analyses found consistent associations between the 5-HTTLPR short allele and neuroticism, a trait related to anxiety, hostility, and depression, on the NEO Personality Inventory Scales (Schinka *et al.*, 2004; Sen *et al.*, 2004).

The 5-HTTLPR is postulated to produce alterations in anxiety-related traits by driving allele-specific SERT promoter activity, giving rise to a 40% variation in SERT mRNA levels in heterologous expression systems (Heils *et al.*, 1996; Lesch *et al.*, 1996). Furthermore, 40% decreases in SERT protein expression in postmortem human brain and [^{3}H]5-HT uptake in human lymphoblasts and platelets are reported to be associated with the short allele (Greenberg *et al.*, 1999; Lesch *et al.*, 1996; Little *et al.*, 1998). However, recent studies on human SERT binding by PET in vivo and in postmortem frontal cortex, as well as on SERT mRNA levels in human raphe tissue, are not in agreement with earlier findings (Lim *et al.*, 2006; Mann *et al.*, 2000; Parsey *et al.*, 2006a). In each of these cases, the authors hypothesized that the effects of the 5-HTTLPR to reduce SERT expression might be limited to developmental periods. The results of the animal studies described above involving perinatal administration of serotonin reuptake inhibiting antidepressants further suggest that genetically driven decreases in SERT expression, whether constitutive or limited to key periods of development, might have their greatest influence during early life in humans and animals. In any case, many studies in humans suggest that reduced SERT expression and function, whether present throughout life or limited to development, contribute to increases in adult anxiety-related behavior and susceptibility to major depressive disorder observed (Caspi *et al.*, 2003; Grabe *et al.*, 2005; Neumeister *et al.*, 2002, 2006; Parsey *et al.*, 2006b; Pezawas *et al.*, 2005; Zalsman *et al.*, 2006).

Drawing conclusions from the extensive literature on the effects of chronic antidepressant treatment on adaptive responses in the presynaptic serotonergic system is more difficult. There appears to be some consensus across studies that long-term administration of antidepressants, and in particular SSRIs, leads to a decrease in SERT. However, it is not yet clear whether this involves a downregulation of protein expression and/or a redistribution of SERT from the plasma membrane. The majority of studies also point to decreased tissue 5-HT levels occurring in response to chronic antidepressant treatment. By contrast, we examined approximately 50 microdialysis papers utilizing various regimens of antidepressant administration and discovered that almost half of these reported no change in dialysate 5-HT levels, as opposed to the often hypothesized increases in dialysate 5-HT reported in the other half of the studies. We were unable to rectify these differences by considering brain region, drugs or drug class, dose, route of administration, or washout period. In fact, even when zero net flux microdialysis was used in mice to correct for in vivo probe recovery, a single study on antidepressant treatment concluded that increases in extracellular 5-HT were not present in hippocampus or frontal cortex following continuous delivery of therapeutic levels of paroxetine (Gardier *et al.*, 2003). These results contrast with our findings using zero net flux in SERT-deficient mice where increases in extracellular 5-HT were detected in SERT+/− mice, as well as SERT−/− mice (Mathews *et al.*, 2004). Finally, the findings of two immunocytochemical studies that reported on changes in forebrain axon densities following chronic antidepressant treatment were in opposition to each other (Williams *et al.*, 2005; Zhou *et al.*, 2006). Neither study specifically examined the hippocampus so comparisons cannot be made to the data we report here on decreased axonal innervation occurring in some but not all subregions of hippocampus in mice lacking SERT.

There is a wide range of drug administration protocols that has been utilized in the studies discussed above, and this likely contributes to some of the conflicting findings. It will be important for future studies to consider closely the methods of drug delivery employed. There is some evidence that administration by osmotic minipump to achieve continuous delivery in rodents leads to more consistent results. This was particularly evident in the studies on the effects of chronic antidepressant treatment on SERT levels. Serum or plasma drug levels resulting from different administration paradigms and drug doses will need to be investigated further to ensure that human therapeutic levels are reached, as demonstrated by the work of Hirano and coworkers (2005), among others. However, the ultimate test of drug efficacy across species will lie in demonstrating that reuptake is effectively blocked for a period of weeks in experimental animals.

These considerations should be extended to studies aimed at investigating the effects of antidepressants during critical developmental periods. Here, much additional work needs to be done to investigate adaptive responses in the presynaptic serotonergic system following disruption of SERT function in pre- and early postnatal periods, particularly regarding the possible persistence of these responses into adulthood. Elucidating these types of changes will help us to understand the mechanisms underlying lasting alterations in exploratory behavior and a depressive-like endophenotype (Andersen *et al.*, 2002; Ansorge *et al.*, 2004, 2008; Hansen *et al.*, 1997; Hilakivi and Hilakivi, 1987; Mirmiran *et al.*, 1981; Popa *et al.*, 2008; Velazquez-Moctezuma and Diaz Ruiz, 1992; Vogel *et al.*, 1990). These, as well as the many other factors enumerated above, point to the need for the development of conditional SERT-deficient mice. This type of model, similar to what has been done for 5-HT1A receptors (Gross *et al.*, 2002), will allow better controlled investigations of the powerful adaptive forces evoked by long-term loss of serotonin reuptake, as well as the critical temporal windows modulating its pleotropic effects.

ACKNOWLEDGMENTS

The authors would like to thank Dr. Erica L. Unger for preliminary work on 5-HT immunocytochemistry in SERT-deficient mice and Dr. Dennis L. Murphy for insightful feedback on the manuscript. The authors also gratefully acknowledge funding from the National Institute of Mental Health (MH064756 and MH067713).

REFERENCES

Altamura C, Dell'Acqua M L, Moessner R, Murphy D L, Lesch K P, Persico A M (2007). Altered neocortical cell density and layer thickness in serotonin transporter knockout mice: a quantitation study. *Cereb Cortex* **17**: 1394–401.

Amargos-Bosch M, Artigas F, Adell A (2005). Effects of acute olanzapine after sustained fluoxetine on extracellular monoamine levels in the rat medial prefrontal cortex. *Eur J Pharmacol* **516**: 235–8.

Andersen S L, Dumont N L, Teicher M H (2002). Differences in behavior and monoamine laterality following neonatal clomipramine treatment. *Dev Psychobiol* **41**: 50–7.

Andrews A M, Ladenheim B, Epstein C J, Cadet J L, Murphy D L (1996). Transgenic mice with high levels of superoxide dismutase activity are protected from the neurotoxic effects of 2′-NH2-MPTP on serotonergic and noradrenergic nerve terminals. *Mol Pharmacol* **50**: 1511–9.

Ansorge M S, Morelli E, Gingrich J A (2008). Inhibition of serotonin but not norepinephrine transport during development produces delayed, persistent perturbations of emotional behaviors in mice. *J Neurosci* **28**: 199–207.

Ansorge M S, Zhou M, Lira A, Hen R, Gingrich J A (2004). Early-life blockade of the 5-HT transporter alters emotional behavior in adult mice. *Science* **306**: 879–81.

Arborelius L, Nomikos G G, Hertel P, *et al.* (1996). The 5-HT1A receptor antagonist (S)-UH-301 augments the increase in extracellular concentrations of 5-HT in the frontal cortex produced by both acute and chronic treatment with citalopram. *Naunyn Schmiedebergs Arch Pharmacol* **353**: 630–40.

Bel N, Artigas F (1993). Chronic treatment with fluvoxamine increases extracellular serotonin in frontal cortex but not in raphe nuclei. *Synapse* **15**: 243–5.

Bel N, Artigas F (1996). In vivo effects of the simultaneous blockade of serotonin and norepinephrine transporters on serotonergic function. Microdialysis studies. *J Pharmacol Exp Ther* **278**: 1064–72.

Bengel D, Jöhren O, Andrews A M, *et al.* (1997). Cellular localization and expression of the serotonin transporter in mouse brain. *Brain Res* **778**: 338–45.

Bengel D, Murphy D L, Andrews A M, *et al.* (1998). Altered brain serotonin homeostasis and locomotor insensitivity to 3,4-methylenedioxymethamphetamine ("Ecstasy") in serotonin transporter-deficient mice. *Mol Pharmacol* **53**: 649–55.

Benmansour S, Cecchi M, Morilak D A, *et al.* (1999). Effects of chronic antidepressant treatments on serotonin transporter function, density, and mRNA level. *J Neurosci* **19**: 10 494–501.

Benmansour S, Owens W A, Cecchi M, Morilak D A, Frazer A (2002). Serotonin clearance in vivo is altered to a greater extent by antidepressant-induced downregulation of the serotonin transporter than by acute blockade of this transporter. *J Neurosci* **22**: 6766–72.

Blakely R D, Defelice L J, Galli A (2005). Biogenic amine neurotransmitter transporters: just when you thought you knew them. *Physiology (Bethesda)* **20**: 225–31.

Bosker F J, Cremers T I, Jongsma M E, Westerink B H, Wikstrom H V, den Boer J A (2001). Acute and chronic effects of citalopram on postsynaptic 5-hydroxytryptamine(1A) receptor-mediated feedback: a microdialysis study in the amygdala. *J Neurochem* **76**: 1645–53.

Bosker F J, Klompmakers A A, Westenberg H G (1995a). Effects of single and repeated oral administration of fluvoxamine on extracellular serotonin in the median raphe nucleus and dorsal hippocampus of the rat. *Neuropharmacology* **34**: 501–8.

Bosker F J, van Esseveldt K E, Klompmakers A A, Westenberg H G (1995b). Chronic treatment with fluvoxamine by osmotic minipumps fails to induce persistent functional changes in central 5-HT1A and 5-HT1B receptors, as measured by in vivo microdialysis in dorsal hippocampus of conscious rats. *Psychopharmacology (Berl)* **117**: 358–63.

Brunello N, Riva M, Volterra A, Racagni G (1987). Effect of some tricyclic and nontricyclic antidepressants on [3H]imipramine binding and serotonin uptake in rat cerebral cortex after prolonged treatment. *Fundam Clin Pharmacol* **1**: 327–33.

Burnet P W, Michelson D, Smith M A, Gold P W, Sternberg E M (1994). The effect of chronic imipramine administration on the densities of 5-HT1A and 5-HT2 receptors and the abundances of 5-HT receptor and transporter mRNA in the cortex, hippocampus and dorsal raphe of three strains of rat. *Brain Res* **638**: 311–24.

Caccia S, Fracasso C, Garattini S, Guiso G, Sarati S (1992). Effects of short- and long-term administration of fluoxetine on the monoamine content of rat brain. *Neuropharmacology* **31**: 343–7.

Cases O, Vitalis T, Seif I, De Maeyer E, Sotelo C, Gaspar P (1996). Lack of barrels in the somatosensory cortex of monoamine oxidase A-deficient mice: role of a serotonin excess during the critical period. *Neuron* **16**: 297–307.

Caspi A, Sugden K, Moffitt T E, *et al.* (2003). Influence of life stress on depression: moderation by a polymorphism in the 5-HTT gene. *Science* **301**: 386–9.

Castren E (2004). Neurotrophic effects of antidepressant drugs. *Curr Opin Pharmacol* **4**: 58–64.

Ceglia I, Acconcia S, Fracasso C, Colovic M, Caccia S, Invernizzi R W (2004). Effects of chronic treatment with escitalopram or citalopram on extracellular 5-HT in the prefrontal cortex of rats: role of 5-HT1A receptors. *Br J Pharmacol* **142**: 469–78.

Cheetham S C, Viggers J A, Slater N A, Heal D J, Buckett W R (1993). [3H]paroxetine binding in rat frontal cortex strongly correlates with [3H]5-HT uptake: effect of administration of various antidepressant treatments. *Neuropharmacology* **32**: 737–43.

Chefer V I, Zapata A, Shippenberg T S, Bungay P M (2006). Quantitative no-net-flux microdialysis permits detection of increases and decreases in dopamine uptake in mouse nucleus accumbens. *J Neurosci Meth* **155**: 187–93.

Dawson L A, Nguyen H Q, Smith D I, Schechter L E (2000). Effects of chronic fluoxetine treatment in the presence and absence of (+/−)pindolol: a microdialysis study. *Br J Pharmacol* **130**: 797–804.

Dawson L A, Nguyen H Q, Smith D L, Schechter L E (2002). Effect of chronic fluoxetine and WAY-100635 treatment on serotonergic neurotransmission in the frontal cortex. *J Psychopharmacol* **16**: 145–52.

Donovan S L, Mamounas L A, Andrews A M, Blue M E, McCasland J S (2002). GAP-43 is critical for normal development of the serotonergic innervation in forebrain. *J Neurosci* **22**: 3543–52.

Durand M, Berton O, Aguerre S, *et al.* (1999). Effects of repeated fluoxetine on anxiety-related behaviors, central serotonergic systems, and the corticotropic axis axis in SHR and WKY rats. *Neuropharmacology* **38**: 893–907.

Fabre V, Beaufour C, Evrard A, *et al.* (2000). Altered expression and functions of serotonin 5-HT1A and 5-HT1B receptors in knock-out mice lacking the 5-HT transporter. *Eur J Neurosci* **12**: 2299–310.

Ferrer A, Artigas F (1994). Effects of single and chronic treatment with tranylcypromine on extracellular serotonin in rat brain. *Eur J Pharmacol* **263**: 227–34.

Fredricson Overo K (1982). Kinetics of citalopram in test animals; drug exposure in safety studies. *Prog Neuropsychopharmacol Biol Psychiatry* **6**: 297–309.

Gardier A M, David D J, Jego G, *et al.* (2003). Effects of chronic paroxetine treatment on dialysate serotonin in 5-HT1B receptor knockout mice. *J Neurochem* **86**: 13–24.

Gartside S E, Leitch M M, Young A H (2003). Altered glucocorticoid rhythm attenuates the ability of a chronic SSRI to elevate forebrain 5-HT: implications for the treatment of depression. *Neuropsychopharmacology* **28**: 1572–8.

Gobbi M, Crespi D, Foddi M C, *et al.* (1997). Effects of chronic treatment with fluoxetine and citalopram on 5-HT uptake, 5-HT1B autoreceptors, 5-HT3 and 5-HT4 receptors in rats. *Naunyn Schmiedebergs Arch Pharmacol* **356**: 22–8.

Golembiowska K, Dziubina A (2000). Effect of acute and chronic administration of citalopram on glutamate and aspartate release in the rat prefrontal cortex. *Pol J Pharmacol* **52**: 441–8.

Gould G G, Altamirano A V, Javors M A, Frazer A (2006). A comparison of the chronic treatment effects of venlafaxine and other antidepressants on serotonin and norepinephrine transporters. *Biol Psychiatry* **59**: 408–14.

Gould G G, Javors M A, Frazer A (2007). Effect of chronic administration of duloxetine on serotonin and norepinephrine transporter binding sites in rat brain. *Biol Psychiatry* **61**: 210–5.

Grabe H J, Lange M, Wolff B, *et al.* (2005). Mental and physical distress is modulated by a polymorphism in the 5-HT transporter gene interacting with social stressors and chronic disease burden. *Mol Psychiatry* **10**: 220–4.

Graham D, Tahraoui L, Langer S Z (1987). Effect of chronic treatment with selective monoamine oxidase inhibitors and specific 5-hydroxytryptamine uptake inhibitors on [3H]paroxetine binding to cerebral cortical membranes of the rat. *Neuropharmacology* **26**: 1087–92.

Greenberg B D, Li Q, Lucas F R, *et al.* (2000). Association between the serotonin transporter promoter polymorphism and personality traits in a primarily female population sample. *Am J Med Genet* **96**: 202–16.

Greenberg B D, Tolliver T J, Huang S J, Li Q, Bengel D, Murphy D L (1999). Genetic variation in the serotonin transporter promoter region affects serotonin uptake in human blood platelets. *Am J Med Genet* **88**: 83–7.

Gross C, Zhuang X, Stark K, *et al.* (2002). Serotonin1A receptor acts during development to establish normal anxiety-like behavior in the adult. *Nature* **416**: 396–400.

Gundlah C, Hjorth S, Auerbach S B (1997). Autoreceptor antagonists enhance the effect of the reuptake inhibitor citalopram on extracellular 5-HT: this effect persists after repeated citalopram treatment. *Neuropharmacology* **36**: 475–82.

Gur E, Dremencov E, Lerer B, Newman M E (1999a). Venlafaxine: acute and chronic effects on 5-hydroxytryptamine levels in rat brain in vivo. *Eur J Pharmacol* **372**: 17–24.

Gur E, Dremencov E, Van De Kar L D, Lerer B, Newman M E (2002a). Effects of chronically administered venlafaxine on 5-HT receptor activity in rat hippocampus and hypothalamus. *Eur J Pharmacol* **436**: 57–65.

Gur E, Lerer B, Newman M E (1999b). Chronic clomipramine and triiodothyronine increase serotonin levels in rat frontal cortex in vivo: relationship to serotonin autoreceptor activity. *J Pharmacol Exp Ther* **288**: 81–7.

Gur E, Lifschytz T, Lerer B, Newman M E (2002b). Effects of triiodothyronine and imipramine on basal 5-HT levels and 5-HT(1) autoreceptor activity in rat cortex. *Eur J Pharmacol* **457**: 37–43.

Gur E, Lifschytz T, Van De Kar L D, Lerer B, Newman M E (2004). Effects of triiodothyronine on 5-HT(1A) and 5-HT(1B) autoreceptor activity, and postsynaptic 5-HT(1A) receptor activity, in rat hypothalamus: lack of interaction with imipramine. *Psychoneuroendocrinology* **29**: 1172–83.

Hajos-Korcsok E, McTavish S F, Sharp T (2000). Effect of a selective 5-hydroxytryptamine reuptake inhibitor on brain extracellular noradrenaline: microdialysis studies using paroxetine. *Eur J Pharmacol* **407**: 101–7.

Hansen H H, Sanchez C, Meier E (1997). Neonatal administration of the selective serotonin reuptake inhibitor Lu 10–134-C increases forced swimming-induced immobility in adult rats: a putative animal model of depression? *J Pharmacol Exp Ther* **283**: 1333–41.

Heils A, Teufel A, Petri S, *et al.* (1996). Allelic variation of human serotonin transporter gene expression. *J Neurochem* **66**: 2621–4.

Hervas I, Vilaro M T, Romero L, Scorza M C, Mengod G, Artigas F (2001). Desensitization of 5-HT(1A) autoreceptors by a low chronic fluoxetine dose effect of the concurrent administration of WAY-100635. *Neuropsychopharmacology* **24**: 11–20.

Hiemke C, Hartter S (2000). Pharmacokinetics of selective serotonin reuptake inhibitors. *Pharmacol Ther* **85**: 11–28.

Hilakivi L A, Hilakivi I (1987). Increased adult behavioral 'despair' in rats neonatally exposed to desipramine or zimeldine: an animal model of depression? *Pharmacol Biochem Behav* **28**: 367–9.

Hirano K, Seki T, Sakai N, *et al.* (2005). Effects of continuous administration of paroxetine on ligand binding site and expression of serotonin transporter protein in mouse brain. *Brain Res* **1053**: 154–61.

Hjorth S, Auerbach S B (1994). Lack of 5-HT1A autoreceptor desensitization following chronic citalopram treatment, as determined by in vivo microdialysis. *Neuropharmacology* **33**: 331–4.

Hjorth S, Auerbach S B (1999). Autoreceptors remain functional after prolonged treatment with a serotonin reuptake inhibitor. *Brain Res* **835**: 224–8.

Holmes A, Lit Q, Murphy D L, Gold E, Crawley J N (2003a). Abnormal anxiety-related behavior in serotonin transporter null mutant mice: the influence of genetic background. *Genes Brain Behav* **2**: 365–80.

Holmes A, Yang R J, Lesch K P, Crawley J N, Murphy D L (2003b). Mice lacking the serotonin transporter exhibit 5-HT(1A) receptor-mediated abnormalities in tests for anxiety-like behavior. *Neuropsychopharmacology* **28**: 2077–88.

Homberg J R, Olivier J D, Smits B M, *et al.* (2007). Characterization of the serotonin transporter knockout rat: a selective change in the functioning of the serotonergic system. *Neuroscience* **146**: 1662–76.

Horschitz S, Hummerich R, Schloss P (2001). Down-regulation of the rat serotonin transporter upon exposure to a selective serotonin reuptake inhibitor. *Neuroreport* **12**: 2181–4.

Hrdina P D (1987). Regulation of high- and low-affinity [3H]imipramine recognition sites in rat brain by chronic treatment with antidepressants. *Eur J Pharmacol* **138**: 159–68.

Hrdina P D, Vu T B (1993). Chronic fluoxetine treatment upregulates 5-HT uptake sites and 5-HT2 receptors in rat brain: an autoradiographic study. *Synapse* **14**: 324–31.

Hwang E C, Magnussen I, Van Woert M H (1980). Effects of chronic fluoxetine administration on serotonin metabolism. *Res Commun Chem Pathol Pharmacol* **29**: 79–98.

Iceta R, Mesonero J E, Alcalde A I (2007). Effect of long-term fluoxetine treatment on the human serotonin transporter in Caco-2 cells. *Life Sci* **80**: 1517–24.

Invernizzi R, Bramante M, Samanin R (1995). Extracellular concentrations of serotonin in the dorsal hippocampus after acute and chronic treatment with citalopram. *Brain Res* **696**: 62–6.

Invernizzi R, Bramante M, Samanin R (1996). Role of 5-HT1A receptors in the effects of acute chronic fluoxetine on extracellular serotonin in the frontal cortex. *Pharmacol Biochem Behav* **54**: 143–7.

Invernizzi R W, Parini S, Sacchetti G, *et al.* (2001). Chronic treatment with reboxetine by osmotic pumps facilitates its effect on extracellular noradrenaline and may desensitize alpha(2)-adrenoceptors in the prefrontal cortex. *Br J Pharmacol* **132**: 183–8.

Jennings K A, Loder M K, Sheward W J, *et al.* (2006). Increased expression of the 5-HT transporter confers a low-anxiety phenotype linked to decreased 5-HT transmission. *J Neurosci* **26**: 8955–64.

Johnson D A, Grant E J, Ingram C D, Gartside S E (2007). Glucocorticoid receptor antagonists hasten and augment neurochemical responses to a selective serotonin reuptake inhibitor antidepressant. *Biol Psychiatry* **62**: 1228–35.

Keck M E, Sartori S B, Welt T, *et al.* (2005). Differences in serotonergic neurotransmission between rats displaying high or low anxiety/depression-like behavior: effects of chronic paroxetine treatment. *J Neurochem* **92**: 1170–9.

Kehr J (1993). A survey on quantitative microdialysis: theoretical models and practical implications. *J Neurosci Meth* **48**: 251–61.
Kihara T, Ikeda M (1995). Effects of duloxetine, a new serotonin and norepinephrine uptake inhibitor, on extracellular monoamine levels in rat frontal cortex. *J Pharmacol Exp Ther* **272**: 177–83.
Kim D K, Tolliver T J, Huang S J, *et al.* (2005). Altered serotonin synthesis, turnover and dynamic regulation in multiple brain regions of mice lacking the serotonin transporter. *Neuropharmacology* **49**: 798–810.
Kitaichi Y, Inoue T, Nakagawa S, Izumi T, Koyama T (2005). Effect of milnacipran on extracellular monoamine concentrations in the medial prefrontal cortex of rats pre-treated with lithium. *Eur J Pharmacol* **516**: 219–26.
Koed K, Linnet K (1997). The serotonin transporter messenger RNA level in rat brain is not regulated by antidepressants. *Biol Psychiatry* **42**: 1177–80.
Kovachich G B, Aronson C E, Brunswick D J (1992). Effect of repeated administration of antidepressants on serotonin uptake sites in limbic and neocortical structures of rat brain determined by quantitative autoradiography. *Neuropsychopharmacology* **7**: 317–24.
Kreiss D S, Lucki I (1995). Effects of acute and repeated administration of antidepressant drugs on extracellular levels of 5-hydroxytryptamine measured in vivo. *J Pharmacol Exp Ther* **274**: 866–76.
Kuroda Y, Watanabe Y, McEwen B S (1994). Tianeptine decreases both serotonin transporter mRNA and binding sites in rat brain. *Eur J Pharmacol* **268**: R3–5.
Lau T, Horschitz S, Berger S, Bartsch D, Schloss P (2008). Antidepressant-induced internalization of the serotonin transporter in serotonergic neurons. *Faseb J* **22**: 1702–14.
Lesch K P, Aulakh C S, Wolozin B L, Tolliver T J, Hill J L, Murphy D L (1993). Regional brain expression of serotonin transporter mRNA and its regulation by reuptake inhibiting antidepressants. *Brain Res Mol Brain Res* **17**: 31–5.
Lesch K P, Bengel D, Heils A, *et al.* (1996). Association of anxiety-related traits with a polymorphism in the serotonin transporter gene regulatory region. *Science* **274**: 1527–31.
Li Q, Ma L, Innis R B, *et al.* (2004). Pharmacological and genetic characterization of two selective serotonin transporter ligands: 2-[2-(dimethylaminomethyl-phenylthio)]-5-fluoromethylphenylamine (AFM) and 3-amino-4-[2-(dimethyl-aminomethyl-phenylthio)]benzonitrile (DASB). *J Pharmacol Exp Ther* **308**: 481–6.
Lifschytz T, Gur E, Lerer B, Newman M E (2004). Effects of triiodothyronine and fluoxetine on 5-HT1A and 5-HT1B autoreceptor activity in rat brain: regional differences. *J Neurosci Methods* **140**: 133–9.
Lim J E, Papp A, Pinsonneault J, Sadee W, Saffen D (2006). Allelic expression of serotonin transporter (SERT) mRNA in human pons: lack of correlation with the polymorphism SERTLPR. *Mol Psychiatry* **11**: 649–62.
Lira A, Zhou M, Castanon N, *et al.* (2003). Altered depression-related behaviors and functional changes in the dorsal raphe nucleus of serotonin transporter-deficient mice. *Biol Psychiatry* **54**: 960–71.
Lisboa S F, Oliveira P E, Costa L C, Venancio E J, Moreira E G (2007). Behavioral evaluation of male and female mice pups exposed to fluoxetine during pregnancy and lactation. *Pharmacology* **80**: 49–56.
Little K Y, McLaughlin D P, Zhang L, *et al.* (1998). Cocaine, ethanol, and genotype effects on human midbrain serotonin transporter binding sites and mRNA levels. *Am J Psychiatry* **155**: 207–13.
Lonnroth P, Jansson P A, Smith U (1987). A microdialysis method allowing characterization of intercellular water space in humans. *Am J Physiol* **253**: E228–31.

Lopez J F, Chalmers D T, Vazquez D M, Watson S J, Akil H (1994). Serotonin transporter mRNA in rat brain is regulated by classical antidepressants. *Biol Psychiatry* **35**: 287–90.

Luellen B A, Bianco L E, Schneider L M, Andrews A M (2007). Reduced brain-derived neurotrophic factor is associated with a loss of serotonergic innervation in the hippocampus of aging mice. *Genes Brain Behav* **6**: 482–90.

Luellen B A, Szapacs M E, Materese C K, Andrews A M (2006). The neurotoxin 2′-NH2-MPTP degenerates serotonin axons and evokes increases in hippocampal BDNF. *Neuropharmacology* **50**: 297–308.

Malagie I, Deslandes A, Gardier A M (2000). Effects of acute and chronic tianeptine administration on serotonin outflow in rats: comparison with paroxetine by using in vivo microdialysis. *Eur J Pharmacol* **403**: 55–65.

Mamounas L A, Altar C A, Blue M E, Kaplan D R, Tessarollo L, Lyons W E (2000). BDNF promotes the regenerative sprouting, but not survival, of injured serotonergic axons in the adult rat brain. *J Neurosci* **20**: 771–82.

Mamounas L A, Blue M E, Siuciak J A, Altar C A (1995). Brain-derived neurotrophic factor promotes the survival and sprouting of serotonergic axons in rat brain. *J Neurosci* **15**: 7929–39.

Mamounas L A, Molliver M E (1988). Evidence for dual serotonergic projections to neocortex: axons from the dorsal and median raphe nuclei are differentially vulnerable to the neurotoxin *p*-chloroamphetamine (PCA). *Exp Neurol* **102**: 23–36.

Mamounas L A, Mullen C A, O'Hearn E, Molliver M E (1991). Dual serotoninergic projections to forebrain in the rat: morphologically distinct 5-HT axon terminals exhibit differential vulnerability to neurotoxic amphetamine derivatives. *J Comp Neurol* **314**: 558–86.

Mann J J, Huang Y Y, Underwood M D, *et al.* (2000). A serotonin transporter gene promoter polymorphism (5-HTTLPR) and prefrontal cortical binding in major depression and suicide. *Arch Gen Psychiatry* **57**: 729–38.

Mathews T A, Fedele D E, Coppelli F M, Avila A M, Murphy D L, Andrews A M (2004). Gene dose-dependent alterations in extraneuronal serotonin but not dopamine in mice with reduced serotonin transporter expression. *J Neurosci Methods* **140**: 169–81.

Melzacka M, Rurak A, Adamus A, Daniel W (1984). Distribution of citalopram in the blood serum and in the central nervous system of rats after single and multiple dosage. *Pol J Pharmacol Pharm* **36**: 675–82.

Mirmiran M, van de Poll N E, Corner M A, van Oyen H G, Bour H L (1981). Suppression of active sleep by chronic treatment with chlorimipramine during early postnatal development: effects upon adult sleep and behavior in the rat. *Brain Res* **204**: 129–46.

Mirza N R, Nielsen E O, Troelsen K B (2007). Serotonin transporter density and anxiolytic-like effects of antidepressants in mice. *Prog Neuropsychopharmacol Biol Psychiatry* **31**: 858–66.

Mitchell S N, Greenslade R G, Cooper J (2001). LY393558, a 5-hydroxytryptamine reuptake inhibitor and 5-HT(1B/1D) receptor antagonist: effects on extracellular levels of 5-hydroxytryptamine in the guinea pig and rat. *Eur J Pharmacol* **432**: 19–27.

Montanez S, Owens W A, Gould G G, Murphy D L, Daws L C (2003). Exaggerated effect of fluvoxamine in heterozygote serotonin transporter knockout mice. *J Neurochem* **86**: 210–9.

Moret C, Briley M (1996). Effects of acute and repeated administration of citalopram on extracellular levels of serotonin in rat brain. *Eur J Pharmacol* **295**: 189–97.

Murphy D L, Lerner A, Rudnick G, Lesch K P (2004). Serotonin transporter: gene, genetic disorders, and pharmacogenetics. *Mol Interv* **4**: 109–23.

Nakayama K, Katsu H, Ando T, Nakajo R (2003). Possible alteration of tryptophan metabolism following repeated administration of sertraline in the rat brain. *Brain Res Bull* **59**: 293–7.

Neumaier J F, Root D C, Hamblin M W (1996). Chronic fluoxetine reduces serotonin transporter mRNA and 5-HT1B mRNA in a sequential manner in the rat dorsal raphe nucleus. *Neuropsychopharmacology* **15**: 515–22.

Neumeister A, Hu X Z, Luckenbaugh D A, *et al.* (2006). Differential effects of 5-HTTLPR genotypes on the behavioral and neural responses to tryptophan depletion in patients with major depression and controls. *Arch Gen Psychiatry* **63**: 978–86.

Neumeister A, Konstantinidis A, Stastny J, *et al.* (2002). Association between serotonin transporter gene promoter polymorphism (5HTTLPR) and behavioral responses to tryptophan depletion in healthy women with and without family history of depression. *Arch Gen Psychiatry* **59**: 613–20.

Newman M E, Gur E, Dremencov E, Garcia F, Lerer B, Van de Kar L D (2000). Chronic clomipramine alters presynaptic 5-HT(1B) and postsynaptic 5-HT(1A) receptor sensitivity in rat hypothalamus and hippocampus, respectively. *Neuropharmacology* **39**: 2309–17.

Newman M E, Shalom G, Ran A, Gur E, Van de Kar L D (2004). Chronic fluoxetine-induced desensitization of 5-HT1A and 5-HT1B autoreceptors: regional differences and effects of WAY-100635. *Eur J Pharmacol* **486**: 25–30.

Numis A L, Unger E L, Sheridan D L, Chisnell A C, Andrews A M (2004). The role of membrane and vesicular monoamine transporters in the neurotoxic and hypothermic effects of 1-methyl-4-(2′-aminophenyl)-1,2,3,6-tetrahydropyridine (2′-NH(2)-MPTP). *Mol Pharmacol* **66**: 718–27.

Olson Cosford R J, Vinson A P, Kukoyi S, Justice J B, Jr. (1996). Quantitative microdialysis of serotonin and norepinephrine: pharmacological influences on in vivo extraction fraction. *J Neurosci Meth* **68**: 39–47.

Owen J C, Whitton P S (2005). Effects of amantadine and budipine on antidepressant drug-evoked changes in extracellular 5-HT in the frontal cortex of freely moving rats. *Br J Pharmacol* **145**: 587–92.

Owen J C, Whitton P S (2006). Chronic treatment with antidepressant drugs reversibly alters NMDA mediated regulation of extracellular 5-HT in rat frontal cortex. *Brain Res Bull* **70**: 62–7.

Page M E, Lucki I (2002). Effects of acute and chronic reboxetine treatment on stress-induced monoamine efflux in the rat frontal cortex. *Neuropsychopharmacology* **27**: 237–47.

Parsey R V, Hastings R S, Oquendo M A, *et al.* (2006a). Effect of a triallelic functional polymorphism of the serotonin-transporter-linked promoter region on expression of serotonin transporter in the human brain. *Am J Psychiatry* **163**: 48–51.

Parsey RV, Hastings R S, Oquendo M A (2006b). Lower serotonin transporter binding potential in the human brain during major depressive episodes. *Am J Psychiatry* **163**: 52–8.

Parsons L H, Justice J B, Jr. (1994). Quantitative approaches to in vivo brain microdialysis. *Crit Rev Neurobiol* **8**: 189–220.

Perez X A, Andrews A M (2005). Chronoamperometry to determine differential reductions in uptake in brain synaptosomes from serotonin transporter knockout mice. *Anal Chem* **77**: 818–26.

Perez X A, Bianco L E, Andrews A M (2006). Filtration disrupts synaptosomes during radiochemical analysis of serotonin uptake: comparison with chronoamperometry in SERT knockout mice. *J Neurosci Meth* **154**: 245–55.

Persico A M, Baldi A, Dell'Acqua M L, *et al.* (2003). Reduced programmed cell death in brains of serotonin transporter knockout mice. *Neuroreport* **14**: 341–4.

Persico A M, Mengual E, Moessner R, *et al.* (2001). Barrel pattern formation requires serotonin uptake by thalamocortical afferents, and not vesicular monoamine release. *J Neurosci* **21**: 6862–73.

Pezawas L, Meyer-Lindenberg A, Drabant E M, *et al.* (2005). 5-HTTLPR polymorphism impacts human cingulate–amygdala interactions: a genetic susceptibility mechanism for depression. *Nat Neurosci* **8**: 828–34.

Pineyro G, Blier P, Dennis T, de Montigny C (1994). Desensitization of the neuronal 5-HT carrier following its long-term blockade. *J Neurosci* **14**: 3036–47.

Popa D, Lena C, Alexandre C, Adrien J (2008). Lasting syndrome of depression produced by reduction in serotonin uptake during postnatal development: evidence from sleep, stress, and behavior. *J Neurosci* **28**: 3546–54.

Qian Y, Galli A, Ramamoorthy S, Risso S, DeFelice L J, Blakely R D (1997). Protein kinase C activation regulates human serotonin transporters in HEK-293 cells via altered cell surface expression. *J Neurosci* **17**: 45–57.

Ramamoorthy S, Blakely R D (1999). Phosphorylation and sequestration of serotonin transporters differentially modulated by psychostimulants. *Science* **285**: 763–6.

Ramamoorthy S, Giovanetti E, Qian Y, Blakely R D (1998). Phosphorylation and regulation of antidepressant-sensitive serotonin transporters. *J Biol Chem* **273**: 2458–66.

Ravary A, Muzerelle A, Darmon M, *et al.* (2001). Abnormal trafficking and subcellular localization of an *N*-terminally truncated serotonin transporter protein. *Eur J Neurosci* **13**: 1349–62.

Rebsam A, Seif I, Gaspar P (2002). Refinement of thalamocortical arbors and emergence of barrel domains in the primary somatosensory cortex: a study of normal and monoamine oxidase a knock-out mice. *J Neurosci* **22**: 8541–52.

Ren-Patterson R F, Cochran L W, Holmes A, Lesch K P, Lu B, Murphy D L (2006). Gender-dependent modulation of brain monoamines and anxiety-like behaviors in mice with genetic serotonin transporter and BDNF deficiencies. *Cell Mol Neurobiol* **26**: 755–80.

Rossi D V, Burke T F, McCasland M, Hensler J G (2008). Serotonin-1A receptor function in the dorsal raphe nucleus following chronic administration of the selective serotonin reuptake inhibitor sertraline. *J Neurochem* **105**: 1091–9.

Rutter J J, Gundlah C, Auerbach S B (1994). Increase in extracellular serotonin produced by uptake inhibitors is enhanced after chronic treatment with fluoxetine. *Neurosci Lett* **171**: 183–6.

Sacchetti G, Bernini M, Bianchetti A, Parini S, Invernizzi R W, Samanin R (1999). Studies on the acute and chronic effects of reboxetine on extracellular noradrenaline and other monoamines in the rat brain. *Br J Pharmacol* **128**: 1332–8.

Salichon N, Gaspar P, Upton A L, *et al.* (2001). Excessive activation of serotonin (5-HT) 1B receptors disrupts the formation of sensory maps in monoamine oxidase A and 5-ht transporter knock-out mice. *J Neurosci* **21**: 884–96.

Sayer T J, Hannon S D, Redfern P H, Martin K F (1999). Diurnal variation in 5-HT1B autoreceptor function in the anterior hypothalamus in vivo: effect of chronic antidepressant drug treatment. *Br J Pharmacol* **126**: 1777–84.

Schinka J A, Busch R M, Robichaux-Keene N (2004). A meta-analysis of the association between the serotonin transporter gene polymorphism (5-HTTLPR) and trait anxiety. *Mol Psychiatry* **9**: 197–202.

Schmitt A, Mossner R, Gossmann A, *et al.* (2003). Organic cation transporter capable of transporting serotonin is up-regulated in serotonin transporter-deficient mice. *J Neurosci Res* **71**: 701–9.

Sen S, Burmeister M, Ghosh D (2004). Meta-analysis of the association between a serotonin transporter promoter polymorphism (5-HTTLPR) and anxiety-related personality traits. *Am J Med Genet* **127B**: 85–9.

Shen H W, Hagino Y, Kobayashi H, *et al.* (2004). Regional differences in extracellular dopamine and serotonin assessed by in vivo microdialysis in mice lacking dopamine and/or serotonin transporters. *Neuropsychopharmacology* **29**: 1790–9.

Sora I, Hall F S, Andrews A M, *et al.* (2001). Molecular mechanisms of cocaine reward: combined dopamine and serotonin transporter knockouts eliminate cocaine place preference. *Proc Natl Acad Sci USA* **98**: 5300–5.

Spurlock G, Buckland P, O'Donovan M, McGuffin P (1994). Lack of effect of antidepressant drugs on the levels of mRNAs encoding serotonergic receptors, synthetic enzymes and 5HT transporter. *Neuropharmacology* **33**: 433–40.

Stuart J N, Hummon A B, Sweedler J V (2004). The chemistry of thought: neurotransmitters in the brain. *Anal Chem* **76**: 121A–128A.

Swan M C, Najlerahim A R, Bennett J P (1997). Expression of serotonin transporter mRNA in rat brain: presence in neuronal and non-neuronal cells and effect of paroxetine. *J Chem Neuroanat* **13**: 71–6.

Szabo S T, de Montigny C, Blier P (1999). Modulation of noradrenergic neuronal firing by selective serotonin reuptake blockers. *Br J Pharmacol* **126**: 568–71.

Tachibana K, Matsumoto M, Koseki H, *et al.* (2006). Electrophysiological and neurochemical characterization of the effect of repeated treatment with milnacipran on the rat serotonergic and noradrenergic systems. *J Psychopharmacol* **20**: 562–9.

Tjurmina O A, Armando I, Saavedra J M, Goldstein D S, Murphy D L (2002). Exaggerated adrenomedullary response to immobilization in mice with targeted disruption of the serotonin transporter gene. *Endocrinology* **143**: 4520–6.

Trigo J M, Renoir T, Lanfumey L, *et al.* (2007). 3,4-Methylenedioxymethamphetamine self-administration is abolished in serotonin transporter knockout mice. *Biol Psychiatry* **62**: 669–79.

Velazquez-Moctezuma J, Diaz Ruiz O (1992). Neonatal treatment with clomipramine increased immobility in the forced swim test: an attribute of animal models of depression. *Pharmacol Biochem Behav* **42**: 737–9.

Vitalis T, Cases O, Callebert J, *et al.* (1998). Effects of monoamine oxidase A inhibition on barrel formation in the mouse somatosensory cortex: determination of a sensitive developmental period. *J Comp Neurol* **393**: 169–84.

Vogel G, Neill D, Hagler M, Kors D (1990). A new animal model of endogenous depression: a summary of present findings. *Neurosci Biobehav Rev* **14**: 85–91.

Watanabe Y, Sakai R R, McEwen B S, Mendelson S (1993). Stress and antidepressant effects on hippocampal and cortical 5-HT1A and 5-HT2 receptors and transport sites for serotonin. *Brain Res* **615**: 87–94.

Wegener G, Bandpey Z, Heiberg I L, Mork A, Rosenberg R (2003). Increased extracellular serotonin level in rat hippocampus induced by chronic citalopram is augmented by subchronic lithium: neurochemical and behavioral studies in the rat. *Psychopharmacology (Berl)* **166**: 188–94.

Wegerer V, Moll G H, Bagli M, Rothenberger A, Ruther E, Huether G (1999). Persistently increased density of serotonin transporters in the frontal cortex of rats treated with fluoxetine during early juvenile life. *J Child Adolesc Psychopharmacol* **9**: 13–24; discussion 25–6.

Wendland J R, Martin B J, Kruse M R, Lesch K P, Murphy D L (2006). Simultaneous genotyping of four functional loci of human SLC6A4, with a reappraisal of 5-HTTLPR and rs25531. *Mol Psychiatry* **11**: 224–6.

Whittington R A, Virag L (2006). Isoflurane decreases extracellular serotonin in the mouse hippocampus. *Anesth Analg* **103**: 92–8, table of contents.

Wightman R M (2006). Detection technologies. Probing cellular chemistry in biological systems with microelectrodes. *Science* **311**: 1570–4.

Wikell C, Apelqvist G, Hjorth S, Kullingsjo J, Bergqvist P B, Bengtsson F (2002). Effects on drug disposition, brain monoamines and behavior after chronic treatment with the antidepressant venlafaxine in rats with experimental hepatic encephalopathy. *Eur Neuropsychopharmacol* **12**: 327–36.

Williams S M, Bryan-Lluka L J, Pow D V (2005). Quantitative analysis of immunolabeling for serotonin and for glutamate transporters after administration of imipramine and citalopram. *Brain Res* **1042**: 224–32.

Zalsman G, Huang Y Y, Oquendo M A, *et al.* (2006). Association of a triallelic serotonin transporter gene promoter region (5-HTTLPR) polymorphism with stressful life events and severity of depression. *Am J Psychiatry* **163**: 1588–93.

Zhao S, Edwards J, Carroll J, *et al.* (2006). Insertion mutation at the C-terminus of the serotonin transporter disrupts brain serotonin function and emotion-related behaviors in mice. *Neuroscience* **140**: 321–34.

Zhou F C, Lesch K P, Murphy D L (2002). Serotonin uptake into dopamine neurons via dopamine transporters: a compensatory alternative. *Brain Res* **942**: 109–19.

Zhou L, Huang K X, Kecojevic A, Welsh A M, Koliatsos V E (2006). Evidence that serotonin reuptake modulators increase the density of serotonin innervation in the forebrain. *J Neurochem* **96**: 396–406.

QIAN LI

2

Cellular and molecular alterations in animal models of serotonin transporter disruption: a comparison between developmental and adult stages

ABSTRACT

Serotonin transporter (SERT, 5-HTT) plays an important role in the regulation of emotional states. It is a target for the most widely used class of antidepressants, selective serotonin reuptake inhibitors (SSRIs), and is also related to a genetic factor underlying the pathogenesis of affective disorders. Humans with lower SERT expression genotypes show a higher neuroticism score and are more sensitive to stress, suggesting that low SERT expression during development may be a trigger for affective disorders. On the other hand, repeated administration of SSRIs reduces the stress response and treats affective disorders. These observations suggest that disruption of SERT function early in life and in adulthood produces different phenotypes. Thus, understanding the cellular and molecular mechanisms underlying these phenotypes will help us to understand the pathogenesis of affective disorders and develop better therapeutic approaches for their treatment. Animal models with altered SERT function provide useful tools for the studies concerning this purpose. This chapter is intended to overview current available data concerning the cellular and molecular alterations in the models in which SERT functions are disrupted during different developmental stages. We will focus on a comparison between constitutive SERT knock-out mice and repeated administration of SSRIs in adulthood. Furthermore, studies concerning the prenatal administration of SSRIs and genomic manipulation of SERT expression in adulthood are also discussed.

Experimental Models in Serotonin Transporter Research, eds. A. V. Kalueff and J. L. LaPorte. Published by Cambridge University Press.

INTRODUCTION

The serotonin (5-HT) transporter (SERT, 5-HTT) functions as a 5-HT reuptake site to take extracellular 5-HT back into the nerve terminals and, therefore, terminates the action of 5-HT. Thus, the function of SERT is critical for controlling 5-HT activity, which plays an important role in emotional regulation. In fact, SERT is not only the target for the most widely used antidepressants, selective serotonin reuptake inhibitors (SSRIs), but may also be a genetic factor for the pathogenesis of affective disorders. SSRIs bind to SERT and block the 5-HT reuptake sites, which results in an increase of 5-HT concentration in the synaptic cleft and, therefore, prolongs the effect of 5-HT on 5-HT receptors. However, it is unlikely that the antidepressant effects of SSRIs are directly mediated by the blockade of SERT because their therapeutic effects usually require 3–4 weeks of repeated administration. Although the therapeutic mechanisms of SSRIs are still unknown, it is believed that they are mediated by the adaptive changes in the serotonergic systems induced by the increased 5-HT concentration in the synaptic cleft [1, 2].

Several polymorphisms and mutations have been found in the SERT promoter and coding regions [3], such as a polymorphism in 5-HTT-linked promoter region (5-HTTLPR) [4–6]. Studies have demonstrated that individuals carrying the lower SERT expression genotypes may be associated with anxiety-related personality, such as neuroticism [6–8], and are more sensitive to stress. Several recent studies revealed that the number of stressful life events is correlated with the severity and number of episodes of major depression in the individuals carrying lower SERT expression genotypes [9–11]. These data suggest that reduction in the SERT function early in life may contribute to the development of personality traits that potentially trigger affective disorders later in life. Thus, a question arises as to why reduction in the SERT function early in life produces the personal traits that may trigger affective disorders, whereas blockade of SERT function in adult and perhaps adolescence initiates the therapeutic effect for treatment of affective disorders. To answer this question, it is necessary to study the cellular and molecular alterations when SERT function is disrupted early in life and adulthood. In the present chapter, we will compare the cellular and molecular changes in the genetic and pharmacological animal models in which SERT function is disrupted early in life with those in which disruption of SERT function occurs in adulthood.

Several animal models for studying the SERT function are available, generated by either genetic or pharmacological approaches. These

Table 2.1. *Applications of animal models for SERT studies*

Models	Application
Early in life	
SERT knock-out mice	The genetic variance of SERT on early development
Prenatal and postnatal administration of SSRIs	Administration of SSRIs during pregnancy and nursery on development of offspring
Adulthood	
Administration of SSRIs	The mechanisms mediating the therapeutic action of SSRIs
Manipulation of SERT expression	The functions of SERT

animal models can be divided into developmental models and adulthood models based on the developmental stages when the disruption of SERT function occurs. The developmental models include constitutive SERT knock-out mice, prenatal and postnatal administration of SSRIs, in which the SERT function is disrupted before or during the first 8 weeks after birth. The adulthood models include repeated administration of SSRIs and reduction of SERT expression using genomic approaches, such as administration of small interfering RNA (siRNA) and antisense oligos for the SERT gene, in adulthood (>8 weeks). Each of these models is useful to test certain conditions in which the SERT function is disrupted, as shown in Table 2.1. Among these models, SERT knock-out mice and repeated administration of SSRIs have been particularly well studied, and the present chapter will focus on these models. Also, since SERT knock-out rats will be discussed in a separate chapter in this book, we exclude this model in the present chapter.

DEVELOPMENTAL MODELS

Animal models in this category include constitutive SERT knock-out mice and rats and prenatal and postnatal administration of SSRIs. SERT expression appears as early as embryonic day 12, the same time as 5-HT appears [12, 13]. In the early developmental period, 5-HT and SERT are expressed in both serotonergic neurons and other non-serotonergic neurons, such as thalamic and hypothalamic neurons [13]. It is known that 5-HT serves as a neurotrophic factor during early development [14–16]. Thus, it can be expected that disruption of SERT function early in life results in an increase of extracellular 5-HT concentrations and could consequently affect the development of numerous systems, resulting in adaptive changes not only in the serotonergic system but also in other systems, such as the hypothalamic–pituitary–adrenal (HPA) axis. These adaptive changes could be structurally and "permanently" stored throughout life, which may alter the personality of individuals.

SERT knock-out mice

To date, three lines of constitutive SERT knock-out mice have been reported with deletions at the second exon [17], the first exon [18], and the C-terminus [19], respectively. Although most of the studies have been conducted in the mice where the second exon of SERT was deleted, the phenotypes reported from all three lines of SERT knock-out mice are consistent. The homozygous SERT knock-out mice had no detectable SERT binding sites, whereas the heterozygous have about 50% reduction in SERT binding sites [17]. Consistently, 5-HT uptake is completely absent in homozygous SERT knock-out mice (SERT−/−) [17], while about 60% reduction of 5-HT uptake was found in heterozygous SERT knock-out mice (SERT+/−) [20]. Furthermore, the extracellular 5-HT concentration is also increased about 6–8 times in the striatum of SERT−/− mice relative to their SERT+/+ littermates [21, 22]. In contrast, 5-HT content in the brain tissue is significantly reduced in SERT−/− mice, whereas only slight reduction of 5-HT content in the brain was observed in SERT+/− mice [17]. A compensatory increase in the rate of synthesis and a decreased rate of degradation of 5-HT were measured in the brain of SERT knock-out mice [23].

Behavioral studies demonstrated that SERT knock-out mice are more anxious, more sensitive to stress, less aggressive, and have increased antidepressant-like behavior [18, 24–26]. This suggests that constitutive deficiency or reduction of SERT function produces emotional alterations. These phenotypes in SERT knock-out mice, especially in heterozygous SERT knock-out mice (SERT+/−), are similar with those in humans with lower SERT expression genotypes [27–30]. This suggests that SERT knock-out mice can be used as a model to study the mechanisms underlying emotional alterations induced by genetic variation in SERT function in humans.

Alterations in 5-HT receptors

At least 15 5-HT receptors have been identified [31, 32]. Alterations in the concentration of 5-HT in the synaptic cleft may produce adaptive changes in these receptors, including alterations in their expression, post-translational modifications and their signal transduction systems. Currently, several 5-HT receptors have been characterized in SERT knock-out mice, including 5-HT_{1A}, 5-HT_{1B}, 5-HT_{2A}, 5-HT_{2C} and 5-HT_3 receptors.

5-HT_{1A} receptors

5-HT_{1A} receptors are known to play a role in the regulation of anxiety behaviors [33–35]. Studies have demonstrated that deletion of 5-HT_{1A} receptors increases anxiety-like behaviors in mice [36–38]. Since behavioral studies found that SERT knock-out mice are more anxious than their SERT+/+ littermates [18, 24, 26, 29, 39], we hypothesized that 5-HT_{1A} receptors are desensitized in SERT knock-out mice. Studies demonstrated that the density of 5-HT_{1A} receptors is region-specifically reduced in the hypothalamus, amygdala, septum, and dorsal raphe of SERT knock-out mice [21, 39, 40]. These changes were observed in all three strains of the SERT knock-out mice (CD1, C57/B6 and sv129), suggesting the reduction in the density is due to absence of SERT. Consistently, the functions of 5-HT_{1A} receptors in SERT knock-out mice are desensitized. The hormonal responses and the hypothermic response to 5-HT_{1A} receptor agonists, the markers of the function of 5-HT_{1A} receptor in the hypothalamus and dorsal raphe nucleus, respectively, were decreased in SERT knockout mice [39, 41]. Furthermore, 5-HT_{1A} agonist-induced reduction in the firing rate of 5-HT neurons is blunted in SERT knock-out mice [42, 43], suggesting a desensitization of 5-HT_{1A} autoreceptors.

To determine the mechanisms mediating the reduction of 5-HT_{1A} receptor function, the expression of 5-HT_{1A} receptors and their G-protein coupling were examined by in situ hybridization, competitive RT-PCR, and 8-OH-DPAT stimulated ^{35}S-GTP-γ-S binding [21, 40]. The reduction of 5-HT_{1A} mRNA was only detected in the dorsal raphe of SERT knock-out mice, but not in the other brain regions. Additionally, the results from these studies suggest that the reduction in the functions of 5-HT_{1A} receptors is not due to a decrease in G-protein coupling [40]. Furthermore, G-proteins (G_i and G_o proteins) that are coupled to 5-HT_{1A} receptors are not decreased in the hypothalamus and midbrain of SERT knock-out mice. Indeed, some of them are even increased (Table 2.2), suggesting a compensatory effect for the reduction in 5-HT_{1A} receptors [40]. Together, these data suggest that the alteration of 5-HT_{1A} receptors in SERT knock-out mice may be mediated by regulations at post-transcriptional, translational and/or post-translational levels.

Table 2.2. *Comparison of the alterations in the serotonergic system and G-proteins among animal models that SERT is disrupted in different life stages*

Alterations		SERT knock-out mice		Early-life exposure to SSRIs*		Repeated administration of SSRIs	
		Alteration	Regions/response#	Alteration	Regions/response	Alteration	Regions/response
SERT	Density	↓50% or 100%[a]	Entire body	↑[1] (E) ↓(E)	Hippo, Amy, LH DMN[h]	↓	Hippo, Amy, CTX, Str, Tha, MB[k]
5-HT receptors							
5-HT_{1A}	Density	↓ F>M	RN, Hypo, Amy Sep[b]			0[l]	
	Function	↓ F>M	Firing, Oxy, Cort, Hypothermia[b]	↑ (P)	Hypothermia[i]	↓ F>M	Firing, Oxy, Cort[l]
5-HT_{1B}	Density	↓	SN[c]				
	Function	↓	5-HT outflow[c]			↓	FCX, Hypo[m]
5-$HT_{2A/2C}$	Density	5-HT_{2A}:↑ 5-HT_{2A}:↓ 5-HT_{2C}:↑	Hypo, Sep; Str Amy, ChP[d]	↓[2](E)	Hypo[j]	↑	Hypo(activated)[n]
	Function		↑ Oxy[d]	↓ (E)	ACTH, Cort[j], IP_3 in CTX[j]	↑↓	ACTH, Oxy[o]
5-HT_3	Density	↑	CTX, Hippo[e]			0[p]	
	mRNA	↓	Hippo, Int[e]				
	Function	↓	Int[e]				

G proteins					
G_s				↓	MB[q]
	G_{i1}	↓	MB[f]	↓	Hypo, MB, FCX[r]
G_i	G_{i2}	0[f]		↓	MB, FCX[r]
	G_{i3}	0[f]		↓	Hypo, MB[r]
	G_z	↑	Hypo[f]	↓	Hypo[r]
G_o		↓	MB[f]	↓	Hypo, MB[r]
$G_{q/11}$		0[g]		0[s]	
G_{12}				↑	CTX, Str[q]

Abbreviations: Amy: amygdala; ChP: choroid plexus; Cort: corticosterone; CTX: cortex; DMN: dorsomedial nucleus of hypothalamus; FCX: frontal cortex; Hippo: hippocampus; Hypo: hypothalamus; Int, intestine; LH: lateral hypothalamus; MB: middle brain; Oxy: oxytocin response to agonists; RN: Raphe nuclei; Sep: septum; Str: striatum; SN: substantia nigra; Tha: thalamus; F>M: female more extensive than male.

[*]Include prenatal (E) and postnatal (P) exposure to SSRIs.

[#]Brain regions where changes were observed or responses to agonists (functions).

[1]Only in prepubescent offspring.

[2]Only in adult offspring.

↑Increase; ↓ Decrease; 0 No change; ↑↓ Biphase time course.

[a][17]; [b][21, 40, 41, 44]; [c][21]; [d][55, 56]; [e][74–76]; [f][40]; [g][55]; [h][86, 87]; [i][95]; [j][89, 90]; [k][99, 100, 102, 103]; [l][110–116; 126–129]; [m][136, 137]; [n][139]; [o][94]; [p][164]; [q][147]; [r][126; 128; 129]; [s][94; 139].

It is interesting that the desensitization of 5-HT_{1A} receptors is more extensive in female than male SERT knock-out mice. This is consistent with the observation that increase in anxiety-like behaviors are more substantial in female than male SERT knock-out mice [24, 39]. However, the reduction in 5-HT_{1A} mRNA does not appear to be different between the genders, suggesting the reduction of 5-HT_{1A} receptors is not mediated by transcriptional regulation [40]. Bouali *et al.* reported that gonadectomy diminishes the gender differences in desensitization of 5-HT_{1A} receptors in the dorsal raphe neurons of SERT knock-out mice [44]. They found that in SERT knock-out mice, but not SERT+/+ mice, testosterone prevented and estradiol produced the desensitization of 5-HT_{1A} receptors in the dorsal raphe of SERT knock-out mice. These data demonstrated that sex hormones play an important role in regulation of 5-HT_{1A} receptors in SERT knock-out mice. Estrogen synergizes, whereas testosterone prevents, the desensitization of 5-HT_{1A} receptors induced by reduction in SERT function. Although gonadectomy did not alter the function of 5-HT_{1A} receptors in the dorsal raphe of normal mice [44], several studies have found that estrogen desensitizes 5-HT_{1A} receptors in ovariectomized rats and monkeys [45–49].

Considering that SERT knock-out mice have constitutively deficient or reduced SERT function, a time course (postnatal day 1 to 8 weeks) of alteration in the density of 5-HT_{1A} receptors during postnatal development was determined in SERT knock-out mice. The study demonstrated that the reduction in the density of 5-HT_{1A} receptors was more extensive in the first week after birth, suggesting that the reduction in expression of 5-HT_{1A} receptors may occur during prenatal development. The most dramatic changes between genotypes were observed in the amygdala and dorsal raphe of SERT knock-out mice (Li, in preparation). Since 5-HT plays an important role during development and 5-HT_{1A} receptors are the earliest developing 5-HT receptors [50–52], one can speculate that the increase in extracellular concentrations of 5-HT due to a deficit of SERT in the early developmental stage would alter the expression of 5-HT_{1A} receptors. This early reduction in 5-HT_{1A} receptors may account for the similarity of the behavioral alterations between SERT knock-out mice and 5-HT_{1A} receptor knock-out mice. To overcome the decreased 5-HT_{1A} receptors, compensatory changes are developed during later developmental and adult stages, such as increasing 5-HT_{1A} receptor-coupled G-protein concentrations and maintaining 5-HT_{1A} mRNA levels. As a result, the degree of the reduction in the density of 5-HT_{1A} receptors is attenuated in adult SERT knockout mice. Furthermore, because the expression of 5-HT_{1A} receptors in the hippocampus and cortex do not peak until postnatal 3 weeks [53] (and our observation), the density of 5-HT_{1A} receptors in these brain regions is not altered in SERT knock-out mice.

The next question is whether the reduction in 5-HT_{1A} receptors mediates an increased stress response and anxiety-like behaviors observed in SERT knock-out mice. To address this question, recombinant adenoviruses containing 5-HT_{1A} sense or antisense sequences were used to manipulate 5-HT_{1A} receptors [54]. Injection with recombinant adenovirus containing 5-HT_{1A} sense sequence into the hypothalamus of SERT knock-out mice restored the density of 5-HT_{1A} receptors in the medial hypothalamus. The restoration of 5-HT_{1A} receptors normalized the sensitivity to stress in SERT knock-out mice. These data suggest that the reduction of 5-HT_{1A} receptors in the medial hypothalamus of SERT knock-out mice contributes to their increased sensitivity to stress. Although the restoration of hypothalamic 5-HT_{1A} receptors did not affect the increased anxiety-like behaviors [54], injection of adenovirus containing 5-HT_{1A} sense sequence into the amygdala normalized the increased anxiety-like behaviors in SERT knockout mice (Li, unpublished data). These results suggest that 5-HT_{1A} receptors in the amygdala, but not in the hypothalamus, mediate the regulation of anxiety-like behaviors.

5-HT_{1B} receptors

5-HT_{1B} receptors can be further divided into autoreceptors, located in the serotonergic nerve terminals, and postsynaptic receptors in several brain regions, such as the basal ganglia. The brain regions containing the highest density of 5-HT_{1B} receptors are the striatum and substantia nigra. Fabre *et al.* [21] reported that the density of 5-HT_{1B} receptors in the substantia nigra of SERT+/− and SERT−/− are reduced by about 17% and 29%, respectively, relative to their SERT+/+ littermates. The reduction in the density of 5-HT_{1B} receptors was not observed in the globus pallidus of SERT knock-out mice. 5-HT_{1B} agonist-stimulated GTP-γ-S binding was decreased in the substantia nigra of SERT knock-out mice to the same degree as the density of 5-HT_{1B} receptors [21]. These data suggest that the decreased 5-HT_{1B} agonist-stimulated GTP-γ-S binding represents a reduction in the density of 5-HT_{1B} receptors, but not a reduction of G-protein coupling of 5-HT_{1B} receptors.

5-HT_{2A} receptors

5-HT_{2A} receptors are distributed in most brain regions, with the highest density in the cortex. The alteration in the function of 5-HT_{2A}

receptors may be related to psychotic disorders. Interestingly, the density of 5-HT$_{2A}$ receptors in SERT knock-out mice is altered in opposite directions in different brain regions. Using 5-HT$_{2A}$ receptor antagonist (^{3}H-MDL 100907) and agonist (^{125}I-DOI in the presence of 5-HT$_{2C}$ receptor antagonist) binding, we and Rioux *et al.* found that the density of 5-HT$_{2A}$ receptors in the ventral striatum and claustrum was significantly reduced in SERT+/− and SERT−/− mice [55, 56]. On the other hand, the density of 5-HT$_{2A}$ receptors in the septum and hypothalamus is significantly increased in SERT knock-out mice [55]. Although we did not observe an alteration in the density of 5-HT$_{2A}$ receptors in the cortex with ^{125}I-DOI binding, Rioux *et al.* reported a decrease in 5-HT$_{2A}$ binding sites in the cortex of SERT knock-out mice using a ^{3}H-MDL 100907 binding assay [56]. These different observations may result from the fact that antagonist binding (^{3}H-MDL 100907) measures the total number of 5-HT$_{2A}$ receptors, whereas agonist binding (^{125}I-DOI) measures the high affinity (G-protein-coupled) 5-HT$_{2A}$ receptors. It is possible that the total number of 5-HT$_{2A}$ receptors is reduced, but the 5-HT$_{2A}$ receptors in a high affinity state are not changed in the cortex of SERT knock-out mice. The differential alterations of 5-HT$_{2A}$ receptors in SERT knock-out mice suggest that the regulation of 5-HT$_{2A}$ receptors may be different between the brain regions. Studies have demonstrated that stimulation of 5-HT$_{2A}$ receptors in the hypothalamus potentiates the stress-induced adrenocorticotropic hormone (ACTH) response, while stimulation of 5-HT$_{1A}$ receptors inhibits the stress-induced ACTH response [57]. It is possible that the increase in 5-HT$_{2A}$ receptors and decrease in 5-HT$_{1A}$ receptors in SERT knock-out mice contribute to their increased sensitivity to stress.

5-HT$_{2C}$ receptors

The highest density of 5-HT$_{2C}$ receptors is present in the choroid plexus. The amygdala, lateral habenular nucleus, and thalamus contain a relatively high density of 5-HT$_{2C}$ receptors [55, 58, 59]. In contrast to 5-HT$_{1A}$ receptors, stimulation of 5-HT$_{2C}$ receptors produces an anxiogenic effect [34, 60]. The expression of 5-HT$_{2C}$ receptors can be regulated by RNA editing and alternative splicing [61–64]. It has been demonstrated that fluoxetine, a SERT inhibitor, and stress can trigger the RNA editing and alter the ratio of 5-HT$_{2C}$ isomers, resulting in alterations of 5-HT$_{2C}$ functions [65–67]. Therefore, we hypothesized that 5-HT$_{2C}$ receptors may be altered in SERT knock-out mice. Using autoradiography of ^{125}I-DOI binding in the presence of MDL 100907, a 5-HT$_{2A}$ antagonist, to block

5-HT_{2A} binding sites, we demonstrated that the density of 5-HT_{2C} receptors in the choroid plexus and amygdala is significantly increased in SERT knock-out mice [55]. This elevation was not observed in other brain regions. Furthermore, mRNA levels of 5-HT_{2C} receptors in the amygdala were not changed, whereas 5-HT_{2C} mRNA was reduced in the choroid plexus and lateral habenular nucleus. These data suggest that the increase in the density of 5-HT_{2C} receptors in the amygdala is not due to an increase in their gene expression or mRNA stability. The alteration may occur at post-transcriptional and post-translational levels.

It is particularly interesting that 5-HT_{2C} receptors are increased in the amygdala, which controls fear and anxiety behaviors. Therefore, the increase in 5-HT_{2C} receptors and decrease in 5-HT_{1A} receptors in the amygdala of SERT knock-out mice may be related to the increased anxiety-like behavior of these mice. On the other hand, it is unlikely that the later onset of obesity observed in SERT knock-out mice [30] is due to alterations in 5-HT_{2C} receptors, since reductions in 5-HT_{2C} receptors, which are associated with obesity, are not detected in SERT knock-out mice [68–70].

5-HT$_3$ *receptors*

5-HT_3 receptors are the only ligand-gated ion channel receptors in the 5-HT receptor family. They are located in both central nervous system and peripheral tissues. Studies showed that administration of 5-HT_3 antagonists produces an anxiolytic effect, suggesting that 5-HT_3 receptors are related to regulation of anxiety behaviors [71–73]. Using autoradiography with *S*-methoxyl-(^{3}H) zacopride, a 5-HT_3 antagonist, binding assay, Mossner *et al.* reported that the density of 5-HT_3 receptors was significantly increased in the frontal cortex, parietal cortex, and hippocampal CA3 region of SERT knock-out mice [74]. However, 5-HT_{3A} mRNA levels were found to be reduced in the hippocampal CA1 region [74]. The frontal cortex innervates the amygdala to control fear and anxiety behaviors. The increased density of 5-HT_3 receptors in the frontal cortex may contribute to the increased anxiety-like behaviors in SERT knock-out mice, although there is no evidence that 5-HT_3 receptors in the frontal cortex are indeed related to the regulation of anxiety-like behaviors.

5-HT_3 receptors are also located in the enteric neurons and epithelial cells of the gastrointestinal system. These receptors may play a role in control of intestinal motility. Studies have found increased colon motility and subsequently increased water content in stool of SERT knock-out mice [75]. It was hypothesized that adaptive changes of 5-HT receptors in the gastrointestinal system of SERT knock-out mice may be responsible for these alterations [75, 76]. Liu *et al.* examined the expression and the function of 5-HT_3 receptors in the intestinal epithelial cell and enteric neurons of SERT knock-out mice [76]. A reduction of 5-HT_{3B} mRNA was detected, although the mRNA level of 5-HT_{3A} receptors was normal. Furthermore, the 5-HT-evoked fast inward current in myenteric neurons, a 5-HT_3 receptor-mediated response, is reduced in SERT−/− mice, suggesting a desensitization of 5-HT_3 receptors [76]. The desensitization of intestinal 5-HT_3 receptors may be related to the increased intestinal motility and watery stools in SERT knock-out mice.

Impaired hypothalamic–pituitary–adrenal gland (HPA) axis

Besides increased anxiety-like behaviors, SERT knock-out mice also showed increased sensitivity to stress. Minor stressors, such as handling or saline injection, increase ACTH secretion in SERT+/− and SERT−/− mice [41]. The ACTH response to placement in an elevated plus maze, a psychological stressor, is significantly higher in SERT+/− mice than that in SERT+/+ mice [28]. Although decreased 5-HT_{1A} receptors and increased 5-HT_{2A} receptors in the hypothalamus of SERT knock-out mice may play certain roles as discussed above, it is unlikely that they are primary reasons for the increased sensitivity to stress. It is known that the activity of the HPA axis is related to stress responses. Studies have found that although the ACTH response to stress is increased in SERT knock-out mice, corticosterone responses were not significantly altered in most cases [41, 42]. These data led to the hypothesis that the HPA axis in SERT knock-out mice is impaired. Our recent studies (Li, in preparation) demonstrated that the HPA axis in SERT knock-out mice is altered. The overall basal activity of the HPA axis in the SERT knock-out mice was reduced, demonstrated by the decreased corticotrophin releasing factor (CRF) expression and low basal plasma corticosterone concentration [41, 42]. The reduction of CRF may induce an upregulation of CRF type 1 receptor (CRF R1), resulting in an increase in the function and the density of CRF R1 in the pituitary of SERT−/− mice. Under stressed conditions, the HPA axis in SERT+/− and SERT−/− mice is over-activated. Stress for only 5 min via placement in an elevated plus maze significantly increased CRF mRNA in the paraventricular nucleus (PVN) of both SERT+/− and SERT−/− mice relative to that in the non-stressed condition. This is consistent with our previous reports that minor stress, such as saline injection, produced a significant increase of ACTH release in SERT+/− and SERT−/− mice [41, 54]. To determine whether the hypersensitivity of the HPA axis to stress in SERT knock-out mice is due to a reduction in the glucocorticoid receptor-mediated feedback regulation, the protein and mRNA levels of glucocorticoid receptors (GR) in the HPA axis were examined in SERT knock-out mice. The GR expression was significantly reduced in all three organs of the HPA axis (the hypothalamus, pituitary, and adrenal cortex) of SERT+/− and SERT−/− mice. These results suggest that the HPA axis and its feedback regulation are impaired in SERT+/− and SERT−/− mice, which could account for their increased sensitivity to stress.

The next question is how disruption of SERT function early in life impairs the HPA axis and GR-related feedback regulation. No data are available currently regarding the mechanisms that mediate alterations of HPA axis and its feedback regulation. It is possible that epigenetic and post-transcriptional regulation of CRF and GR expression are involved. Understanding these mechanisms is particularly important, because the hypersensitivity of the HPA axis to stress is also observed in humans carrying the lower SERT expression genotype. A recent study reported that psychological stress, such as public speaking, significantly increased plasma ACTH and cortisol levels in individuals with lower SERT expression genotypes [77]. These data suggest that the sensitivity of the HPA axis response to stress is increased in individuals with lower SERT expression genotypes. Since increased activity of HPA axis is known to be involved in the pathophysiology of affective disorders, the increased sensitivity of HPA axis response to stress could be a trigger for the development of affective disorders in these individuals when they suffer stressful events. Therefore, studying the mechanisms by which reduced SERT function during development influences the sensitivity of HPA axis response to stress will provide significant insight into our understanding of the etiology of affective disorders and, thus, in the development of better approaches to prevent and treat affective disorders.

Besides the alterations in the serotonergic system and HPA axis systems, several changes in other neurotransmitter systems are also observed in SERT knock-out mice (see review [28] for more complete information).

Prenatal and maternal administration of SSRIs

SSRIs are prescription drugs used for the treatment of depression during pregnancy and lactation. Thus, it is important to understand whether these medications affect the development of offspring. Although data are still controversial, some clinical studies have indicated that prenatal and lactating exposure to SSRIs may increase the risk for perinatal problems and heart and pulmonary diseases [78–80]. However, only a few studies on the behaviors of children who are prenatally exposed to SSRIs have been reported [79, 81–82]. Most of these studies were conducted in childhood and no data are available on the mental status of these offspring in adulthood. It is particularly difficult to conduct studies on the effects of emotional behavior in humans since the genetic and environmental factors have major inputs on these behaviors. Furthermore, few data are available regarding the cellular and molecular alterations induced by prenatal and postnatal exposure to SSRIs in humans. Several animal studies reveal that prenatal and lacteal exposure of SSRIs may alter locomotor activity, depression-like and impulsive behaviors of the offspring in adulthood [81, 83, 84]. Therefore, it is necessary to establish animal models for studying the effects of prenatal and postnatal exposure of SSRIs on the mental development.

In comparison to studies conducted in adult animals, few animal studies on the effects of prenatal and lacteal exposure to SSRIs have been reported. Two studies have found that the density of 5-HT transporters were altered by in utero exposure to fluoxetine [85, 86]. Cabrera-Vera *et al.* reported that in utero exposure of fluoxetine from embryonic days 13 to 20 altered the density of SERT in the nuclei of the hypothalamus, hippocampus, and amygdala of prepubescent (postnatal day 28) offspring [85] differentially. Although Cabrera-Vera *et al.* did not detect any change in the cortex, Montero *et al.* reported a reduction in the density of SERT in the cortex of offspring in postnatal day 25 that were prenatally exposed to fluoxetine in the last 15 days of gestation [86]. Both studies reported that alterations in the density of SERT were only observed in the prepubescent but not adult offspring. Similarly, 5-HT content was reduced in the frontal cortex of prepubescent but not adult prenatal fluoxetine-exposed offspring [87]. On the other hand, a reduction in the 5-HT content was found in the midbrain of adult offspring that were exposed to fluoxetine during pregnancy [87]. These data suggest that adaptive changes in the SERT expression and 5-HT metabolism occurred during development to compensate for the effects of blockade of SERT by SSRI treatment.

Only two studies concerning alterations in serotonergic receptors in the offspring following prenatal SSRI exposure have been reported. Both studies found that prenatal fluoxetine exposure produced a desensitization of 5-$HT_{2A/2C}$ receptors, although the data were slightly different. Cabrera *et al.* reported that prenatal fluoxetine exposure from embryonic days 13 to 20 significantly reduced the density of 5-$HT_{2A/2C}$ receptors in the hypothalamus, but not in the frontal cortex of adult offspring [88]. Consistently, the ACTH response to 5-$HT_{2A/2C}$ receptor agonist, DOI, was decreased, suggesting that 5-$HT_{2A/2C}$ receptors in the hypothalamus are desensitized. However, the reduction in 5-$HT_{2A/2C}$ receptors was not observed in prepubescent offspring [88]. On the other hand, Romero *et al.* found that exposure to fluoxetine from gestation days 6 to 21 decreased 5-HT-induced increase of inositol phosphate accumulation in the cortex of 25-day-old offspring [89], suggesting a desensitization of 5-HT_2 receptors. The different observations between these studies could be due to the different duration of prenatal fluoxetine exposure and testing points.

Only a few studies have been reported on SSRI treatment of the postnatal or prepubescent animals, especially on the cellular and molecular alterations after the postnatal SSRI treatments. Landry *et al.* [90] reported that administration of fluoxetine to prepubescent rats (5 weeks of age) for 2 weeks reduced oxytocin response to a 5-$HT_{2A/2C}$ receptor agonist, DOI (15 min after the injection), suggesting a desensitization of 5-HT_{2A} receptors in the hypothalamus [91, 92]. This is similar to the observation in adult rats (see below) [93]. On the other hand, administration of SSRIs in the early postnatal stage may produce alterations similar to SERT knock-out mice. Popa *et al.* compared several behavioral alterations between SERT knock-out mice and mice treated with escitalopram (an SSRI) during postnatal days 5–20 [94]. They found that several behaviors, such as sleep abnormalities and increased depression-like behavior, were similar between SERT knock-out mice and postnatal SSRI-treated mice. Also, Ansorge *et al.* found that administration of fluoxetine during postnatal days 4–20 significantly increased anxiety-like behavior in adult-stage mice, which is consistent with the observation in SERT knock-out mice [26, 95]. The increased anxiety-like behavior was not observed in mice treated with SSRI at 9 weeks of age. However, the increased anxiety-like behavior was not observed in postnatal escitalopram-treated mice [94]. These inconsistent results could be due to the possibility that the alteration in anxiety-like behavior requires disruption of SERT function earlier than postnatal day 5. However, it could also be due to the difference in the SSRIs and the strains of mice used in these experiments. These data suggest that the developmental stage at which an SSRI is given is critical for determining the subsequent alterations in emotions. It will be interesting to understand the cellular and molecular alterations behind these behavioral changes.

Currently, there are too few data for us to compare the cellular and molecular alterations between mice exposed to SSRIs prenatally and postnatally and SERT knock-out mice. We can expect that the response in these two models will be somewhat different. In SERT knock-out mice, the function of SERT is constitutively reduced or absent through the entire life, whereas early life exposure to SSRIs only partially blocks SERT function for a period after administration. As discussed above, prenatal exposure to SSRIs produced a desensitization of 5-HT_{2A} receptors in the hypothalamus [96], whereas the 5-HT_{2A} receptors in the hypothalamus was increased in SERT knock-out mice [55]. On the other hand, the function of 5-HT_{2A} receptors in the cortex was reduced in rats exposed to SSRIs prenatally [89], which is similar to the decrease in the density of 5-HT_{2A} receptors in the cortex of SERT knock-out mice [56]. This could account for the attenuation of aggressive behavior observed in both prenatal SSRI-treated rats [83, 84] and SERT knock-out mice [25]. Furthermore, Popa *et al.* have recently reported that administration of escitalopram during postnatal days 5–20 did not produce the desensitization of 5-HT_{1A} receptors as determined by hypothermic response to 5-HT_{1A} agonist, 8-OH-DPAT, which have been observed in SERT knock-out mice [94]. These data suggest that the mechanisms underlying the alterations induced by prenatal and early postnatal administration of SSRIs may be different from those in SERT knock-out mice. Therefore, understanding these mechanisms is important for developing better approaches to prevent disruption of normal mental development of children exposed prenatally and postnatally to SSRIs.

ADULT MODELS

The animal models in this category include models in which fSERT function is disrupted using pharmacological approaches and genomic approaches in adult animals. The pharmacological models are used mainly to study the mechanisms of drug action, such as the therapeutic mechanisms of SSRIs. The genomic models use SERT antisense or siRNA to reduce the SERT expression [97, 98]. These models avoid developmental adaptations caused by constitutive SERT knock-out. Therefore, they are useful tools for studying the function of SERT during adulthood. By comparison with the pharmacological approach, the results from the genomic approach can verify whether a drug effect is mediated by SERT. However, only two studies using these models have been reported. Both studies used non-viral delivery techniques and obtained about 30–40% reduction of SERT expression. More studies are needed to evaluate these techniques. Furthermore, other techniques should be tested. The inducible SERT knock-out mice are another option. Currently, no data have been reported using inducible SERT knock-out mice.

Repeated SSRI administration model

Most studies using this model were intended to investigate the therapeutic mechanisms of these drugs. Although it is known that the pharmacologic mechanism underlying the effects of SSRIs is blockade of 5-HT reuptake from synaptic cleft back to nerve terminals, their pharmacotherapeutic mechanisms in treatment of affective disorders are still not fully understood. Although blockade of the transporter following drug administration occurs rapidly, there is a 2–3-week delay in the improvement of clinical symptoms after the administration of SSRIs. Therefore, it is hypothesized that the therapeutic effects of SSRIs are mediated by the adaptive changes induced by the blockade of 5-HT reuptake. Therefore, once we know what these adaptive changes are, we can develop novel approaches to achieve more rapid therapeutic effects. Studies with this model have focused on the alterations in the 5-HT receptors and signal transduction pathways, which could relate to the adaptive changes.

Alteration in 5-HT transporter and receptors

5-HT transporters

Several studies have found that chronic treatment with SSRIs attenuates the density of 5-HT transporters in the brain [98–101]. Furthermore, Hirano *et al.* reported that the protein level of SERT was reduced after chronic administration of paroxetine for 21 days in most brain regions [102]. However, the SERT mRNA was not altered by repeated administration of SSRIs [99]. These results suggest that chronic SSRI-induced alterations in the density of SERT may be mediated by post-transcriptional regulation of SERT expression and/or alteration in the rate of SERT turnover.

5-HT$_{1A}$ receptors

The effects of SSRIs on 5-HT$_{1A}$ receptors have been studied extensively. It is hypothesized that the action of somatodendritic 5-HT$_{1A}$ receptors is related to the delay of SSRI-mediated improvement of clinical symptoms [103, 104]. When an SSRI is administered initially, the increased 5-HT in the synaptic cleft of 5-HT neurons activates somatodendritic 5-HT_{1A} receptors and, consequently, inhibits 5-HT neuron firing. As a result, the 5-HT release is reduced and the 5-HT concentration in the synaptic cleft is not increased even when the 5-HT reuptake is blocked by SSRI. After a repeated administration of SSRI, the somatodendritic 5-HT_{1A} receptors are desensitized, resulting in reactivation of the 5-HT neurons and an increase of 5-HT release. The increased 5-HT concentration in the synaptic cleft then activates the postsynaptic 5-HT receptors, resulting in adaptive changes of the postsynaptic 5-HT receptors and signal transduction pathways. These adaptive changes alter the emotional states and improve the clinical symptoms. To test this hypothesis, numerous studies have been conducted in last decade.

The first question asked was whether the increase in the 5-HT level in the synaptic cleft is delayed after the administration of SSRIs. Several studies have demonstrated that basal and SSRI-induced increases in the extracellular 5-HT concentrations are increased after the chronic administration of SSRIs, relative to acute administration [105–107]. The second question is whether somatodendritic 5-HT_{1A} receptors are desensitized after administration of SSRI. Several studies have reported that repeated administration of SSRIs produces a desensitization of 5-HT_{1A} receptors in the dorsal and medial raphe nuclei where the 5-HT_{1A} autoreceptors are located [108–111]. Most of these studies demonstrated that the function of the 5-HT_{1A} autoreceptors is reduced by repeated injection of SSRIs using parameters, such as 5-HT_{1A} agonist-induced reduction in 5-HT release [109–112] or G-protein coupling of 5-HT_{1A} receptors [113, 114]. However, the density of 5-HT_{1A} receptors in the raphe nuclei is not found to be changed in most of these studies. For example, Hensler *et al.* [114] demonstrated that 8-OH-DPAT-induced GTP-γ-S binding was attenuated in chronic SSRI-treated rats, but neither 5-HT_{1A} receptor agonist nor antagonist binding sites is altered after chronic treatment with fluoxetine or sertraline. This is consistent with our previous results that repeated administration of fluoxetine and paroxetine for 2 days–4 weeks did not alter the density of 5-HT_{1A} receptors in the dorsal and medial raphe [115]. These data suggest that desensitization of 5-HT_{1A} autoreceptors induced by repeated administration of SSRIs may be mediated by alterations in the G-protein coupling and signal transduction pathways. A recent study suggested that desensitization of 5-HT_{1A} receptors in the dorsal raphe may be mediated by G-protein-coupled inwardly rectifying potassium channel (GIRK) [111]. Evidence has shown that GIRK is associated with 5-HT_{1A} receptors and can be inhibited by chronic treatment of SSRIs [116–118]. Understanding the mechanisms underlying the SSRI-induced desensitization of 5-HT_{1A} receptors will help us to improve the therapeutic effects of SSRIs. Indeed, clinical studies have found that a combination of 5-HT_{1A} antagonists and SSRIs reduced the delay of clinical improvement relative to SSRIs alone [119–123].

The third question is which postsynaptic 5-HT receptors are altered by repeated administration of SSRIs. SSRI-induced alterations in postsynaptic receptors may be related to their therapeutic effects. Therefore, understanding the changes in the postsynaptic 5-HT receptors may lead us to find the more direct targets that are related to affective disorders. Numerous studies have investigated 5-HT receptors and their signal transduction pathways, as will be discussed in the sections below.

Postsynaptic 5-HT_{1A} receptors are distributed in most brain regions. Repeated administration of SSRIs produces a desensitization of 5-HT_{1A} receptors in several brain regions, such as frontal cortex and hypothalamus. For example, Kantor *et al.* found that repeated administration of fluoxetine attenuated the hypothermic response to a 5-HT_{1A} agonist, suggesting a desensitization of hypothalamic 5-HT_{1A} receptors [124]. We have demonstrated that repeated, but not acute, administration of fluoxetine or paroxetine reduces 5-HT_{1A} agonist-induced increases in secretion of several hormones, including oxytocin, ACTH, and corticosterone. Because these hormonal responses to 5-HT_{1A} agonists are mediated by 5-HT_{1A} receptors in the PVN, the results suggest a desensitization of 5-HT_{1A} receptors in the PVN [125–127]. Furthermore, desensitization of 5-HT_{1A} receptors in the hypothalamus induced by the repeated administration of fluoxetine is more extensive in female than male rats [128] and is sustained for more than 60 days [129]. On the other hand, a few studies reported that repeated administration of SSRIs increases the function of 5-HT_{1A} receptors. For example, Zanoveli *et al.* recently reported that chronic treatment with fluoxetine and sertraline sensitized 5-HT_{1A} receptors in dorsal pariaqueductal gray (DPAG) [130]. Also, Beck *et al.* found an increase in the 5-HT_{1A} receptor-mediated inhibitory effects in the hippocampus of rats treated with chronic fluoxetine [131]. These data suggest that the effects of SSRIs on 5-HT_{1A}-mediated functions occur in a brain region-specific manner. However, unlike in SERT knock-out mice, alterations in the density of 5-HT_{1A} receptors were not detected in most studies [113, 115]. Furthermore, unlike 5-HT_{1A} autoreceptors in the raphe nuclei, a reduction in the G-protein-coupling of 5-HT$_{1A}$ receptors was also not detected in most studies [113, 115, 132], although Castro *et al.* reported an increase of 8-OH-DPAT-stimulated GTP-γ-S binding in the hippocampus of chronic fluoxetine-treated rats [114]. These data suggest that desensitization of postsynaptic 5-HT$_{1A}$ receptors may be mediated by alterations downstream of 5-HT$_{1A}$ receptors in their signaling pathways. Supporting this hypothesis, it was found that G$_i$ and G$_o$ proteins that couple to 5-HT$_{1A}$ receptors were changed by repeated administration of SSRIs. We found that G$_{i1/2}$ proteins were reduced in the hypothalamus and G$_o$ proteins were increased in the hippocampus of rats treated with fluoxetine and paroxetine [125, 127]. G$_z$ protein, a pertussis toxin-insensitive G$_i$ protein, is also reduced by repeated injection with fluoxetine [128], which may be responsible for the SSRI-induced desensitization of 5-HT$_{1A}$ receptor-mediated hormone secretions [133]. On the other hand, G$_{i/o}$ proteins may be related to 5-HT$_{1A}$ receptor-mediated activation of mitogen activated protein kinase (MAPK) signal pathway in the hypothalamus [134], which is not desensitized by repeated administration of SSRIs, but is required for G$_z$ protein-mediated desensitization of 5-HT$_{1A}$ receptors in the PVN [133]. These data suggest that different G-proteins coupled to 5-HT$_{1A}$ receptors can direct 5-HT$_{1A}$ receptors to undergo different signal transduction pathways and consequently display different functions. It is possible that SSRI-treatment not only alters G-protein levels but also induces a redistribution of G-proteins coupled to 5-HT$_{1A}$ receptors, which provokes alterations in the function of 5-HT$_{1A}$ receptors.

Altogether, although both the SERT knock-out model and repeated SSRI administration in adult models produce a desensitization of 5-HT$_{1A}$ receptors in various brain regions, including both autoreceptors and postsynaptic receptors, the mechanisms underlying the desensitization may be different between these two models. In the SERT knock-out model, desensitization of 5-HT$_{1A}$ receptors is mediated by a reduction in the expression of 5-HT$_{1A}$ receptors, which could result from the epigenetic regulation of 5-HT$_{1A}$ receptor expression during early development. In the adult SSRI model, desensitization of 5-HT$_{1A}$ receptors may be mediated by the alterations in their signal transduction pathways.

Other 5-HT receptors

5-HT$_{1B}$ receptor is another 5-HT autoreceptor. It is located on the nerve terminal and controls local 5-HT release. Several studies have reported that repeated administration of fluoxetine produces a desensitization of 5-HT_{1B} receptors in the frontal cortex and hypothalamus [135, 136]. Anthony *et al.* reported that chronic treatments of fluoxetine and paroxetine, but not sertraline, reduce 5-HT_{1B} mRNA in the dorsal raphe [137]. These data suggest that the expression of 5-HT_{1B} receptors may be altered by repeated administration of SSRIs. However, the alteration appears to be brain region-specific.

The effects of repeated administration of SSRI on 5-HT_{2A} receptors are more complicated. The data from the literature are not consistent, even contradictory. For example, Damjanoska *et al.* reported that chronic fluoxetine produces a biphasic time course on hormonal response to 5-$HT_{2A/2C}$ receptor agonist, DOI [93]. Chronic fluoxetine attenuated the oxytocin and ACTH responses to DOI at 15 min post-DOI administration, but potentiated the ACTH and corticosterone response to DOI at 30 min post-DOI injection. On the other hand, 5-HT_{2A} receptor binding studies revealed that the high affinity, but not total number of 5-HT_{2A} receptors in the hypothalamus, are increased by repeated administration of fluoxetine [138]. This chronic fluoxetine-induced alteration in the 5-HT_{2A} receptor binding sites was not observed in the frontal cortex [138]. These data suggest that repeated administration of SSRI-induced alterations in the 5-HT_{2A} receptors is in a brain region-specific manner. They may be mediated by alterations in the G-protein coupling and signal transduction pathways of 5-HT_{2A} receptors.

Like 5-HT_{2A} receptors, the data concerning the effects of repeated administration with SSRIs on 5-HT_{2C} receptors are not consistent. Studies have found that repeated administration of SSRIs produces a desensitization of 5-HT_{2C} receptors [139, 140]. On the other hand, chronic citalopram and fluoxetine increased action of 5-HT_{2C} receptors in the choroid plexus [141, 142]. These inconsistent data could result from differential regulation of 5-HT_{2C} receptors among brain regions. Two studies have demonstrated that chronic fluoxetine alters the RNA editing of 5-HT_{2C} receptors [65, 66]. However, since fluoxetine has relatively high affinity for 5-HT_{2C} receptors, it is unclear whether the alterations in RNA editing are mediated by the blockade of SERT. 5-HT_{2C} receptors are involved in the anxiogenic effect and related to several affective disorders, such as obsessive compulsive disorder. Therefore, the reduction in the activity of 5-HT_{2C} receptors may have therapeutic relevance. Several studies have demonstrated that 5-HT_{2C} antagonists facilitated the effects of SSRIs [143, 144], which may be mediated by blockade of 5-HT_{2C} receptor-induced activation of GABAergic system [145]. Thus, understanding the mechanisms that mediate the involvement of 5-HT_{2C}

receptors in the antidepressant effects of SSRIs may provide additional approaches to improve the therapeutic efficiency of SSRIs.

Alterations in G-proteins and signal transduction pathways

As most studies reported, alterations in the function of 5-HT receptors induced by repeated administration with SSRIs are not accompanied by changes in the density of 5-HT receptors. These observations suggest that the effects of SSRIs may be mediated by alterations in downstream mechanisms, such as G-protein coupling and signal transduction pathways.

Studies have demonstrated that repeated administration of fluoxetine and paroxetine gradually and dose-dependently reduces G_i and G_o proteins in the hypothalamus and midbrain [125, 127, 128]. However, in the frontal cortex, only paroxetine, but not fluoxetine, reduced G_i proteins [125, 127]. The SSRI-induced reduction of G_i and G_o proteins in the hypothalamus and midbrain may be related to the desensitization of 5-HT_1 receptors. On the other hand, G_q and G_{11} proteins that couple to 5-HT_2 receptors were not altered in the hypothalamus by chronic SSRIs [93, 138], although the expression of G_q and G_{12} proteins are increased in the striatum and frontal cortex [146]. Instead, chronic SSRIs increase 5-HT-induced phospholipase C (PLC) activity [93, 147] and phospholipase A (PLA) activity [149] in the frontal cortex. Since PLC and PLA are related to the signaling of 5-$HT_{2A/2C}$ receptors, the SSRI-induced alterations in the PLC and PLA may contribute to the sensitization of 5-HT_{2A} receptors in the frontal cortex. These data suggest that the desensitization of 5-HT_{1A} and 5-HT_{1B} receptors by chronic treatment with SSRIs may be related to alteration of G_i/G_o proteins, whereas alteration in the 5-HT_{2A} receptors may be mediated by the changes in the signal transduction pathways. Since the changes in the G-protein levels are only observed in the membrane but not in cytosol [128], they could result from a redistribution of G-proteins [149].

Besides the G-proteins, repeated administration of SSRIs also alters protein kinases and transcription factors. Using microarray techniques, two studies reported that chronic SSRIs reduced the expression of several protein kinases, including protein kinase C (PKC), stress-activated protein kinase, cAMP-dependent protein kinase, Janus protein kinase and phosphofructokinase M [150, 151]. Also, phosphorylated extracellular signal-regulated kinase 1&2 (pERK1/2, pMAPK44/42) was reduced by chronic treatment with fluoxetine, suggesting an attenuation in the activity of MAPK signal transduction pathway [152, 153]. Furthermore, several transcription factors, such as cAMP response element binding protein (CREB) and the brain-derived neurotrophic factor (BDNF) were upregulated by chronic SSRI treatments [153–156]. Consistently, the BDNF receptors (TrkB) are also activated by administration of SSRI [147]. Moreover, a recent study reported that the phosphorylation of two translation factors, eukaryotic initiation factor 4E (eIF4E) and eukaryotic elongation factor 2 (eEF2) were increased by chronic treatment with fluoxetine [157]. These data suggest that repeated administration with SSRIs may not only alter the transcriptional regulation, but also affect the translational regulation. Interestingly, results from recent studies reveal that epigenetic regulation may be involved in the antidepressant effect of fluoxetine [158, 159]. Cassel *et al.* found that chronic fluoxetine increases methyl-CpG-binding proteins, which results in recruiting histone deacetylase (HDAC) and consequently reduces gene transcription [158]. On the other hand, Schroeder *et al.* demonstrated that co-administration of fluoxetine with a deacetylase inhibitor enhanced the antidepressant-like behaviors and increased BDNF in the hippocampus [159]. Although these data are not consistent, one can expect that the epigenetic alterations induced by chronic SSRIs may be cell-specific.

HPA axis

Unlike SERT knock-out mice in which sensitivity to stress is increased, repeated administration of SSRIs in adulthood reduces the sensitivity to stress and reverses stress-induced behaviors [111, 160, 161]. However, stress-induced increases in the HPA axis activity are not attenuated by chronic SSRIs [161, 162]. For example, Zhang *et al.* demonstrated that chronic fluoxetine reduced the conditional fear, i.e. produced an anxiolytic effect, but did not alter stress-induced increases of ACTH and corticosterone secretion [161]. Consistently, Stout *et al.* found that chronic treatments with antidepressants did not affect plasma ACTH and corticosterone in basal and stressed conditions. However, they reported that chronic antidepressants reduced acute stress-induced increases of CRF hnRNA and chronic stress-induced accumulation of CRF mRNA in the medial eminence [162]. These data suggest that repeated administration of SSRIs reduces the sensitivity of HPA axis to stress, but may not alter the basal activity of HPA axis. These observations are opposite to those in SERT knock-out mice, which showed an increased sensitivity of the HPA axis to stress and impaired HPA axis, suggesting that the alterations in the HPA axis of SERT knock-out mice may result from the reduction or lack of SERT during early development.

Adult genomic model

A drawback of the repeated SSRI administration model is that SSRI may have other effects than their high affinity for SERT. In this aspect, selective manipulation of SERT expression using a genomic approach is advantageous. Currently, only two studies have been reported which reduce the expression of SERT with a plasmid containing SERT antisense sequence [97] or a SERT siRNA [98] using non-viral approaches. Both studies produced about 30–40% reduction of the density of SERT and similar effects as SSRIs. These results suggest that selective manipulation of SERT in the adult animal is a useful approach for studies of the function of SERT.

REMARKS AND CONCLUSIONS

As summarized in Table 2.2, interruption of SERT function during different stages of life differentially affects serotonergic systems. The alterations induced by constitutive reduction or deficit of SERT may be mediated by the mechanisms related to changes in the regulation of gene expression. Because 5-HT functions as a neurotrophic factor during early development, alterations in the concentration of 5-HT by disruption of SERT expression early in life may induce a reprogramming of gene expression, such as via epigenetic changes. Thus, these changes may not only occur in genes related to the serotonergic system, but could also affect other genes. Importantly, these changes may be carried throughout the life span and result in emotional alterations later in life. For example, SERT knock-out mice are more sensitive to stress than their SERT normal littermates throughout their lifetime. Similarly, humans with lower SERT expression genotypes also have higher sensitivity to stress. On the other hand, blockade of SERT by chronic administration of SSRIs in adulthood produces changes in the serotonergic systems through alterations in the G-protein coupling and signal transduction pathways. Since G-proteins and signal transduction pathways can be shared by various receptors in the cells, the alterations in the G-proteins and signal transduction pathways could affect multiple neurotransmitter receptors. Furthermore, some receptors, such as 5-HT_{1A} receptors, can couple to different G-proteins that activate different signal transduction pathways. Redistribution of the G proteins coupled to the receptors alters the activation of signal transduction pathways. These alterations in the G-protein coupling and signal transduction pathways may result in functional changes in various neurotransmitter systems and may be related to the therapeutic effects of SSRIs. Unlike developmental models, the changes induced in adult models are reversible and usually sustained for several weeks, although recent studies reveal that treatment with SSRIs may also lead to epigenetic changes [158, 163]. These epigenetic alterations may last longer, even through the rest of life.

In conclusion, the animal models whereby SERT is disrupted in different stages of life are useful tools for studying SERT functions under various conditions. Constitutive SERT knock-out mice, especially SERT+/− mice, can be applied in studies to understand the effects of genetic variance of SERT on mental development. By studying this model, we can address questions, such as what genes are epigenetically altered when the SERT function is constitutively interrupted, what are the mechanisms underlying these epigenetic changes, and how the genetic × environmental factors affect the mental development. Furthermore, study is necessary on the effects of prenatal and postnatal exposure to SSRIs on mental development, as SSRIs are the first-line medication for women with depression during pregnancy and lactation. If necessary, we can develop novel approaches to prevent the influence of interrupting SERT function early in life on mental development. On the other hand, studies on SSRI-induced alterations in animals will have a significant impact on our understanding of the therapeutic mechanisms of SSRIs. The questions that should be further addressed could be which signal pathways and transcription factors are critical for the therapeutic effect of SSRIs, and whether targeting these signal transduction pathways and transcription factors will produce an earlier therapeutic effect. This knowledge will aid in the development of better approaches to treat affective disorders.

ACKNOWLEDGMENTS

The author thanks Drs. Nancy A. Muma and Dania V. Rossi in the University of Kansas who kindly provided feedback for the chapter. The chapter was partly supported by USPHS MH72938 to Qian Li.

REFERENCES

1. Bourin M, David D J P, Jolliet P, Gardier A (2002). Mechanism of action of antidepressants and therapeutic perspectives. *Therapie* **57**: 385–96.

2. Artigas F, Bel N, Casanovas J M, Romero L (1996). Adaptative changes of the serotonergic system after antidepressant treatments. *Adv Exp Med Biol* **398**: 51–9.
3. Murphy D L, Lerner A, Rudnick G, Lesch K P (2004). Serotonin transporter: gene, genetic disorders, and pharmacogenetics. *Molec Interv* **4**: 109–23.
4. Hu X, Oroszi G, Chun J, Smith T L, Goldman D, Schuckit M A (2005). An expanded evaluation of the relationship of four alleles to the level of response to alcohol and the alcoholism risk. *Alcohol Clin Exp Res* **29**: 8–16.
5. Nakamura M, Ueno S, Sano A, Tanabe H (2000). The human serotonin transporter gene linked polymorphism (5-HTTLPR) shows ten novel allelic variants. *Mol Psychiatry* **5**: 32–8.
6. Lesch K P, Bengel D, Heils A, *et al.* (1996). Association of anxiety-related traits with a polymorphism in the serotonin transporter gene regulatory region. *Science* **274**: 1527–31.
7. Heils A, Teufel A, Petri S, *et al.* (1996). Allelic variation of human serotonin transporter gene expression. *J Neurochem* **66**: 2621–4.
8. Greenberg B D, Li Q, Lucas F R, *et al.* (2000). Association between the serotonin transporter promoter polymorphism and personality traits in a primarily female population sample. *Am J Med Genetics* **96**: 202–16.
9. Caspi A, Sugden K, Moffitt T E, *et al.* (2003). Influence of life stress on depression: moderation by a polymorphism in the 5-HTT gene. *Science* **301**: 386–9.
10. Zalsman G, Huang Y Y, Oquendo M A, *et al.* (2006). Association of a triallelic serotonin transporter gene promoter region (5-HTTLPR) polymorphism with stressful life events and severity of depression. *Am J Psychiatry* **163**: 1588–93.
11. Roy A, Hu X Z, Janal M N, Goldman D (2007). Interaction between childhood trauma and serotonin transporter gene variation in suicide. *Neuropsychopharmacology* **32**: 2046–52.
12. Bruning G, Liangos O, Baumgarten H G (1997). Prenatal development of the serotonin transporter in mouse brain. *Cell Tissue Res* **289**: 211–21.
13. Zhou F C, Sari Y, Zhang J K (2000). Expression of serotonin transporter protein in developing rat brain. *Dev Brain Res* **119**: 33–45.
14. Azmitia E C (2001a). Neuronal instability: implications for Rett's syndrome. *Brain Dev* **23** (Suppl 1): S1–10.
15. Buznikov G A, Lambert H W, Lauder J J (2001). Serotonin and serotonin-like substances as regulators of early embryogenesis and morphogenesis. *Cell Tissue Res* **305**: 177–86.
16. Whitaker-Azmitia PM (2001). Serotonin and brain development: role in human developmental diseases. *Brain Res Bull* **56**: 479–85.
17. Bengel D, Murphy D L, Andrews A M, *et al.* (1998). Altered brain serotonin homeostasis and locomotor insensitivity to 3,4-methylenedioxymethamphetamine ("ecstasy") in serotonin transporter-deficient mice. *Molec Pharmacol* **53**: 649–55.
18. Lira A, Zhou M M, Castanon N, *et al.* (2003). Altered depression-related behaviors and functional changes in the dorsal raphe nucleus of serotonin transporter-deficient mice. *Biol Psychiatry* **54**: 960–71.
19. Zhao S, Edwards J, Carroll J, *et al.* (2006). Insertion mutation at the C-terminus of the serotonin transporter disrupts brain serotonin function and emotion-related behaviors in mice. *Neuroscience* **140**: 321–34.
20. Perez X A, Andrews A M (2005). Chronoamperometry to determine differential reductions in uptake in brain synaptosomes from serotonin transporter knockout mice. *Analyt Chem* **77**: 818–26.
21. Fabre V, Beaufour C, Evrard A, *et al.* (2000a). Altered expression and functions of serotonin 5-HT1A and 5-HT1B receptors in knock-out mice lacking the 5-HT transporter. *Eur J Neurosci* **12**: 2299–310.

22. Mathews TA, Fedele D E, Coppelli F M, Avila A M, Murphy D L, Andrews A M (2004). Gene dose-dependent alterations in extraneuronal serotonin but not dopamine in mice with reduced serotonin transporter expression. *J Neurosci Met* **140**: 169–81.
23. Kim D K, Tolliver T J, Huang S J, *et al.* (2005). Altered serotonin synthesis, turnover and dynamic regulation in multiple brain regions of mice lacking the serotonin transporter. *Neuropharmacology* **49**: 798–810.
24. Holmes A, Yang R J, Lesch K P, Crawley J N, Murphy D L (2003a). Mice lacking the serotonin transporter exhibit 5-HT1A receptor-mediated abnormalities in tests for anxiety-like behavior. *Neuropsychopharmacology* **28**: 2077–88.
25. Holmes A, Murphy D L, Crawley J N (2002). Reduced aggression in mice lacking the serotonin transporter. *Psychopharmacology* **161**: 160–7.
26. Ansorge M S, Zhou M M, Lira A, Hen R, Gingrich J A (2004). Early-life blockade of the 5-HT transporter alters emotional behavior in adult mice. *Science* **306**: 879–81.
27. Kalueff A V, Ren-Patterson R F, Murphy D L (2007). The developing use of heterozygous mutant mouse models in brain monoamine transporter research. *Trends Pharmacol Sci* **28**: 122–7.
28. Li Q (2006). Cellular and molecular alterations in mice with deficient and reduced serotonin transporters. *Mol Neurobiol* **34**: 51–66.
29. Holmes A, Murphy D L, Crawley J N (2003b). Abnormal behavioral phenotypes of serotonin transporter knockout mice: parallels with human anxiety and depression. *Biol Psychiatry* **54**: 953–9.
30. Murphy D L, Lesch K P (2008). Targeting the murine serotonin transporter: insights into human neurobiology. *Nat Rev Neurosci* **9**: 85–96.
31. Hoyer D, Hannon J P, Martin G R (2002). Molecular, pharmacological and functional diversity of 5-HT receptors. *Pharmacol Biochem Behav* **71**: 533–54.
32. Hoyer D, Clarke D E, Fozard J R, *et al.* (1994). VII. International Union of Pharmacology classification of receptors for 5-hydroxytryptamine (serotonin). *Pharmacol Rev* **46**: 157–204.
33. den Boer J A, Bosker F J, Slaap B R (2000). Serotonergic drugs in the treatment of depressive and anxiety disorders. *Human Psychopharmacol Clin Exp* **15**: 315–36.
34. Graeff F G, Guimaraes F S, De Andrade T G, Deakin J F (1996). Role of 5-HT in stress, anxiety, and depression. *Pharmacol Biochem Behav* **54**: 129–41.
35. Griebel G (1995). 5-Hydroxytryptamine-interacting drugs in animal models of anxiety disorders: more than 30 years of research. *Pharmacol Ther* **65**: 319–95.
36. Groenink L, Pattij T, de Jongh R, *et al.* (2003). 5-HT1A receptor knockout mice and mice overexpressing corticotropin-releasing hormone in models of anxiety. *Eur J Pharmacol* **463**: 185–97.
37. Olivier B, Pattij T, Wood S J, Oosting R, Sarnyai Z, Toth M (2001). The 5-HT1A receptor knockout mouse and anxiety. *Behav Pharmacol* **12**: 439–50.
38. Gingrich J A, Hen R (2001). Dissecting the role of the serotonin system in neuropsychiatric disorders using knockout mice. *Psychopharmacology* **155**: 1–10.
39. Holmes A, Li Q, Murphy D L, Gold E, Crawley JN (2003a). Abnormal anxiety-related behavior in serotonin transporter null mutant mice: the influence of genetic background. *Genes Brain Behav* **2**: 365–80.
40. Li Q, Wichems C, Heils A, Lesch K P, Murphy D L (2000). Reduction in the density and expression, but not G-protein coupling, of serotonin receptors (5-HT1A) in 5-HT transporter knock-out mice: gender and brain region differences. *J Neurosci* **20**: 7888–95.

41. Li Q, Wichems C, Heils A, Van de Kar L D, Lesch K P, Murphy D L (1999). Reduction of 5-hydroxytryptamine (5-HT)(1A)-mediated temperature and neuroendocrine responses and 5-HT(1A) binding sites in 5-HT transporter knockout mice. *J Pharmacol Exp Ther* **291**: 999–1007.
42. Lanfumey L, La Cour C M, Froger N, Hamon M (2000). 5-HT-HPA interactions in two models of transgenic mice relevant to major depression. *Neurochem Res* **25**: 1199–206.
43. Gobbi G, Murphy D L, Lesch K P, Blier P (2001). Modifications of the serotonergic system in mice lacking serotonin transporters: an in vivo electrophysiological study. *J Pharmacol Exp Ther* **296**: 987–95.
44. Bouali S, Evrard A, Chastanet M, Lesch K P, Hamon M, Adrien J (2003). Sex hormone-dependent desensitization of 5-HT1A autoreceptors in knockout mice deficient in the 5-HT transporter. *Eur J Neurosci* **18**: 2203–12.
45. Bethea C L, Gundlah C, Mirkes S J (2000). Ovarian steroid action in the serotonin neural system of macaques. *Novartis Found Symp* **230**: 112–30.
46. Carrasco G A, Barker S A, Zhang Y, *et al.* (2004). Estrogen treatment increases the levels of regulator of G protein signaling-Z1 in the hypothalamic paraventricular nucleus: possible role in desensitization of 5-hydroxytryptamine (1A) receptors. *Neuroscience* **127**: 261–7.
47. D'Souza D N, Zhang Y H, Damjanoska K J, *et al.* (2004). Estrogen reduces serotonin-1A receptor-mediated oxytocin release and G alpha(i/o/z) proteins in the hypothalamus of ovariectomized rats. *Neuroendocrinology* **80**: 31–41.
48. Le Saux M, Di Paolo T (2005). Changes in 5-HT1A receptor binding and G-protein activation in the rat brain after estrogen treatment: comparison with tamoxifen and raloxifene. *J Psychiatry Neurosci* **30**: 110–17.
49. Lu N Z, Bethea C L (2002). Ovarian steroid regulation of 5-HT1A receptor binding and G protein activation in female monkeys. *Neuropsychopharmacology* **27**: 12–24.
50. Azmitia E C, Whitaker-Azmitia P M (1997). Development and adult plasticity of serotoninergic neurons and their target cells. In Baumgarten H G, Gothert M, editors. *Serotoninergic neurons and 5-HT receptors in the CNS*. Berlin: Springer, pp. 1–39.
51. Azmitia E C (2001b). Modern views on an ancient chemical: serotonin effects on cell proliferation, maturation, and apoptosis. *Brain Res Bull* **56**: 413–24.
52. Whitaker-Azmitia P M (2005). Behavioral and cellular consequences of increasing serotonergic activity during brain development: a role in autism? *Int J Devel Neurosci* **23**: 75–83.
53. Gross C, Zhuang X X, Stark K, *et al.* (2002). Serotonin(1A) receptor acts during development to establish normal anxiety-like behavior in the adult. *Nature* **416**: 396–400.
54. Li Q, Holmes A, Ma L, Van de Kar L D, Garcia F, Murphy D L (2004). Medial hypothalamic 5-hydroxytryptamine (5-HT)1A receptors regulate neuroendocrine responses to stress and exploratory locomotor activity: application of recombinant adenovirus containing 5-HT1A sequences. *J Neurosci* **24**: 10 868–77.
55. Li Q, Wichems C H, Ma L, Van de Kar L D, Garcia F, Murphy D L (2003). Brain region-specific alterations of 5-HT2A and 5-HT2C receptors in serotonin transporter knockout mice. *J Neurochem* **84**: 1256–65.
56. Rioux A, Fabre V, Lesch K P, *et al.* (1999). Adaptive changes of serotonin 5-HT2A receptors in mice lacking the serotonin transporter. *Neurosci Lett* **262**: 113–16.
57. Saphier D, Farrar G E, Welch J E (1995). Differential inhibition of stress-induced adrenocortical responses by 5-HT1A agonists and by 5-HT2 and 5-HT3 antagonists. *Psychoneuroendocrinology* **20**: 239–57.

58. Pompeiano M, Palacios J M, Mengod G (1994). Distribution of the serotonin 5-HT$_2$ receptor family mRNAs: comparison between 5-HT$_{2A}$ and 5-HT$_{2C}$ receptors. *Mol Brain Res* **23**: 163–78.
59. Hartig P R, Hoffman B J, Kaufman M J, Hirata F (1990). The 5-HT1C receptor. *Ann NY Acad Sci* **600**: 149–66.
60. Broocks A, Bandelow B, George A, *et al.* (2000). Increased psychological responses and divergent neuroendocrine responses to m-CPP and ipsapirone in patients with panic disorder. *Int Clin Psychopharmacol* **15**: 153–61.
61. Burns C M, Chu H, Rueter S M, *et al.* (1997). Regulation of serotonin-2C receptor G-protein coupling by RNA editing. *Nature* **387**: 303–08.
62. Niswender C M, Sanders-Bush E, Emeson R B (1998). Identification and characterization of RNA editing events within the 5-HT2C receptor. *Ann NY Acad Sci* **861**: 38–48.
63. Wang Q, O'Brien P J, Chen C X, Cho D S, Murray J M, Nishikura K (2000). Altered G protein-coupling functions of RNA editing isoform and splicing variant serotonin2C receptors. *J Neurochem* **74**: 1290–300.
64. Canton H, Emeson R B, Barker E L, *et al.* (1996). Identification, molecular cloning, and distribution of a short variant of the 5-hydroxytryptamine2C receptor produced by alternative splicing. *Mol Pharmacol* **50**: 799–807.
65. Englander M T, Dulawa S C, Bhansali P, Schmauss C (2005). How stress and fluoxetine modulate serotonin 2C receptor pre-mRNA editing. *J Neurosci* **25**: 648–51.
66. Gurevich I, Tamir H, Arango V, Dwork A J, Mann J J, Schmauss C (2002b). Altered editing of serotonin 2C receptor pre-mRNA in the prefrontal cortex of depressed suicide victims. *Neuron* **34**: 349–56.
67. Gurevich I, Englander M T, Adlersberg M, Siegal N B, Schmauss C (2002a). Modulation of serotonin 2C receptor editing by sustained changes in serotonergic neurotransmission. *J Neurosci* **22**: 10 529–32.
68. Heisler L K, Chu H M, Tecott L H (1998). Epilepsy and obesity in serotonin 5-HT2C receptor mutant mice. *Ann NY Acad Sci* **861**: 74–8.
69. Nonogaki K, Strack A M, Dallman M F, Tecott L H (1998). Leptin-independent hyperphagia and type 2 diabetes in mice with a mutated serotonin 5-HT2C receptor gene. *Nat Med* **4**: 1152–6.
70. Vickers S P, Clifton P G, Dourish C T, Tecott L H (1999). Reduced satiating effect of d-fenfluramine in serotonin 5-HT(2C) receptor mutant mice. *Psychopharmacology (Berl)* **143**: 309–14.
71. Bloom F E, Morales M (1998). The central 5-HT3 receptor in CNS disorders. *Neurochem Res* **23**: 653–9.
72. Delagrange P, Misslin R, Seale T W, Pfeiffer B, Rault S, Renard P (1999). Effects of S-21007, a potent 5-HT3 partial agonist, in mouse anxiety. *Acta Pharmacol Sin* **20**: 805–12.
73. Ye J H, Ponnudurai R, Schaefer R (2001). Ondansetron: a selective 5-HT3 receptor antagonist and its applications in CNS-related disorders. *CNS Drug Rev* **7**: 199–213.
74. Mossner R, Schmitt A, Hennig T, *et al.* (2004). Quantitation of 5HT3 receptors in forebrain of serotonin transporter deficient mice. *J Neural Transm* **111**: 27–35.
75. Chen J J, Li Z S, Pan H, *et al.* (2001). Maintenance of serotonin in the intestinal mucosa and ganglia of mice that lack the high-affinity serotonin transporter: abnormal intestinal motility and the expression of cation transporters. *J Neurosci* **21**: 6348–61.
76. Liu M T, Rayport S, Jiang Y, Murphy D L, Gershon M D (2002). Expression and function of 5-HT3 receptors in the enteric neurons of mice lacking the serotonin transporter. *Am J Physiol-Gastroint Liver Physiol* **283**: G1398–411.

77. Jabbi M, Korf J, Kema I P, *et al.* (2007). Convergent genetic modulation of the endocrine stress response involves polymorphic variations of 5-HTT, COMT and MAOA. *Mol Psychiatry* **12**: 483–90.
78. Oberlander T F, Warburton W, Misri S, Aghajanian J, Hertzman C (2006). Neonatal outcomes after prenatal exposure to selective serotonin reuptake inhibitor antidepressants and maternal depression using population-based linked health data. *Arch Gen Psychiatry* **63**: 898–906.
79. Gentile S (2005b). SSRIs in pregnancy and lactation – emphasis on neurodevelopmental outcome. *CNS Drugs* **19**: 623–33.
80. Gentile, S (2005a). The safety of newer antidepressants in pregnancy and breastfeeding. *Drug Safety* **28**: 137–52.
81. Bairy K L, Madhyastha S, Ashok K P, Bairy I, Malini S (2007). Developmental and behavioral consequences of prenatal fluoxetine. *Pharmacology* **79**: 1–11.
82. Oberlander T F, Misri S, Fitzgerald C E, Kostaras X, Rurak D, Riggs W (2004). Pharmacologic factors associated with transient neonatal symptoms following prenatal psychotropic medication exposure. *J Clin Psychiatry* **65**: 230–7.
83. Coleman F H, Christensen H D, Gonzalez C L, Rayburn W F (1999). Behavioral changes in developing mice after prenatal exposure to paroxetine (Paxil). *Am J Obstet Gynecol* **181**: 1166–71.
84. Lisboa S F, Oliveira P E, Costa L C, Venancio E J, Moreira E G (2007). Behavioral evaluation of male and female mice pups exposed to fluoxetine during pregnancy and lactation. *Pharmacology* **80**: 49–56.
85. Cabrera-Vera T M, Battaglia G (1998). Prenatal exposure to fluoxetine (Prozac) produces site-specific and age-dependent alterations in brain serotonin transporters in rat progeny: evidence from autoradiographic studies. *J Pharmacol Exp Therap* **286**: 1474–481.
86. Montero D, de Ceballos M L, Del Rio J (1990). Down-regulation of 3H-imipramine binding sites in rat cerebral cortex after prenatal exposure to antidepressants. *Life Sci* **46**: 1619–26.
87. Cabrera-Vera T M, Garcia F, Pinto W, Battaglia G (1997). Effect of prenatal fluoxetine (Prozac) exposure on brain serotonin neurons in prepubescent and adult male rat offspring. *J Pharmacol Exp Ther* **280**: 138–45.
88. Cabrera T M, Battaglia G (1994). Delayed decreases in brain 5-hydroxytryptamine2A/2C receptor density and function in male rat progeny following prenatal fluoxetine. *J Pharmacol Exp Ther* **269**: 637–45.
89. Romero G, Toscano E, Del Rio J (1994). Effect of prenatal exposure to antidepressants on 5-HT-stimulated phosphoinositide hydrolysis and 5-HT2 receptors in rat brain. *Gen Pharmacol* **25**: 851–6.
90. Landry M, Frasier M, Chen Z, *et al.* (2005). Fluoxetine treatment of prepubescent rats produces a selective functional reduction in the 5-HT2A receptor-mediated stimulation of oxytocin. *Synapse* **58**: 102–09.
91. Van de Kar L D, Javed A, Zhang Y H, Serres F, Raap D K, Gray T S (2001). 5-HT2A receptors stimulate ACTH, corticosterone, oxytocin, renin, and prolactin release and activate hypothalamic CRF and oxytocin-expressing cells. *J Neurosci* **21**: 3572–9.
92. Zhang Y H, Damjanoska K J, Carrasco G A, *et al.* (2002). Evidence that 5-HT2A receptors in the hypothalamic paraventricular nucleus mediate neuroendocrine responses to (-)DOI. *J Neurosci* **22**: 9635–42.
93. Damjanoska K J, Van de Kar L D, Kindel G H, *et al.* (2003). Chronic fluoxetine differentially affects 5-hydroxytryptamine (2A) receptor signaling in frontal cortex, oxytocin- and corticotropin-releasing factor-containing neurons in rat paraventricular nucleus. *J Pharmacol Exp Ther* **306**: 563–71.

94. Popa D, Lena C, Alexandre C, Adrien J (2008). Lasting syndrome of depression produced by reduction in serotonin uptake during postnatal development: evidence from sleep, stress, and behavior. *J Neurosci* **28**: 3546–54.
95. Ansorge M S, Morelli E, Gingrich J A (2008). Inhibition of serotonin but not norepinephrine transport during development produces delayed, persistent perturbations of emotional behaviors in mice. *J Neurosci* **28**: 199–207.
96. Cabrera T M, Levy A D, Li Q, Van de Kar L D, Battaglia G (1994). Cocaine-induced deficits in ACTH and corticosterone responses in female rat progeny. *Brain Res Bull* **34**: 93–7.
97. Fabre V, Boutrel B, Hanoun N, *et al.* (2000b). Homeostatic regulation of serotonergic function by the serotonin transporter as revealed by nonviral gene transfer. *J Neurosci* **20**: 5065–75.
98. Thakker D R, Natt F, Husken D, *et al.* (2005). siRNA-mediated knockdown of the serotonin transporter in the adult mouse brain. *Mol Psychiatry* **10**: 782–9.
99. Benmansour S, Cecchi M, Morilak D A, *et al.* (1999). Effects of chronic antidepressant treatments on serotonin transporter function, density, and mRNA level. *J Neurosci* **19**: 10 494–501.
100. Horschitz S, Hummerich R, Schloss P (2001). Structure, function and regulation of the 5-hydroxytryptamine (serotonin) transporter. *Biochem Soc Trans* **29**: 728–32.
101. Mirza N R, Nielsen E O, Troelsen K B (2007). Serotonin transporter density and anxiolytic-like effects of antidepressants in mice. *Prog Neuropsychopharmacol Biol Psychiatry* **31**: 858–66.
102. Hirano K, Seki T, Sakai N, *et al.* (2005). Effects of continuous administration of paroxetine on ligand binding site and expression of serotonin transporter protein in mouse brain. *Brain Res* **1053**: 154–61.
103. Artigas F (1993). 5-HT and antidepressants: new views from microdialysis studies. *Trends Pharmacol Sci* **14**: 262.
104. Blier P, De Montigny C (1994). Current advances and trends in the treatment of depression. *Trends Pharmacol Sci* **15**: 220–6.
105. Dawson L A, Nguyen H Q, Smith D L, Schechter L E (2002). Effect of chronic fluoxetine and WAY-100635 treatment on serotonergic neurotransmission in the frontal cortex. *J Psychopharmacol* **16**: 145–52.
106. Dawson L A, Nguyen H Q, Smith D I, Schechter L E (2000). Effects of chronic fluoxetine treatment in the presence and absence of (+/−)pindolol: a microdialysis study. *Br J Pharmacol* **130**: 797–804.
107. Kreiss D S, Lucki I (1995). Effects of acute and repeated administration of antidepressant drugs on extracellular levels of 5-hydroxytryptamine measured in vivo. *J Pharmacol Exp Ther* **274**: 866–76.
108. Hensler J G (2003). Regulation of 5-HT1A receptor function in brain following agonist or antidepressant administration. *Life Sci* **72**: 1665–82.
109. Hjorth S, Bengtsson H J, Kullberg A, Carlzon D, Peilot H, Auerbach S B (2000). Serotonin autoreceptor function and antidepressant drug action. *J Psychopharmacol* **14**: 177–85.
110. Hervas I, Bel N, Fernandez A G, Palacios J M, Artigas F (1998). In vivo control of 5-hydroxytryptamine release by terminal autoreceptors in rat brain areas differentially innervated by the dorsal and median raphe nuclei. *Naunyn Schmiede Arch Pharmacol* **358**: 315–22.
111. Cornelisse L N, van der Harst J E, Lodder J C, *et al.* (2007). Reduced 5-HT1A and GABAB receptor function in dorsal raphe neurons upon chronic fluoxetine treatment of socially stressed rats. *J Neurophysiol* **98**: 196–204.

112. Rossi D V, Burke T F, McCasland M, Hensler J G (2008). Serotonin-1A receptor function in the dorsal raphe nucleus following chronic administration of the selective serotonin reuptake inhibitor sertraline. *J Neurochem* **105**: 1091–9.
113. Hensler J G (2002). Differential regulation of 5-HT1A receptor-G protein interactions in brain following chronic antidepressant administration. *Neuropsychopharmacology* **26**: 565–73.
114. Castro M E, Diaz A, Del Olmo E, Pazos A (2003). Chronic fluoxetine induces changes in G protein coupling at pre and postsynaptic 5-HT1A receptors in rat brain. *Neuropharmacology* **44**: 93–101.
115. Li Q, Battaglia G, Van de Kar L D (1997a). Autoradiographic evidence for differential G-protein coupling of 5-HT1A receptors in rat brain: lack of effect of repeated injections of fluoxetine. *Brain Res* **769**: 141–51.
116. Kobayashi T, Washiyama K, Ikeda K (2003). Inhibition of G protein-activated inwardly rectifying K+ channels by fluoxetine (Prozac). *Br J Pharmacol* **138**: 1119–28.
117. Kobayashi T, Washiyama K, Ikeda K (2004). Inhibition of G protein-activated inwardly rectifying K+ channels by various antidepressant drugs. *Neuropsychopharmacology* **29**: 1841–51.
118. Levita L, Hammack S E, Mania I, Li X Y, Davis M, Rainnie D G (2004). 5-Hydroxytryptamine(1A)-like receptor activation in the bed nucleus of the stria terminalis: electrophysiological and behavioral studies. *Neuroscience* **128**: 583–96.
119. Artigas F, Adell A, Celada P (2006). Pindolol augmentation of antidepressant response. *Curr Drug Targets* **7**: 139–47.
120. Artigas F, Perez V, Alvarez E (1994). Pindolol induces a rapid improvement of depressed patients treated with serotonin reuptake inhibitors. *Arch Gen Psychiatry* **51**: 248–51.
121. Blier P, Lista A, de Montigny C (1993). Differential properties of presynaptic and postsynaptic 5-hydroxytryptamine(1A) Receptors in the dorsal raphe and hippocampus. 1. Effect of spiperone. *J Pharmacol Exp Ther* **265**: 7–15.
122. Hervas I, Vilaro M T, Romero L, Scorza M C, Mengod G, Artigas F (2001). Desensitization of 5-HT1A autoreceptors by a low chronic fluoxetine dose effect of the concurrent administration of WAY-100635. *Neuropsychopharmacology* **24**: 11–20.
123. Romero L, Casanovas J M, Perez V, Alvarez E, Artigas F (1996). Rapid antidepressant effects with SSRIs and 5-HT1A antagonists. Basic and clinical studies. *J Neurochem* **66**: S35.
124. Kantor S, Graf M, Anheuer Z E, Bagdy G (2001). Rapid desensitization of 5-HT1A receptors in Fawn-Hooded rats after chronic fluoxetine treatment. *Euro Neuropsychopharmacol* **11**: 15–24.
125. Li Q, Muma N A, Battaglia G, Van de Kar L D (1997c). A desensitization of hypothalamic 5-HT1A receptors by repeated injections of paroxetine: reduction in the levels of G(i) and G(o) proteins and neuroendocrine responses, but not in the density of 5-HT1A receptors. *J Pharmacol Exp Ther* **282**: 1581–90.
126. Li Q, Brownfield M S, Levy A D, Battaglia G, Cabrera T M, Van de Kar L D (1994). Attenuation of hormone responses to the 5-HT1A agonist ipsapirone by long-term treatment with fluoxetine, but not desipramine, in male rats. *Biol Psychiatry* **36**: 300–08.
127. Li Q, Muma N A, Van de Kar L D (1996). Chronic fluoxetine induces a gradual desensitization of 5-HT_{1A} receptors: reductions in hypothalamic and midbrain G_i and G_o proteins and in neuroendocrine responses to a 5-HT_{1A} agonist. *J Pharmacol Exp Ther* **279**: 1035–42.

128. Raap D K, Evans S, Garcia F, *et al.* (1999a). Daily injections of fluoxetine induce dose-dependent desensitization of hypothalamic 5-HT1A receptors: reductions in neuroendocrine responses to 8-OH-DPAT and in levels of G(z) and G(i) proteins. *J Pharmacol Exp Ther* **288**: 98–106.
129. Raap D K, Garcia F, Muma N A, Wolf W A, Battaglia G, Van de Kar L D (1999b). Sustained desensitization of hypothalamic 5-hydroxytryptamine(1A) receptors after discontinuation of fluoxetine: inhibited neuroendocrine responses to 8-hydroxy-2-(dipropylamino)tetralin in the absence of changes in G(i/o/z) proteins. *J Pharmacol Exp Ther* **288**: 561–7.
130. Zanoveli J M, Nogueira R L, Zangrossi H, Jr. (2007) Enhanced reactivity of 5-HT1A receptors in the rat dorsal periaqueductal gray matter after chronic treatment with fluoxetine and sertraline: evidence from the elevated T-maze. *Neuropharmacology* **52**: 1188–95.
131. Beck S G, Birnstiel S, Choi K C, Pouliot W A (1997). Fluoxetine selectively alters 5-hydroxytryptamine1A and gamma-aminobutyric acidB receptor-mediated hyperpolarization in area CA1, but not area CA3, hippocampal pyramidal cells. *J Pharmacol Exp Ther* **281**: 115–22.
132. Pejchal T, Foley M A, Kosofsky B E, Waeber C (2002). Chronic fluoxetine treatment selectively uncouples raphe 5-HT1A receptors as measured by [S-35]-GTP gamma S autoradiography. *Br J Pharmacol* **135**: 1115–22.
133. Jia C, Carrasco G A, Garcia F, *et al.* (2006). Treatment with SSRIs or 8-OH-DPAT differentially alters 5-HT_{1A} receptor-mediated phosphorylation of ERK and neuroendocrine responses in rats. *Neuroscience meeting*. **33**. 21/C13. Ref Type: Abstract.
134. Crane J W, Shimizu K, Carrasco G A, *et al.* (2007). 5-HT(1A) receptors mediate (+)8-OH-DPAT-stimulation of extracellular signal-regulated kinase (MAP kinase) in vivo in rat hypothalamus: time dependence and regional differences. *Brain Res* **1183**: 51–9.
135. Lifschytz T, Gur E, Lerer B, Newman M E (2004). Effects of triiodothyronine and fluoxetine on 5-HT1A and 5-HT1B autoreceptor activity in rat brain: regional differences. *J Neurosci Meth* **140**: 133–9.
136. Shalom G, Gur E, Van de Kar L D, Newman M E (2004). Repeated administration of the 5-HT1B receptor antagonist SB-224289 blocks the desensitisation of 5-HT1B autoreceptors induced by fluoxetine in rat frontal cortex. *Naunyn Schmiede Arch Pharmacol* **370**: 84–90.
137. Anthony J P, Sexton T J, Neumaier J F (2000). Antidepressant-induced regulation of 5-HT1B RNA in rat dorsal raphe nucleus reverses rapidly after drug discontinuation. *J Neurosci Res* **61**: 82–7.
138. Li Q, Muma N A, Battaglia G, Van der Kar L D (1997b). Fluoxetine gradually increases [I-125]DOI-labelled 5-HT2A/2C receptors in the hypothalamus without changing the levels of G(q)- and G(11)-proteins. *Brain Res* **775**: 225–8.
139. Bristow L J, O'Connor D, Watts R, Duxon M S, Hutson P H (2000). Evidence for accelerated desensitisation of 5-HT2C receptors following combined treatment with fluoxetine and the 5-HT1A receptor antagonist, WAY 100, 635, in the rat. *Neuropharmacology* **39**: 1222–36.
140. Yamauchi M, Tatebayashi T, Nagase K, Kojima M, Imanishi T (2004). Chronic treatment with fluvoxamine desensitizes 5-HT2C receptor-mediated hypolocomotion in rats. *Pharmacol Biochem Behav* **78**: 683–9.
141. Laakso A, Palvimaki E P, Kuoppamaki M, Syvalahti E, Hietala J (1996). Chronic citalopram and fluoxetine treatments upregulate 5-HT2C receptors in the rat choroid plexus. *Neuropsychopharmacology* **15**: 143–51.
142. Palvimaki E P, Majasuo H, Syvalahti E, Hietala J (2005). Serotonin 5-HT2C receptor-mediated phosphoinositide hydrolysis in rat choroid plexus after fluoxetine and citalopram treatments. *Pharmacol Res* **51**: 419–25.

143. Cremers T I F H, Giorgetti M, Bosker F J, *et al.* (2004). Inactivation of 5-HT2C receptors potentiates consequences of serotonin reuptake blockade. *Neuropsychopharmacology* **29**: 1782–9.
144. Boothman L J, Mitchell S N, Sharp T (2006). Investigation of the SSRI augmentation properties of 5-HT(2) receptor antagonists using in vivo microdialysis. *Neuropharmacology* **50**: 726–32.
145. Cremers T I, Rea K, Bosker F J, *et al.* (2007). Augmentation of SSRI effects on serotonin by 5-HT2C antagonists: mechanistic studies. *Neuropsychopharmacology* **32**: 1550–7.
146. Lesch K P, Hough C J, Aulakh C S, *et al.* (1992). Fluoxetine modulates G protein alpha-S, alpha-Q, and alpha-12 subunit messenger-RNA expression in rat brain. *Eur J Pharmacol Mol Pharmacol* **227**: 233–7.
147. Rantamaki T, Hendolin P, Kankaanpaa A, *et al.* (2007). Pharmacologically diverse antidepressants rapidly activate brain-derived neurotrophic factor receptor TrkB and induce phospholipase-Cgamma signaling pathways in mouse brain. *Neuropsychopharmacology* **32**: 2152–62.
148. Qu Y, Chang L, Klaff J, Seemann R, Greenstein D, Rapoport S I (2006). Chronic fluoxetine upregulates arachidonic acid incorporation into the brain of unanesthetized rats. *Eur Neuropsychopharmacol* **16**: 561–71.
149. Donati R J, Rasenick M M (2003). G protein signaling and the molecular basis of antidepressant action. *Life Sci* **73**: 1–17.
150. Conti B, Maier R, Barr A M, *et al.* (2007). Region-specific transcriptional changes following the three antidepressant treatments electro convulsive therapy, sleep deprivation and fluoxetine. *Mol Psychiatry* **12**: 167–89.
151. Rausch J L, Gillespie C F, Fei Y, *et al.* (2002). Antidepressant effects on kinase gene expression patterns in rat brain. *Neurosci Lett* **334**: 91–4.
152. Fumagalli F, Molteni R, Calabrese F, Frasca A, Racagni G, Riva M A (2005). Chronic fluoxetine administration inhibits extracellular signal-regulated kinase 1/2 phosphorylation in rat brain. *J Neurochem* **93**: 1551–60.
153. Morinobu S, Russel D S, Sugawara S, Takahashi M, Fujimaki K (2000). Regulation of phosphorylation of cyclic AMP response element-binding protein by paroxetine treatments. *Clin Neuropharmacol* **23**: 106–09.
154. Vinet J, Carra S, Blom J M, Brunello N, Barden N, Tascedda F (2004). Chronic treatment with desipramine and fluoxetine modulate BDNF, CaMKKalpha and CaMKKbeta mRNA levels in the hippocampus of transgenic mice expressing antisense RNA against the glucocorticoid receptor. *Neuropharmacology* **47**: 1062–9.
155. Tiraboschi E, Tardito D, Kasahara J, *et al.* (2004). Selective phosphorylation of nuclear CREB by fluoxetine is linked to activation of CaM kinase IV and MAP kinase cascades. *Neuropsychopharmacology* **29**: 1831–40.
156. Koch J M, Kell S, Aldenhoff J B (2003). Differential effects of fluoxetine and imipramine on the phosphorylation of the transcription factor CREB and cell viability. *J Psychiatric Res* **37**: 53–9.
157. Dagestad G, Kuipers S D, Messaoudi E, Bramham C R (2006). Chronic fluoxetine induces region-specific changes in translation factor eIF4E and eEF2 activity in the rat brain. *Eur J Neurosci* **23**: 2814–8.
158. Cassel S, Carouge D, Gensburger C, *et al.* (2006). Fluoxetine and cocaine induce the epigenetic factors MeCP2 and MBD1 in adult rat brain. *Mol Pharmacol* **70**: 487–92.
159. Schroeder F A, Lin CL, Crusio W E, Akbarian S (2007). Antidepressant-like effects of the histone deacetylase inhibitor, sodium butyrate, in the mouse. *Biol Psychiatry* **62**: 55–64.

160. Conley R K, Hutson P H (2007). Effects of acute and chronic treatment with fluoxetine on stress-induced hyperthermia in telemetered rats and mice. *Eur J Pharmacol* **564**: 138–45.
161. Zhang Y H, Raap D K, Garcia F, *et al.* (2000). Long-term fluoxetine produces behavioral anxiolytic effects without inhibiting neuroendocrine responses to conditioned stress in rats. *Brain Res* **855**: 58–66.
162. Stout S C, Owens M J, Nemeroff C B (2002). Regulation of corticotropin-releasing factor neuronal systems and hypothalamic–pituitary–adrenal axis activity by stress and chronic antidepressant treatment. *J Pharmacol Exp Ther* **300**: 1085–92.
163. Csoka A, Bahrick A, Mehtonen O P (2008). Persistent sexual dysfunction after discontinuation of selective serotonin reuptake inhibitors. *J Sex Med* **5**: 227–33.
164. Gobbi M, Crespi D, Foddi M C, *et al.* (1997). Effects of chronic treatment with fluoxetine and citalopram on 5-HT uptake, 5-HT1B autoreceptors, 5-HT3 and 5-HT4 receptors in rats. *Naunyn Schmiede Arch Pharmacol* **356**: 22–8.

ANTONIO M. PERSICO

3

Developmental roles for the serotonin transporter

ABSTRACT

From invertebrates to humans, serotonin (5-HT) exerts structural effects, especially during development. The 5-HT transporter (SERT) directly regulates these effects by maintaining extracellular 5-HT concentrations within a physiological range and possibly by modulating the intracellular redox state of the cell. This chapter addresses 5-HT trophic effects on developing neural and non-neural mammalian cells, and summarizes SERT roles in 5HT-mediated structural effects from basic neurodevelopment to human teratology.

INTRODUCTION

The neurotransmitter serotonin (5-HT) is known to influence behavioral, autonomic, and cognitive functions, including learning and memory, sleep, temperature regulation, appetite, and mood. 5HT also plays a major role in human disorders such as anxiety, fear, depression, obsessive compulsive behavior, autism, and aggression [1, 2]. In addition to triggering a wide variety of electrophysiological effects, 5-HT also exerts important developmental roles in neural and non-neural tissues from early embryogenesis [3–6]. In many regions of the central nervous system (CNS), this dual "functional" and "structural" involvement is interestingly paralleled at the histological and molecular levels by classical synaptic neurotransmission co-existing with paracrine mechanisms typical of "volume" or "mass" transmission [7–9]. Indeed, many serotoninergic presynaptic terminals are not in direct proximity to postsynaptic

Experimental Models in Serotonin Transporter Research, eds. A. V. Kalueff and J. L. LaPorte. Published by Cambridge University Press.

elements [8]. Many 5-HT receptors display CNS distributions necessarily implying the existence of abundant extrasynaptic binding sites [7, 9], and the 5-HT transporter (SERT) is distributed along 5-HT axonal membranes mostly at extrasynaptic, non-junctional sites [10]. Conceivably, the diffusion of 5-HT several microns away from the release site is better suited to exert trophic roles during development and to modulate electrical, metabolic, and neuroplastic responses of populations of surrounding cells in the adult brain than to provide localized information processing. This, however, does not exclude that one-to-one neurochemical messages conveyed by 5-HT neurons to single cells through direct synaptic contacts can also play relevant developmental roles, as shown for 5-HT terminals in cortical layer I establishing synaptic contacts with Cajal–Retzius cells and possibly modulating reelin secretion [11].

During pre- and postnatal development, the growth, differentiation, and plasticity of 5HT-releasing and 5HT-sensing cells appear to be extraordinarily coordinated with the transcriptional activation of genes encoding the molecular machinery underlying 5-HT-mediated morphogenetic effects. In this context, SERT plays a pivotal role by fostering 5-HT entry from the extracellular space into cells, thus terminating 5-HT's effects on its membrane receptors [12]. This chapter reviews current knowledge on the trophic effects exerted by 5-HT on developing neural and non-neural mammalian cells, and summarizes SERT roles in 5HT-mediated structural effects from basic neurodevelopment to potential human teratology.

DEVELOPMENT OF THE SEROTONERGIC SYSTEM

In the CNS, 5-HT neurons are organized into two main groups of midline cell clusters: the rostral and caudal raphe nuclei [13]. The rostral raphe nuclei, located in the midbrain and pons, project throughout the brain, whereas the caudal raphe nuclei are found in the medulla oblongata and project to the spinal cord. Serotonergic neurons differentiate early in neurodevelopment [13–15]. In humans, they appear by week 5 of gestation, grow rapidly through week 10, and assume the cytoarchitectonic organization typical of the raphe nuclei by week 15 [15–18]. In the rat, the superior group, encompassing raphe nuclei B5 to B9, forms at embryonic day 12 (E12, i.e. 10 prior to delivery), whereas the inferior group, composed of raphe nuclei B1 to B3 and the area postrema, forms approximately 2 days later [13, 14]. In the mouse, 5-HT-immunoreactive neurons can be first seen at E11.5 and E12.5 for the rostral and caudal nuclei, respectively [15].

Postnatally, the human CNS undergoes a steady increase in 5-HT levels during the first 2 years after birth, corresponding to a period of extensive development and plasticity. This initial growth subsequently slows down and 5-HT decreases to reach adult levels by 5 years of age [16, 19]. Morphologically, typical 5-HT neurons display long and highly branched axons, connecting each neuron with neuronal, glial, endothelial, and ependymal cells throughout the brain and spinal cord [20]. Also, this highly arborized morphology contributes to sustain widespread 5-HT effects on electrical, metabolic, and neuroplastic responses in groups of cells, particularly during development.

The prenatal establishment of serotonergic neural pathways is accompanied by the transcriptional activation of genes encoding 5-HT transporters and receptors, both in the CNS and peripherally in non-neural tissues. In general, the expression patterns of 5-HT transporters and receptors begin relatively early during development and display a significant degree of plasticity, as shown by the long-term expression changes, sometimes lasting into adulthood, produced by prenatal exposure to 5-HT receptor ligands [21] or to drugs of abuse [22, 23]. The molecular machinery involved in 5-HT uptake and vesicular storage is indeed expressed prenatally by serotonergic growth cones: in rodents, serotonin binding protein- and SERT-like immunoreactivity are detectable at E15, while the vesicular monoamine transporter (VMAT-2) appears at E20 [24]. Subsequently, SERT and VMAT-2 will display transient and variable patterns of gene expression, which at some developmental stages differ dramatically from the central and peripheral distribution of these molecules in the adult [25–27]. Serotonin receptor subtypes have been grouped into seven distinct families based on molecular structure, pharmacological properties, G-protein coupling and second messenger pathways: 5-HT$_1$ (1A, 1B, 1D, 1E and 1F), 5-HT$_2$ (2A, 2B and 2C), 5-HT$_4$ (4A, 4B), 5-HT$_5$ (5A, 5B), 5-HT$_6$ and 5-HT$_7$ families couple to G-proteins, whereas 5-HT$_3$ receptors encompassing two splice variants (3A and 3B) are ligand-gated ion channels [28]. In the prenatal rodent brain, 5-HT receptors are expressed by both neurons and glia along growing serotonergic pathways, with each 5-HT receptor subtype displaying specific developmental expression patterns, depending upon developmental stage and regional receptor distribution [20, 29–36].

Some of the most exciting developments in neuroscience research have taken place in recent years through studies aimed at understanding the molecular mechanisms underlying the differentiation of 5-HT neurons. First, expression of the ETS domain transcription factor Pet-1 in the mouse embryo was found to occur exclusively in neurons that approximately 1 day later would begin displaying a serotonergic phenotype [37]. In addition, Pet-1 response elements are present in the promoter of many serotoninergic genes, including SERT, VMAT, tryptophan hydroxylase (TPH), aromatic L-amino acid decarboxylase, and 5-HT_{1A} receptor [37]. Binding of Pet-1 to these response elements activates the transcription of serotoninergic genes; conversely, Pet-1 knock-out mice display significant decreases in serotoninergic gene expression, including SERT, while as many as 70% of 5-HT neurons fail to differentiate [15]. Interestingly, Pet-1 knock-out mice are viable and display hightened anxiety and aggressive behavior [15]. A second key player in 5-HT neuronal differentiation is the homeobox gene Lmx1b, which is expressed slightly before Pet-1 and does not initiate Pet-1 gene expression, but appears necessary for its sustained expression [38]. Contrary to Pet-1 knock-out mice, Lmx1b knock-out mice are not viable. However, the ability of the Pet-1 enhancer region to specifically direct transgene expression to serotoninergic neurons allowed investigators to restrict the disruption of Lx1b gene expression to Pet-1-expressing cells (i.e. 5-HT neuronal precursors), yielding mice displaying a complete loss of 5-HT neurons [38]. These mice are viable and their locomotor activity appears surprisingly normal, but they show abnormal hypercapnic respiratory responses, impaired thermogenesis, and reduced/enhanced responses to mechanical/inflammatory nociceptive stimuli, respectively [38–40]. These animals indeed represent an impressive experimental model to explore 5-HT roles in physiology at the molecular, electrophysiological, and behavioral levels [41, 42].

STRUCTURAL EFFECTS OF 5-HT DURING EMBRYOGENESIS IN MAMMALIAN TISSUES

Trophic roles for 5-HT arose very early in evolution. Serotonin exerts profound structural effects in a variety of invertebrates, as reviewed elsewhere [6, 43]. In organisms as distant from mammals as plants, the indole ring of the amino acid tryptophan confers light-capturing properties to auxin (which is indolacetic acid, a compound very similar to the 5-HT metabolite 5-hydroxy indolacetic acid, 5-HIAA) to promote bending towards light sources [44–46]. This process involves reorientation, growth and stabilization of cytoskeletal elements, actin filaments and microtubules [44–46]. Therefore, the existence of 5-HT structural effects in mammalian neural and non-neural tissues is not at all surprising. Starting already at cleavage and gastrulation, 5-HT, the SERT and several 5-HT receptors can be coincidently detected in embryos of a wide variety of invertebrate and vertebrate species, including sea urchins, fish, amphibians, rodents, chicks, and *Drosophila* [3, 6, 26, 47, 48]. In this context, the SERT plays a pivotal role by modulating 5-HT extracellular levels and by importing 5-HT into cells (see below).

During embryogenesis, 5-HT profoundly affects neural, craniofacial, cardiac, and limb development by regulating a variety of developmental processes, including cell proliferation, migration, and differentiation, as well as programmed cell death [4, 5, 49]. During specific prenatal critical periods, tissues including the palate and craniofacial mesenchyme, the heart myocardium, endothelium, and vascular smooth muscle transiently express SERT, VMAT, and serotonin binding protein, allowing uptake and vesicular storage of 5-HT in these non-neuronal cells [5, 50–64]. In these same tissues, 5-HT exerts a concentration-dependent influence on cell migration, typically mediated by 5-HT_2 receptor subtypes [5, 51, 52, 54–59, 61]. Consequently, the pan-5-HT_2 receptor antagonist ritanserin causes craniofacial and cardiac dysmorphogenesis in cultured mouse embryos [5, 65, 66]. Meanwhile, 5-HT_{1A} and 5-HT_4 receptors enhance IGF-I production in cultured cranial mesenchymal cells [67]. In addition, the selective serotonin reuptake inhibitor (SSRI) fluoxetine also causes craniofacial and cardiac malformations in cultured mouse embryos [4, 5]. These teratogenetic effects are usually interpreted as secondary to excessive extracellular 5-HT levels yielding 5-HT receptor over-stimulation in craniofacial mesenchyme and endocardial cushions. However, it is also possible that a lack of 5-HT entry into SERT-expressing cells and/or decreased SERT activity per se could contribute to these malformations directly (see below). In this regard, the broad distribution of transient SERT immunoreactivity in mouse embryos [26] suggests that SERT involvement in regulating cell migration and proliferation could also be more widespread than once believed.

The proliferation of neural progenitor cells and their differentiation into postmitotic neurons can be influenced either by direct binding of 5-HT to receptors located on neuronal cells, or by 5-HT stimulating the release of astroglial neurotrophic factors [68]. Similar effects are also seen in non-neural tissues. For example, 5-HT enhances the proliferation of vascular smooth muscle cells and fibroblasts in vitro [53, 60, 62, 63, 65, 69, 70]. Stimulation of cell-cycle progression by 5-HT is mediated by a complex, cell-type specific activation of intracellular pathways. In non-transformed mouse fibroblast LMTK cells, for example, 5-HT activates a cascade including Src, cyclin E/cdk2 and cyclin D1/cdk4, causing retinoblastoma protein phosphorylation and resulting in the passage of the cell-cycle restriction point in G_0 [66].

In other models, reduction in intracellular cAMP produced through 5-HT_1-type receptor activation may be important, since elevated cAMP levels inhibit mitogenesis. In vascular smooth muscle cells, however, these same receptor subtypes surprisingly use reactive oxygen species as second messengers [69]. Regardless of cell-type, one unifying feature of these experimental models is the recurrent cross-talk between 5-HT-activated intracellular cascades and tyrosine kinase-dependent pathways typically activated by "classical" growth factors, with tyrosine phosphorylation of intracellular proteins representing a critical step in 5-HT-stimulated mitogenesis [60]. Importantly, proliferation of vascular smooth muscle cells requires 5-HT internalization through the SERT and cannot be either induced or blocked by 5-HT receptor agonists or antagonists, respectively, acting exclusively on membrane receptors [60]. This points towards intracellular 5-HT effects, possibly mediated at the mitochondrial levels (see below).

Increasing evidence for serotonergic modulation of apoptotic cell death has been provided by in vitro [68, 71, 72], and in vivo studies [73–75]. Many cell culture experiments are consistent with animal models in supporting protective 5-HT effects against both "pathological" apoptosis induced, for example, by ischemia [74], and "physiological" apoptosis occurring during brain development [73, 75]. Some in vitro models support 5-HT_{1A} receptor contributions to the modulation of programmed cell death, through direct activation of the mitogen-activated protein kinase pathway inhibiting caspase 3, as in hippocampal HN2–5 cells [71]. Other in vivo models support indirect 5-HT_{1A}-mediated mechanisms, including neuronal hyperpolarization, reduced glutamate release, and/or enhanced expression of neuroprotective factors, such as astroglial S100β protein [68, 74]. In the case of developmental programmed cell death, 5-HT appears to act through 5-HT_2 receptors, preventing the downregulation of the antiapoptotic proteins Bcl-2 and Bcl-xL [75]. There are also experimental paradigms showing where 5-HT can induce, rather than diminish, apoptosis as demonstrated in cerebellar granule cells [76] and Burkitt lymphoma cells [72]. It is interesting that this effect is blocked by SSRIs and not by antagonists acting upon 5-HT receptors located at the cell membrane. This again indicates that either 5-HT internalization, or at least SERT activation by 5-HT, is also required for this effect [72]. The anti-apoptotic effects documented in SERT knock-out neonatal mice [73] could thus derive not only from enhanced extracellular 5-HT levels [77], over-stimulating one or more 5-HT receptor subtypes, but also from the concomitant blockade of 5-HT internalization due to SERT gene inactivation [78].

STRUCTURAL EFFECTS OF 5-HT IN THE RODENT SOMATOSENSORY CORTEX

The mammalian neocortex represents a complex array of laminar and columnar compartments, largely formed during prenatal brain development by radial and tangential neuronal migration [79, 80]. Serotoninergic afferents reach the cortex at the peak of cortical plate development [81–83], spurring interest in 5-HT roles in neocortical development and plasticity. The rodent somatosensory system, with its one-to-one correspondence between peripheral sense organs and CNS relay stations, offers significant advantages over other sensory systems as an experimental model to assess peripheral and central modulation of cortical development and plasticity. Rodents primarily explore the environment by rhythmically moving their whiskers, while recording the tactile inputs triggered at the level of each whisker follicle by any deflection imposed on the whisker by an external force, such as an object. Each whisker on the rodent snout is somatotopically represented in the trigeminal nucleus into a "barrelette", in the ventro-postero-medial thalamus as a "barreloid", and in the primary somatosensory cortex as a "barrel" [84, 85]. Mouse cortical barrels encompass a hollow center with abundant thalamocortical terminals and few granule cells in layer IV, surrounded by a ring of dense granule cells separated by cell-poor septa [84]. Barrels are clearly visible using common cytochrome oxidase histochemistry, visualizing axonal and dendritic neurites, or with Nissl stainings of cell bodies [84, 86, 87]; also, acetylcholinesterase is transiently found in somatosensory thalamocortical afferents (TCAs) of neonatal rats [88], and can be visualized using standard histochemical methods [89]. TCAs from the ventrobasal (VB) thalamic nucleus are already distributed somatotopically at birth [90, 91] and play an instructive role in cortical barrel field formation, which occurs a few days later [84, 92, 93]. TCA-instructed barrel formation is actually part of a peripheral-to-central maturation cascade, with barrelettes forming prenatally, barrelloids approximately at birth and barrels appearing around postnatal day 4 (P4) in rodents [84]. Peripheral sense organs, namely the vibrissae, play an important role in organizing the barrel field, as demonstrated by the lack of cortical barrel formation following denervation of the corresponding vibrissa follicle during an early postnatal critical period (i.e. P0–P4, where P0 is the day of birth) [87, 94]. Interestingly, local administration of BDNF or NT3, but not NGF, on the sectioned infraorbital nerve leads to recovery of the cortical barrel pattern and rescue from denervation-induced apoptosis [95, 96].

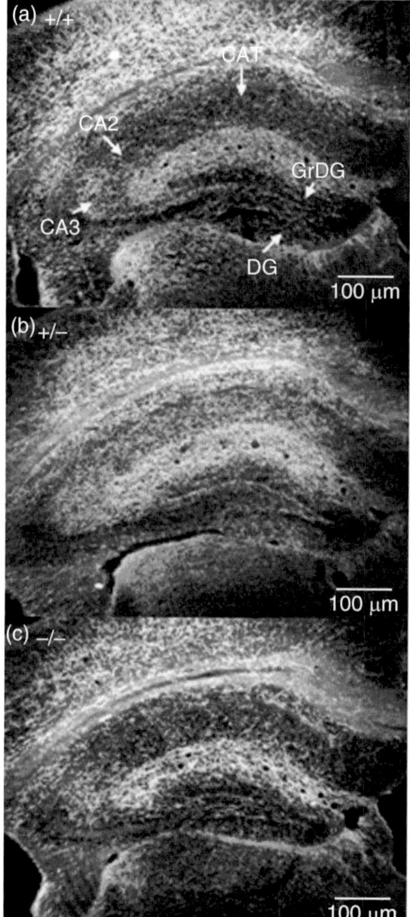

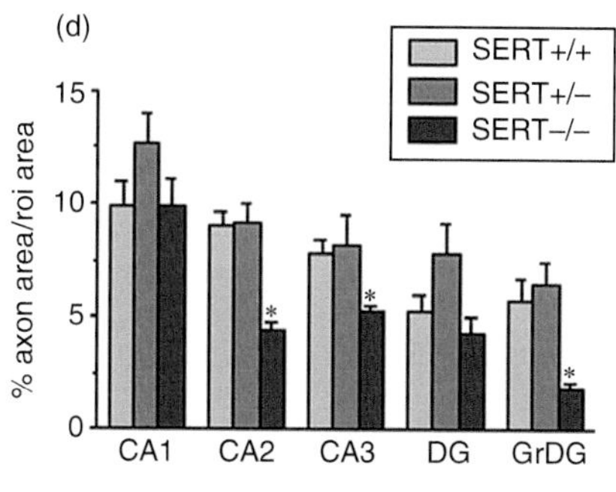

Figure 1.3 Representative darkfield photomicrographs and quantification of 5-HT axons in the hippocampus of 3–4-month-old SERT+/+, SERT+/−, and SERT−/− mice visualized by immunocytochemistry and measured by digitized axon analysis. Serotonin axon innervation is significantly decreased in the CA2 and CA3 subregions and the granular layer of dentate gyrus (GrDG) of the hippocampus in SERT−/− mice (c) compared to SERT+/+ mice (a,d). In d, the data are reported as mean percent axon area/region of interest area ± SEM. DG, dentate gyrus. Probabilities are identified as $^{*}p<0.05$ for differences from SERT+/+ mice.

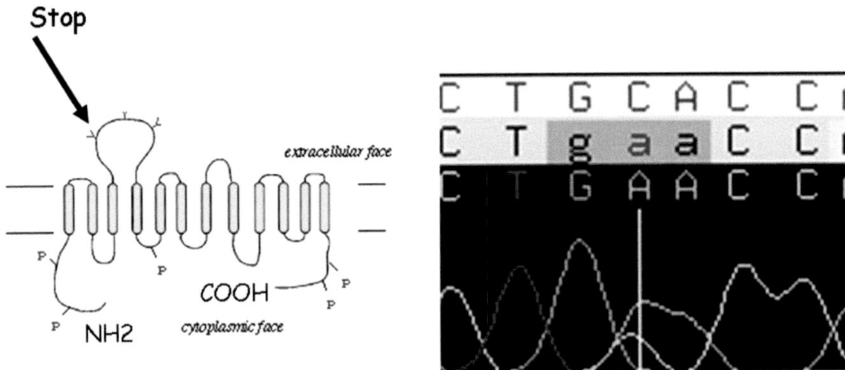

Figure 6.2 Schematic representation of the SERT gene and the induced knock-out mutation (Slc6a4^{1Hubr}) achieved by target-selected mutagenesis. The arrow indicates the location of the ENU-induced C to A mutation that results in the change of amino acid 209 from a cysteine to a stopcodon. Reused from Homberg *et al.*, (2007a), with kind permission of Elsevier Limited.

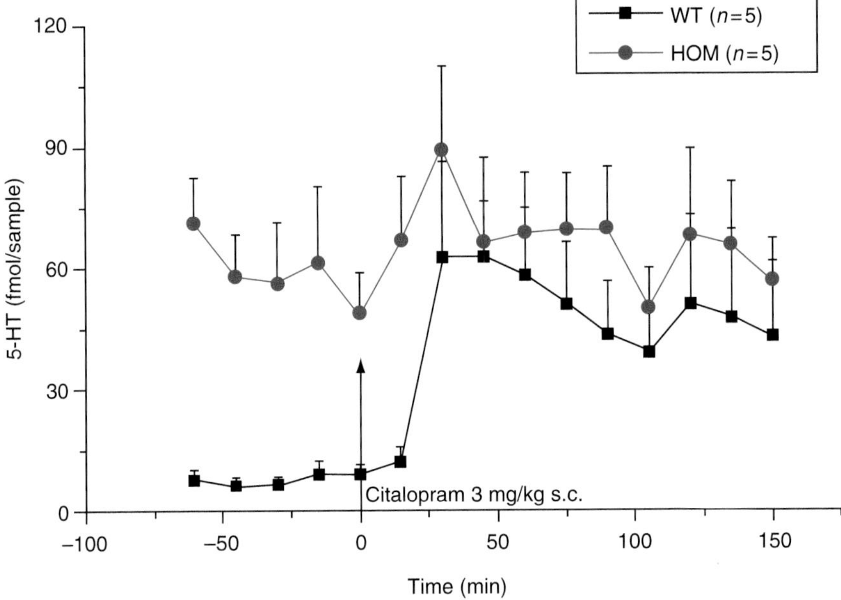

Figure 6.4 Extracellular 5-HT levels in the ventral hippocampus of male SERT+/+ and SERT−/− rats as measured by in vivo microdialysis. Basal dialysate 5-HT levels are ninefold increased in SERT−/− rats. Citalopram (3 mg/kg) increased 5-HT levels in SERT+/+ rats to that of SERT−/− rats, while citalopram had no effect in SERT−/− rats. Data represent mean (± SEM) extracellular 5-HT (fmol/sample). Reused from Homberg *et al.* (2007a), with kind permission of Elsevier Limited.

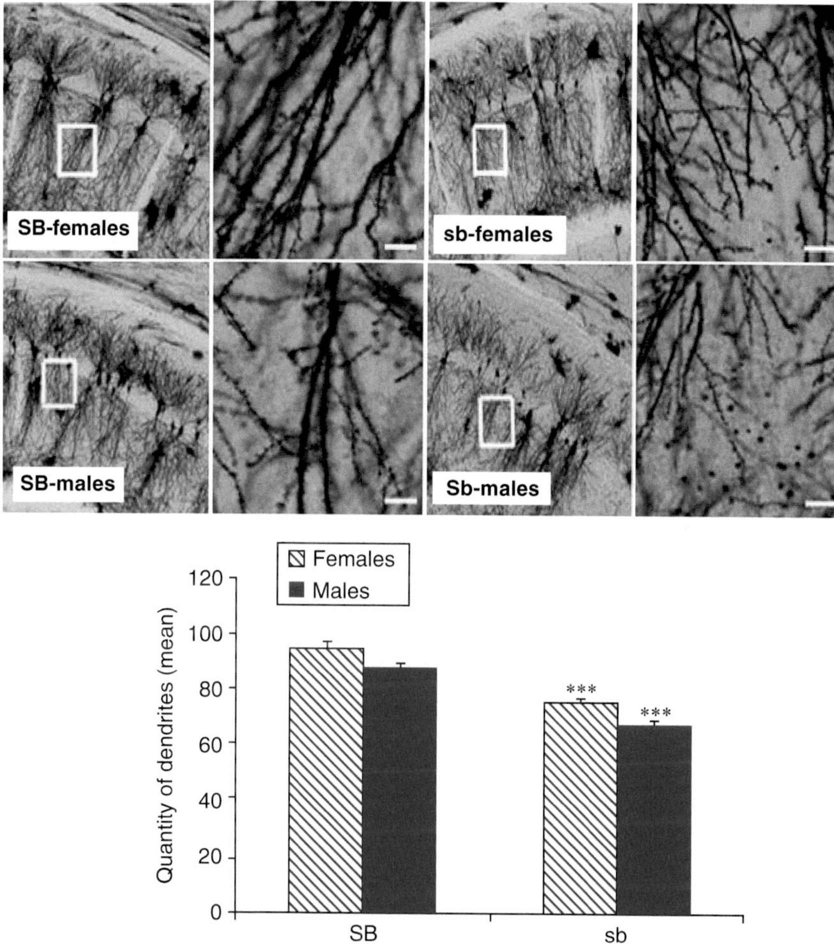

Figure 9.4 Reductions of 5-HT and BDNF affect development of neuronal dendritic branches in sb mice. The morphology of brain neuronal hippocampal near dentate gyrus dendrites and spines was evaluated in 20 fields. (Scale bars = 10 μm). The quantity of dendrites in brain sections with Golgi impregnation. Both genders had significant reductions in sb mice (***$p<0.0001$) compared to SB mice using two-way ANOVA test (see legend for Fig. 9.3 for details).

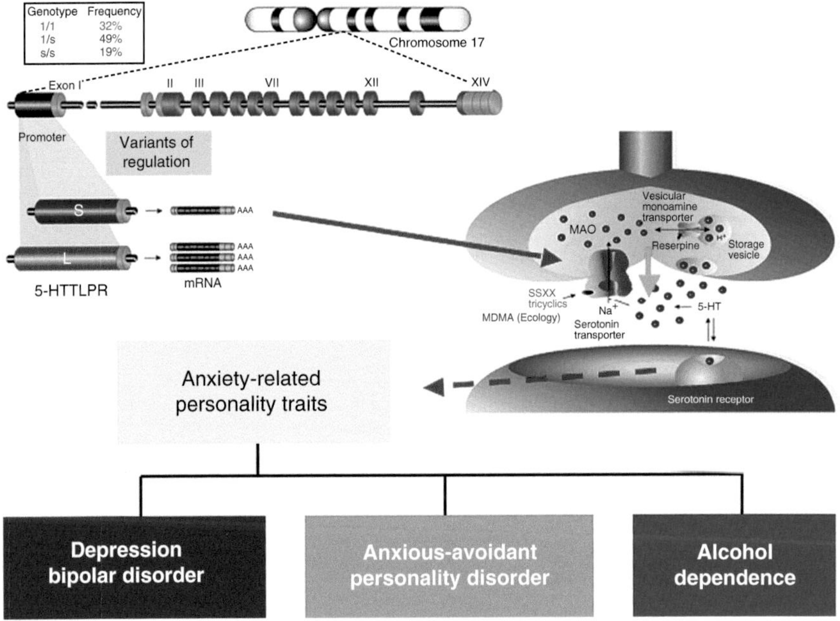

Figure 11.3 Allelic variation of serotonin transporter function in anxiety-related personality, depression and other disorders of emotion regulation.

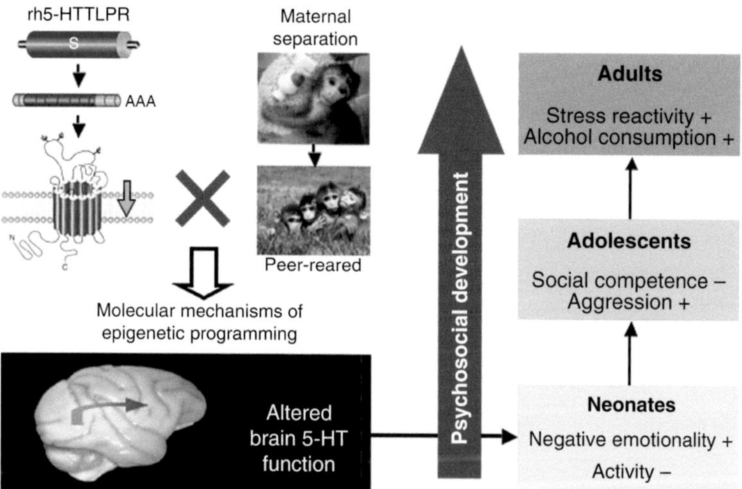

Figure 11.4 Effect of interaction between maternal separation and rh5-HTTLPR genotype on psychosocial development, including brain 5-HT function, emotion regulation, social competence, stress reactivity, behavior, and psychopathology, across the lifespan of rhesus macaques.

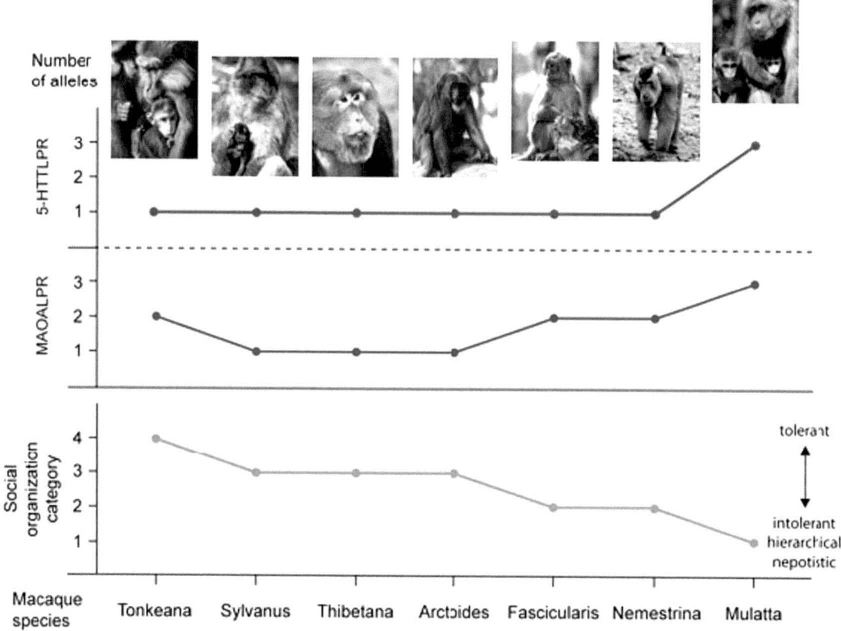

Figure 11.5 Degree of variation in two genes of the 5-HT signaling pathway (5-HT transporter and monoamine oxidase A), aggression and social organization in seven macaque species.

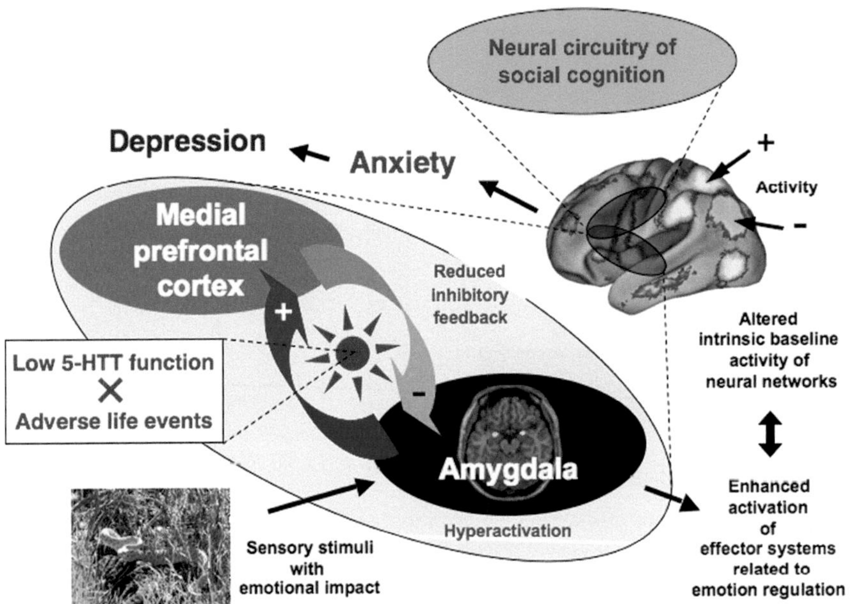

Figure 11.6 Influence of *5-HTT* × life stress interaction on neural networks of emotion regulation. Allelic variation of 5-HTT function is likely to represent a classic susceptibility factor for affective spectrum disorders by biasing the functional reactivity of the amygdala in the context of stressful life experiences and/or deficient cortical regulatory input.

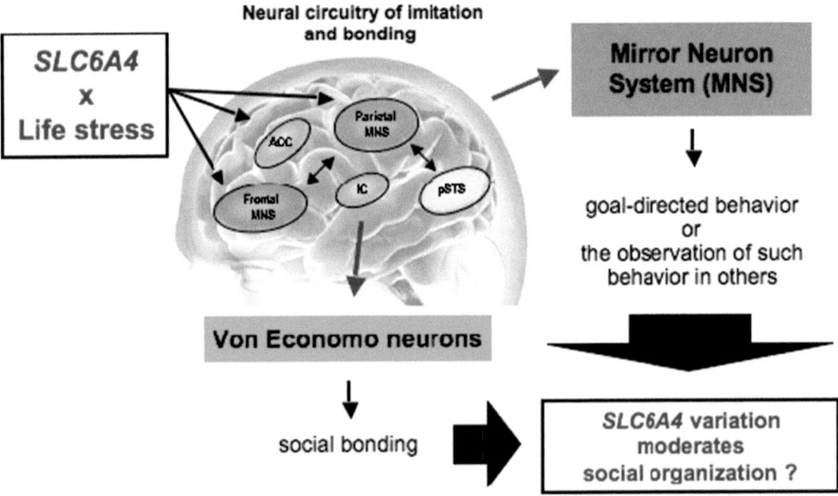

Figure 11.7 Beyond negative emotionality: *5-HTT* variation and neural correlates of social cognition. *5-HTT* × environment interaction may influence neural networks of social cognition and emotion regulation. These interactions are documented in brain regions that comprise the frontal and parietal Mirror Neuron System (MNS) or that contain Von Economo neurons, both of which play a role in social cognition and bonding. ACC, anterior cingulate cortex; IC, insular cortex, pSTS, posterior superior temporal sulcus (visual input to MNS).

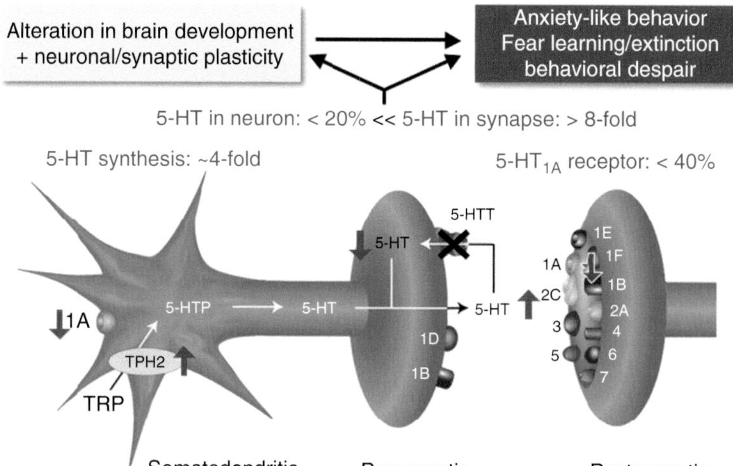

Figure 11.8 Altered brain 5-HT homeostasis in 5-HTT deficient mice: resolving the conundrum of the serotonin hypothesis of depression.

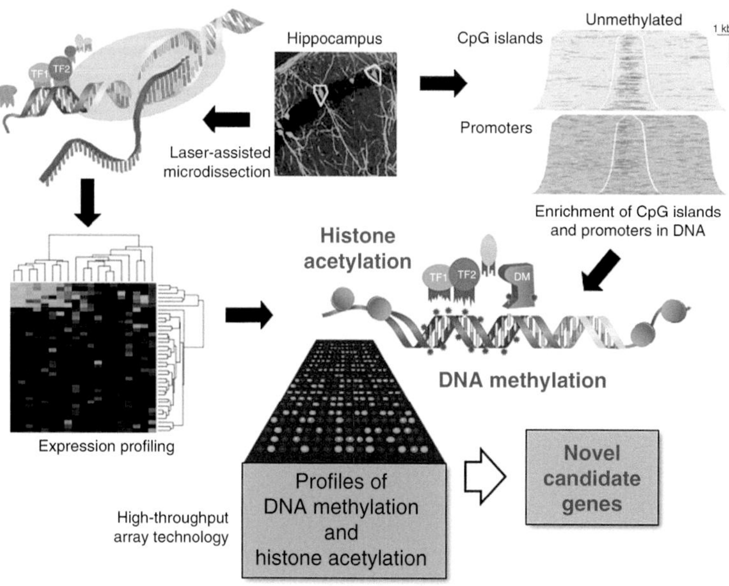

Figure 11.10 Changes in mRNA expression of novel candidate genes associated with altered rearing environment and/or 5-HTT genotype may be identified by microarray-based expression profiling of mRNA extracted from brain region-specific tissue and laser-dissected single neurons in mice from the G×E screen. Whole-genome expression screening methods combined with high-throughput methylation and histone acetylation profiling microarray techniques both genome-wide and of selected genes in mice from the G×E screen promise to identify genes that are epigenetically regulated by rearing environment and *5-HTT* in the mouse. These genes are likely novel candidate susceptibility genes for disorders of emotion regulation and will serve as potential diagnostic and therapeutic targets.

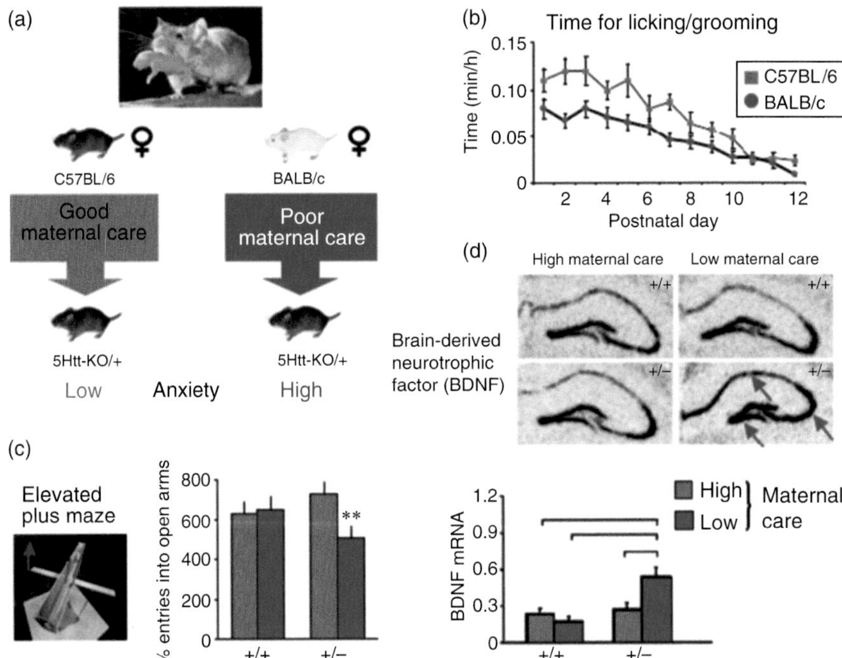

Figure 11.9 a–d Interaction between rearing environment and 5-HTT function: BDNF as a molecular substrate of both *5-HTT* genotype and maternal care (Carola *et al.*, 2008). (a) and (b) To study the molecular mechanisms underlying epigenetic programming by early adverse environment in an animal model amenable to genetic manipulation, an innovative gene × environment interaction screening paradigm (G×E screen) in the mouse was developed. Using this G×E screen it was shown that the effects of adverse rearing environment on anxiety-related behavior is modulated by mutations in 5-HTT in a way that mimics the interaction between early stress and 5-HTT seen in humans. (c) 5-HTT heterozygous null mice experiencing low maternal care showed increased anxiety-like behavior. (d) BDNF mRNA concentrations in hippocampus were elevated exclusively in 5-HTT heterozygous knock-out mice experiencing poor maternal care, suggesting that developmental programming of hippocampal circuits may underlie the *5-HTT*×E risk factor.

However, blockade of sensory input from the vibrissae without sectioning the infraorbital nerve does not affect cortical barrel formation, but induces alterations in barrel cortex plasticity and in neuronal connectivity, especially concerning infra- and supra-granular layers [97–99].

Indirect evidence for 5-HT and SERT involvement in somatosensory thalamocortical development was initially provided by morphological studies performed in a variety of species revealing transient barrel-like distributions of 5-HT, SERT, and 5-HT receptors, including 5-HT_{1B} and 5-HT_{2A}, in the early postnatal primary somatosensory (S1) cortex [25, 26, 83, 88, 90, 100–107]. Surprisingly, layer IV of the S1 cortex of neonatal rodents displays a transient barrel-like 5-HT pattern lasting approximately until P10, which is the result of 5-HT uptake and vesicular storage in thalamocortical neurons. As shown in Figure 3.1, at this developmental stage these neurons transiently express both SERT and VMAT-2 using 5-HT as a "borrowed transmitter", despite their later glutamatergic phenotype [105].

The complex interplay of 5-HT release and uptake by raphe-cortical and thalamocortical endings, respectively, plays a critical role in the formation of somatosensory cortical barrels. The first direct evidence came from MAO-A knock-out mice, where the gene encoding MAO-A was inactivated by the fortuitous integration of an interferon-β transgene, resulting in a 10-fold elevation of brain 5-HT levels [108]. MAO-A knock-out brains displayed a lack of the characteristic barrel-like clustering of layer IV neurons in S1 cortex, despite relatively preserved trigeminal and thalamic patterns [105, 108–110]. TCAs displayed a significant decrease in branching and excessive tangential distributions, suggesting a lack of terminal retraction [111]. Other abnormalities outside the S1 cortex included abnormal segregation of contralateral and ipsilateral retinogeniculate projections [109], and aberrant maturation of the brainstem respiratory network [112]. Although MAO-A metabolizes several monoamines, excess 5-HT is responsible for all of these abnomalities, since barrel formation is restored by the tryptophan hydroxylase inhibitor, *p*-chlorophenylalanine (*p*CPA) [105], which also restores normal development of retinogeniculate projections [109] and of the brainstem respiratory network [112]. Interestingly, denervation-induced plasticity is neither sensitive to 5-HT excess nor to *p*CPA administration [113], again showing that barrel formation and lesion-induced plasticity are separate phenomena, the former implicating TCA instructive roles at the cortical level [84, 92, 93], the latter based on subcortical sites and apparently dependent on neurotrophic factors produced at the level of the whisker pad [95, 96].

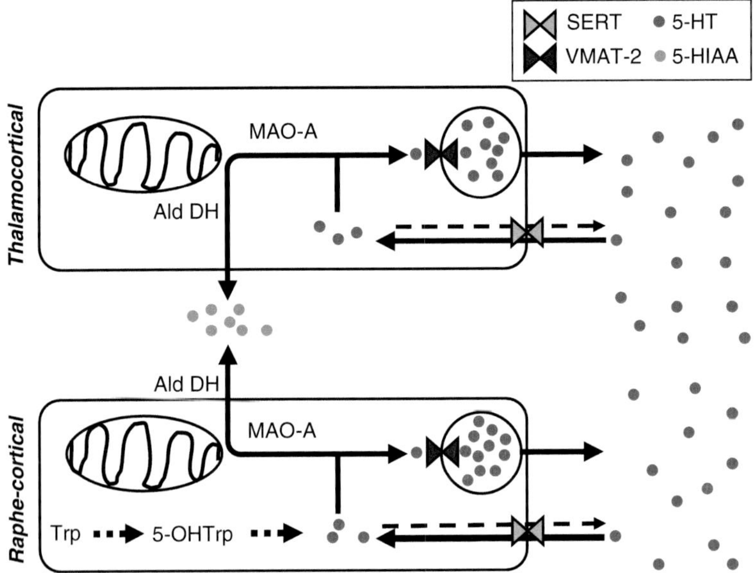

Figure 3.1 Developmental view of cortical serotoninergic and thalamocortical afferents. Serotonergic neurons synthesize 5-HT from tryptophan (Trp) through the rate limiting enzyme tryptophan hydroxylase 2 and an amino acid decarboxylase, which generate 5-hydroxytryptophan (5-OHTrp) and 5-HT, respectively; 5-HT is then either transported into vesicles by VMAT-2 to eventually undergo Ca^{2+}-mediated release, or it is metabolized through deamination by MAO-A, located on the outer mitochondrial membrane, followed by further oxidation to 5-HIAA by an aldehyde dehydrogenase (Ald DH). Neurochemical and paracrine extracellular 5-HT activity is terminated by the SERT, which under certain conditions can also reverse its direction and mediate vesicle-independent neurotransmitter release. In the somatosensory cortex of neonatal rodents, the transient barrel-like 5-HT pattern visible in layer IV is due to 5-HT uptake and vesicular storage in thalamocortical neurons, devoid of 5-HT-synthesizing enzymes but transiently expressing both SERT and VMAT-2.

The SERT knock-out mouse represents another animal model characterized by selective increases in extracellular 5-HT concentration [77, 78, 114, 115]. Since SERT is responsible for the high-affinity reuptake of 5-HT from the synaptic cleft, it plays a central role in the regulation of extracellular 5-HT levels [12]. SERT knock-out mice generated by homologous recombination display:

(a) excessive extracellular 5-HT levels, with 6- and 10-fold increases in striatal and frontal cortical extracellular 5-HT, respectively, recorded by microdialysis in adult mice;
(b) the complete absence of the transient 5-HT-immunostained barrel pattern due to lack of 5-HT uptake into thalamocortical terminals in S1 cortex;
(c) very low 5-HT tissue levels, with 5-HT present only in terminals of 5-HT-synthesizing raphe-cortical neurons sparsely distributed in supragranular and infragranular neocortical layers;
(d) a disrupted segregation of ipsilateral–contralateral retinogeniculate projections in the visual system, though not as severe as that seen in MAO-A knock-out mice;
(e) profound cytoarchitectonic abnormalities present in the S1 cortex of neonates, persisting into adulthood, and characterized by the absence of cortical barrels except for the largest and most caudal whisker barrels of the posteromedial barrel subfield (PMBSF);
(f) reduced developmental programmed cell death; and
(g) increased neuronal cell density and abnormal cortical layer thickness in adult brains, depending on the genetic background [73, 77, 114–116].

A normal barrel pattern can be restored by systemic administration of the 5-HT synthesis inhibitor pCPA during an early postnatal time window, namely P0–P4, corresponding to the critical period of barrel pattern formation [114]. Also, trigeminal barrelettes appear less well organized in SERT knock-out mice and the ventromedial thalamic barreloids which project to the absent anterolateral cortical barrel fields are less defined [114], as occurs in MAO-A knock-out mice (105). Interestingly, this finding parallels prior data demonstrating that lesions of the S1 cortex at P5 abolish or alter somatotopic patterns present at both subcortical relay stations [117].

The results obtained using animal models with an excess of extracellular 5-HT clearly demonstrate the existence of an upper concentration threshold beyond which 5-HT is disruptive to the cytoarchitectonic structure of primary sensory cortices and to the development of sensory afferent pathways, such as the thalamocortical and retinogeniculate projections (for review, see [118] and [119]). To study whether a lower 5-HT concentration threshold is also necessary for appropriate brain development, investigators have employed either 5-HT-depleting neurotoxins, such as parachloroamphetamine and 5,7-dihydroxytryptamine, or 5-HT synthesis inhibitors, such as *p*CPA [90, 104, 120, 121]. Alternatively, the genetic inactivation of VMAT-2 by homologous recombination, eliminates the vesicular uptake and release of 5-HT, resulting in almost undetectable brain 5-HT levels due to the immediate action of MAOs on newly synthesized cytoplasmic 5-HT [122, 123]. In rodents and other species, prenatal or early postnatal pharmacologically induced 5-HT depletion delays or prevents neuronal differentiation, neuritic extension and branching, 5-HT receptor expression patterns, and synapse formation or maintenance [124–129], resulting in smaller-than-normal barrels [104, 120]. The barrels of VMAT-2 knock-out mice are essentially normal in size, but S1 cortical layer IV never reaches a normal stage of differentiation, as evidenced by the presence of densely packed granular neurons in the lower tier [122]. This may occur because development of upper S1 cortical layers is severely delayed and/or reduced in these mice [114, 122].

A major limitation of pharmacological or homologous recombination-based 5-HT depletion models is reduced postnatal survival rates and/or significantly delayed body growth, either due to direct pharmacological effects or indirectly stemming from malnutrition [121]. Only a very small number of VMAT-2 knock-out pups actually survive to reach postnatal day 7 (P7), while displaying variable degrees of hypomorphism [114, 122]. Therefore, in vivo studies conclusively show that 5-HT depletion does not prevent barrel formation, but leave some uncertainty as to whether delayed neuronal or cytoarchitectonic maturation represents a specific 5-HT-mediated effect or is part of an experimentally induced growth retardation. None the less, the neurodevelopmental abnormalities documented in animal models of 5-HT depletion or excess provide compelling evidence that appropriate levels of 5-HT are required for normal cortical development.

CELLULAR MECHANISMS INVOLVED IN DEVELOPMENTAL ROLES OF 5-HT

The critical role played by 5-HT in embryonic and early postnatal development could conceivably be mediated by at least four mechanisms:

(a) 5-HT receptor-mediated modulation of ongoing neural activity;
(b) 5-HT receptor-mediated intracellular effects, not dependent upon changes in neural activity;

(c) activation of the SERT, regardless of 5-HT effects on neural activity and of actual 5-HT entry into SERT-expressing cells;
(d) uptake of 5-HT into SERT-expressing cells and subsequent intracellular effects directly exerted by 5-HT itself, possibly at the cytoskeletal or mitochondrial level.

The evidence is beginning to converge upon "structural", guidance-cue, cAMP-mediated 5-HT effects directly affecting the cytoskeleton, while "functional," neural activity-mediated modulation primarily influences harborization sprouting and pruning. However, areas of uncertainty and much debate still remain, especially given that different mechanisms may likely underlie different neurodevelopmental processes, affecting different neural systems at different times in development.

Despite some controversy, evidence from the visual and somatosensory systems mainly implies molecular guidance cues in pathway establishment, and neural activity in pathway maintenance and plasticity. In the visual system, ocular dominance columns develop prior to the critical period and in the absence of retinal input [130], whereas neural activity is critical for the maintenance and subsequent refinement of neural connections [131–134]. In the somatosensory system, the gross somatotopic patterning of TCA terminals likely results from molecular guidance cues, while their maintenance and refinement, as well as the barrel-like postsynaptic patterning of granule cells in cortical layer IV, is dependent upon activity-mediated *N*-methyl-D-aspartic acid (NMDA) receptor activation [85, 135–137]. Furthermore, the relative weight of molecular guidance cues and neural activity in the two systems may not be identical. Spontaneous waves of neural activity sweep across the mammalian retina well before the onset of vision, and exert profound effects upon the development of the reticulogeniculate pathway [132]. In contrast, no spontaneous activity is recorded in the somatosensory system, and no whisker stimulation-evoked electrical activity can be recorded from the primary somatosensory cortex before P3 or P7, depending on whether it was assessed electrophysiologically or using 2-deoxyglucose respectively [138–140]. Therefore, it is reasonable to expect that guidance cues may play a prominent developmental role, a prediction recently confirmed by studies on the interaction between 5-HT and netrin-1 signaling in determining somatosensory thalamocortical development (see below).

The morphogenetic effects of 5-HT are mediated by multiple receptors [141]. However, several converging lines of evidence strongly support the primary role of 5-HT$_{1B/1D}$ receptors in mediating 5-HT trophic effects, and as direct targets of excessive 5-HT levels in SERT and MAO-A knock-out mouse models. Firstly, reduced TCA branching and disrupted TCA segregation in retinogeniculate and somatosensory thalamocortical pathways of MAO-A knock-out mice are rescued in MAO-A/5-HT$_{1B}$, MAO-A/SERT/5-HT$_{1B}$, and SERT/5-HT$_{1B}$ double or triple knock-outs [115]. Secondly, selective pharmacological activation of 5-HT$_{1B/1D}$ receptors disrupts thalamic afferents and barrel pattern formation [142]. Thirdly, 5-HT$_{1B/1D}$ receptors are transiently expressed between P4 and P16 in thalamocortical neurons, where these receptors exert a presynaptic inhibition on glutamate release from TCA terminals [25, 106, 107, 143]. Fourthly, the 5-HT$_{1B/1D}$ receptor is coupled to the G-protein G_i/G_o, which promotes the opening of voltage-gated K^+ channels and the inhibition of the adenyl cyclase signaling pathway [144]. Interestingly, the spontaneous "barrelless" mutant mice have been shown to lack adenylyl cyclase type I, demonstrating that the cAMP signaling pathway is crucial to barrel formation [145]. Finally, in primary cultures of thalamic neurons, although acting through multiple receptors, serotonergic agonists exert trophic effects with rank-order potency 5-Ht$_{1B/1D}$ > 5-Ht$_{2/1C}$ = 5-Ht$_3$ > 5-Ht$_{1A}$ = vehicle [141, 146].

Since activation of 5-HT$_{1B}$ inhibits neurotransmitter release, reducing excitatory neurotransmission in thalamocortical regions of both the visual and somatosensory systems [115, 143], 5-HT$_{1B}$ receptors were initially viewed as regulators of thalamocortical development through activity-mediated inhibition of glutamate release [85]. It was subsequently shown that the attractant effect exerted on posterior dorsal thalamic neurons by the guidance molecule netrin-1 surprisingly turns into repulsion in the presence of 5-HT, both in vitro and in vivo [147]. This change is mediated by 5-HT$_{1B/1D}$ receptors, through decreased cAMP levels possibly resulting in the netrin-1 receptor DCC (deleted in colorectal cancer) internalization, turning attraction into repulsion [147]. In this context, the transient expression of the SERT by thalamocortical neurons during the development of primary sensory pathways would primarily aim at maintaining physiological levels of extracellular 5-HT, previously released from raphe-cortical fibers, thus allowing thalamocortical afferent growth to proceed following the appropriate guidance cues. Interestingly, 5-HT$_{1B}$ receptor knock-out yields no obvious abnormality in either thalamocortical or retinogeniculate somatotopy [115]. This suggests that either 5-HT$_{1D}$ receptors fully compensate for the lack of 5-HT$_{1B}$ receptors in these animals, or 5-HT$_{1B}$ receptors are relevant mediators only in non-physiological conditions characterized by abnormally elevated extracellular 5-HT levels, such as those encountered in MAO-A and in SERT knock-out mice.

Modulatory 5-HT effects on guidance-cue signaling, such as those exerted on netrin-1, could explain several experimental results that are seemingly incompatible with 5-HT effects being entirely mediated by changes in neural activity. For example, the abnormalities in TCA terminals distribution and barrel cortex cytoarchitectonics present in MAO-A and SERT knock-out mice [115] differ from those of cortex-specific NMDAR1 knock-out mice [136]. Also the blockade of sensory input from the vibrissae with local administration of TTX on the infraorbital nerve or the S1 cortex does not prevent the normal patterning of somatosensory relay stations [97, 148]. Barrel pattern abnormalities induced in vivo by 5,7-DHT administration are TTX-insensitive [149]. Proliferation of vascular smooth muscle cells requires 5-HT internalization through the SERT and cannot be either induced or blocked by agonists or antagonists acting exclusively on 5-HT membrane receptors [60]; this effect is mediated by the stimulation of mitogen-activated protein kinase (MAPK) in response to 5-HT-induced superoxide anion formation [60, 62].

In some cases, 5-HT can induce, and not reduce, apoptosis, as demonstrated with cerebellar granule cells [76] and Burkitt lymphoma cells [72]. As with 5-HT-induced cell proliferation, this effect is dependent on the formation of oxidative metabolites [76]. Furthermore, it is blocked by SSRIs and not by 5-HT receptor antagonists, indicating that either 5-HT internalization or at least SERT activation by 5-HT is required [72]. An initial report has recently shown that pre-implantation mouse embryos express SERT and THP2, and that intracellular 5-HT is highly concentrated in mitochondria, where it increases mitochondrial potentials by 25–40% [150]. This increase in mitochondrial potential should reflect increased proton pumping into the intermembrane space, likely due to enhanced activity of the respiratory chain, which in turn can generate reactive oxygen species [151]. It will be very interesting to assess whether this effect, if confirmed in further studies, stems from 5-HT itself being a charged molecule, or follows "serotonylation" of relevant mitochondrial or cytoplasmic proteins (i.e. a post-translational modification initially discovered in platelets, where small GTPases are rendered constitutively active by transamidation with 5-HT operated by transaminases) [152]. However, enhanced DNA oxidation has also been documented in the hippocampus of SERT knock-out mice [153]. Since hippocampal neurons do not express the SERT, unless 5-HT is being transported by another transporter, oxidative stress may also conceivably stem from an over-stimulation of 5-HT membrane receptors and may not necessarily require 5-HT internalization.

In summary, changes in resting membrane potential and neural activity may not represent an absolute requirement for 5-HT "structural" effects to take place. Intracellular mechanisms that could be activated following 5-HT uptake into TCA terminals include direct modulation of cytoskeletal kinetics, especially through 5-HT/actin interactions [154, 155], "serotonylation" [152], and regulation of intracellular redox state [156–159]. Similarly, layer IV granule cells can sense 5-HT excess/depletion through gap junction-mediated electric coupling, which is significantly downregulated by 5-HT through 5-HT_{2A} receptors in the rat somatosensory cortex [160]. Finally, the possible involvement of the SERT without necessarily requiring 5-HT internalization must also be considered. The SERT participates in a protein complex involving multiple Ser/Thr kinases and phosphatases, such as protein phosphatase 2A; SERT activation by 5-HT counteracts PKC-mediated SERT phosphorylation and internalization, possibly through interactions with integrin αIIbβ3 [161–163]. This mechanism, actively modulating PKC-induced downregulation of the SERT, could also indirectly affect other targets for PKC phosphorylation.

POTENTIAL RELEVANCE TO HUMAN TERATOLOGY

The potential for teratological effects of excessive 5-HT levels is exemplified in human pathology by Brunner syndrome, which is due to point mutations in the MAO-A gene, leading to loss of the catalytic activity of the enzyme [164]. The hallmarks of this disorder are increased aggressiveness and mild mental retardation. Interestingly, MAO-A knock-out mice are also acutely aggressive and their aggressiveness can be prevented by blocking 5-HT synthesis through *p*CPA administration during a critical period limited to the first postnatal days [108].

In contrast to Brunner syndrome, a rare monogenic disease, the use of SSRIs during pregnancy represents an area of major epidemiological concern. On one hand, as many as 5–15% of pregnant women suffer from major depression, which is associated with low birth weight, preterm delivery, and postpartum admission to neonatal intensive care units [165]. On the other hand, the neurodevelopmental effects of 5-HT summarized above raise concern about the potential risk of SSRIs, currently the most frequently prescribed antidepressants, to cause minor craniofacial malformations and, most of all, behavioral teratology. All SSRIs cross the placenta, but only partial SERT blockade results from therapeutic administration of these antidepressants. Consequently, 5-HT concentrations at the synapse in humans taking SSRIs can be anticipated not to be as high as in SERT knock-out mice. None the less, heterozygous SERT knock-out mice do display minor cytoarchitectonic anomalies in S1 cortex, such as enlarged barrel septa [114]. Similar developmental derangements leading to behavioral teratology after prenatal exposure to SSRIs during critical periods in neurodevelopment cannot be excluded. Furthermore, low but detectable serum levels of fluoxetine, sertraline, and citalopram have been found in breast-fed infants, because all SSRIs are secreted into human milk [166]. As an example, a breast-fed infant displays serum levels of citalopram approximately equal to 1/15th the serum levels of his mother [167].

In general, prospective follow-up studies of children exposed prenatally to a variety of antidepressants have shown no increase in major malformations, miscarriage, stillbirth, or prematurity [168–171]. Studies focused on IQ and language development also failed to detect any difference between children exposed prenatally to SSRIs and controls [172]. Therefore, the consensus is that SSRI administration during pregnancy and lactation does not confer teratogenic risk for the newborn [168–171]. Only one study detected a possible increase in minor malformations and preterm delivery in the offspring of mothers treated with fluoxetine during the first or third trimester of pregnancy, respectively [173]. This outcome is quite compatible with the results obtained employing the pregnant sheep as an animal model: by blocking 5-HT uptake in platelets and peripheral organs, such as the gut, fluoxetine causes an acute increase in plasma 5-HT levels, leading to a transient decrease in uterine blood flow which, in turn, reduces delivery of oxygen and nutrients to the fetus, a mechanism typically favoring delayed growth and preterm delivery [174]. Furthermore, studies targeting subtle behavioral teratology in neonates exposed prenatally to SSRIs detected maturation delays in motor development and control [175] and reduced pain sensitivity [176].

Animal studies suffer from several major limitations, such as the use of acute or subacute intravenous antidepressant administration, instead of the prolonged oral regimen typical of human pharmacology. The probability that active compounds or metabolites may persist in the blood of newborn babies has not been thoroughly assessed [177]. Yet, the lack of overt malformations, obvious behavioral changes, or gross differences in brain weight found in SERT knock-out mice, which do display significant cytoarchitectonic abnormalities at the level of the brain, raises concern for changes in neural circuitry and behavioral teratology in humans exposed prenatally to SSRIs. Clinical judgment should be based upon carefully balancing the risk for minor behavioral teratology in the newborn with the risk of maternal relapse into depression and/or suicidal behavior.

CONCLUSIONS

From invertebrates to humans, 5-HT exerts "structural" effects, particularly during development, and SERT directly regulates these effects by maintaining 5-HT concentrations within a physiological range and possibly by modulating at the intracellular level the redox state of the cell. The results summarized in this chapter mainly derive from studies of rodent brain development and plasticity. However, they are in line with in vivo evidence of transiently increased neonatal 5-HT levels in brains of non-rodent species, possibly associated with 5-HT regulation of development and synaptogenesis [125–128], as well as with in vitro studies showing 5-HT effects on cortical synaptogenesis, neurite outgrowth and branching, myelination and glial proliferation in tissue culture [141, 146, 178–181]. The prominent involvement of the SERT, on one hand, raises concern about exposure of human fetuses to pharmacological agents hampering 5-HT uptake and enhancing extracellular 5-HT concentrations. On the other hand, it spurs hope into possible uses of SSRIs during prenatal development to correct dysmorphogenetic conditions. As an example, 5-HT acting through 5-HT_{1A} receptors is capable of reducing apoptotic cell death around the core region of brain ischemic damage [74]. A better understanding of the mechanisms underlying 5-HT "structural" effects may thus prove useful in treating disorders associated with abnormal development or with unbalanced cell proliferation/apoptosis.

ACKNOWLEDGMENTS

The author is supported by the Italian Ministry for University, Scientific Research and Technology, by Autism Speaks (Princeton, NJ), and by the Fondation Jerome Lejeune (Paris, France).

REFERENCES

1. Gingrich J A, Hen R (2001). Dissecting the role of the serotonin system in neuropsychiatric disorders using knockout mice. *Psychopharmacology* **155**: 1–10.
2. Murphy D L, Lesch K P (2008). Targeting the murine serotonin transporter: insights into human neurobiology. *Nat Rev Neurosci* **9**: 85–96.

3. Buznikov G A, Shmukler Y B, Lauder J M (1996). From oocyte to neuron: do neurotransmitters function in the same way throughout development? *Cell Mol Neurobiol* **16**: 537–59.
4. Moiseiwitsch J R (2000). The role of serotonin and neurotransmitters during craniofacial development. *Crit Rev Oral Biol Med* **11**: 230–9.
5. Moiseiwitsch J R, Lambert H W, Lauder J M (2001). Roles for serotonin in non-neural embryonic development. In Kalverboer A, Gramsbergen A, editors. *Brain and behavior in human development.* Amsterdam: Kluwer, pp. 139–52.
6. Buznikov G A, Lambert H W, Lauder J M (2001). Serotonin and serotonin-like substances as regulators of early embryogenesis and morphogenesis. *Cell Tissue Res* **305**: 177–86.
7. Bunin M A, Wightman R M (1999). Paracrine neurotransmission in the CNS: involvement of 5-HT. *Trends Neurosci* **22**: 377–82.
8. Ridet J L, Privat A (2000). Volume transmission. *Trends Neurosci* **23**: 58–9.
9. Zoli M, Jansson A, Sykova E, Agnati L F, Fuxe K (1999). Volume transmission in the CNS and its relevance for neuropsychopharmacology. *Trends Pharmacol Sci* **20**: 142–50.
10. Tao-Cheng J H, Zhou F C (1999). Differential polarization of serotonin transporters in axons versus somadendrites: an immunogold electron microscopy study. *Neuroscience* **94**: 821–30.
11. Janusonis S, Gluncic V, Rakic P (2004). Early serotoninergic projections to Cajal–Retzius cells: relevance for cortical development. *J Neurosci* **24**: 1652–9.
12. Ramamoorthy S, Bauman A L, Moore K R, *et al.* (1993). Antidepressant- and cocaine-sensitive human serotonin transporter: molecular cloning, expression, and chromosomal localization. *Proc Natl Acad Sci USA* **90**: 2542–6.
13. Jacobs B L, Azmitia E C (1992). Structure and function of the brain serotonin system. *Physiol Rev* **72**: 165–229.
14. Lauder J M (1990). Ontogeny of the serotonergic system in the rat: Serotonin as a developmental signal. *Ann NY Acad Sci* **600**: 297–314.
15. Hendricks T J, Fyodorov D V, Wegman L J, *et al.* (2003). Pet-1 ETS gene plays a critical role in 5-HT neuron development and is required for normal anxiety-like and aggressive behavior. *Neuron* **37**: 233–47.
16. Whitaker-Azmitia P M (2001). Serotonin and brain development: role in human developmental diseases. *Brain Res Bull* **56**: 479–85.
17. Sundstrom E, Kolare S, Souverbie F, *et al.* (1993). Neurochemical differentiation of human bulbospinal monoaminergic neurons during the first trimester. *Dev Brain Res* **75**: 1–12.
18. Levallois C, Valence C, Baldet P, Privat A (1997). Morphological and morphometric analysis of serotonin-containing neurons in primary dissociated cultures of human rhombencephalon: a study of development. *Dev Brain Res* **99**: 243–52.
19. Chugani D C, Muzik O, Behen M, *et al.* (1999). Developmental changes in brain serotonin synthesis capacity in autistic and nonautistic children. *Ann Neurol* **45**: 287–95.
20. Verge D, Calas A (2000). Serotonergic neurons and serotonin receptors: gains from cytochemical approaches. *J Chem Neuroanat* **18**: 41–56.
21. Lauder J M, Liu J P, Grayson D R (2000). In utero exposure to serotonergic drugs alters neonatal expression of 5-HT$_{1A}$ receptor transcripts: a quantitative RT- PCR study. *Int J Dev Neurosci* **18**: 171–6.
22. Johns J M, Lubin D A, Lieberman J A, Lauder J M (2002). Developmental effects of prenatal cocaine exposure on 5-HT$_{1A}$ receptors in male and female rat offspring. *Dev Neurosci* **24**: 522–30.
23. Lubin D A, Cannon J B, Black M C, Brown L E, Johns J M (2003). Effects of chronic cocaine on monoamine levels in discrete brain structures of lactating rat dams. *Pharmacol Biochem Behav* **74**: 449–54.

24. Ivgy-May N, Tamir H, Gershon M D (1994). Synaptic properties of serotonergic growth cones in developing rat brain. *J Neurosci* **14**: 1011–29.
25. Mansour-Robaey S, Mechawar N, Radja F, Beaulieu C, Descarries L (1998). Quantified distribution of serotonin transporter and receptors during the postnatal development of the rat barrel field cortex. *Dev Brain Res* **107**: 159–63.
26. Lebrand C, Cases O, Wehrle R, Blakely R D, Edwards R H, Gaspar P (1998). Transient developmental expression of monoamine transporters in the rodent forebrain. *J Comp Neurol* **401**: 506–24.
27. Hansson S R, Mezey E, Hoffman B J (1999). Serotonin transporter messenger RNA expression in neural crest-derived structures and sensory pathways of the developing rat embryo. *Neuroscience* **89**: 243–65.
28. Hoyer D, Hannon J P, Martin G R (2002). Molecular, pharmacological and functional diversity of 5-HT receptors. *Pharmacol Biochem Behav* **71**: 533–54.
29. Roth B L, Hamblin M W, Ciaranello R D (1991). Developmental regulation of 5-HT2 and 5-HT1c mRNA and receptor levels. *Dev Brain Res* **58**: 51–8.
30. Hellendall R P, Schambra U, Liu J, Breese G R, Millhorn D E, Lauder J M (1992). Detection of serotonin receptor transcripts in the developing nervous system. *J Chem Neuroanat* **5**: 299–310.
31. Morilak D A, Ciaranello R D (1993). Ontogeny of 5-hydroxytryptamine2 receptor immunoreactivity in the developing rat brain. *Neuroscience* **55**: 869–80.
32. Zec N, Filiano J J, Panigrahy A, White W F, Kinney H C (1996). Developmental changes in [3H]lysergic acid diethylamide ([3H]LSD) binding to serotonin receptors in the human brainstem. *J Neuropathol Exp Neurol* **55**: 114–26.
33. Borella A, Bindra M, Whitaker-Azmitia P M (1997). Role of the 5-HT$_{1A}$ receptor in development of the neonatal rat brain: preliminary behavioral studies. *Neuropharmacology* **36**: 445–50.
34. Ruiz G, Bancila M, Valenzuela M, Daval G, Kia K H, Verge D (1999). Plasticity of 5-hydroxytryptamine(1B) receptors during postnatal development in the rat visual cortex. *Int J Dev Neurosci* **17**: 305–15.
35. Talley E M, Bayliss D A (2000). Postnatal development of 5-HT$_{1A}$ receptor expression in rat somatic motoneurons. *Dev Brain Res* **122**: 1–10.
36. Rho J M, Storey T W (2001). Molecular ontogeny of major neurotransmitter receptor systems in the mammalian central nervous system: norepinephrine, dopamine, serotonin, acetylcholine, and glycine. *J Child Neurol* **16**: 271–80.
37. Hendricks T, Francis N, Fyodorov D, Deneris E S (1999). The ETS domain factor Pet-1 is an early and precise marker of central serotonin neurons and interacts with a conserved element in serotonergic genes. *J Neurosci* **19**: 10 348–56.
38. Zhao Z Q, Scott M, Chiechio S, *et al.* (2006). Lmx1b is required for maintenance of central serotonergic neurons and mice lacking central serotonergic system exhibit normal locomotor activity. *J Neurosci* **26**: 12 781–8.
39. Zhao Z Q, Chiechio S, Sun Y G, *et al.* (2007). Mice lacking central serotonergic neurons show enhanced inflammatory pain and an impaired analgesic response to antidepressant drugs. *J Neurosci* **27**: 6045–53.
40. Hodges M R, Tattersall G J, Harris M B, *et al.* (2008). Defects in breathing and thermoregulation in mice with near-complete absence of central serotonin neurons. *J Neurosci* **28**: 2495–505.
41. Scott M M, Wylie C J, Lerch J K, *et al.* (2005). A genetic approach to access serotonin neurons for in vivo and in vitro studies. *Proc Natl Acad Sci USA* **102**: 16 472–7.
42. Jensen P, Farago A F, Awatramani R B, Scott M M, Deneris E S, Dymecki S M (2008). Redefining the serotonergic system by genetic lineage. *Nat Neurosci* **11**: 417–9.

43. Whitaker-Azmitia P M, Druse M, Walker P, Lauder J M (1996). Serotonin as a developmental signal. *Behav Brain Res* **73**: 19–29.
44. Harrison M A, Pickard B G (1989). Auxin asymmetry during gravitropism by tomato hypocotyls. *Plant Physiol* **89**: 652–7.
45. Muday G K (2001). Auxins and tropisms. *J Plant Growth Regul* **20**: 226–43.
46. Blancaflor E B (2002). The cytoskeleton and gravitropism in higher plants. *J Plant Growth Regul* **21**: 120–36.
47. Colas J F, Launay J M, Kellermann O, Rosay P, Maroteaux L (1995). *Drosophila* 5-HT2 serotonin receptor: coexpression with fushi-tarazu during segmentation. *Proc Natl Acad Sci USA* **92**: 5441–5.
48. Colas J F, Launay J M, Vonesch J L, Hickel P, Maroteaux L (1999). Serotonin synchronises convergent extension of ectoderm with morphogenetic gastrulation movements in *Drosophila*. *Mech Dev* **87**: 77–91.
49. Levitt P, Harvey J A, Friedman E, Simansky K, Murphy E H (1997). New evidence for neurotransmitter influences on brain development. *Trends Neurosci* **20**: 269–74.
50. Zimmerman E F, Clark R L, Ganguli S, Venkatasubramanian K (1983). Serotonin regulation of palatal cell motility. *J Craniofac Genet Dev Biol* **3**: 371–85.
51. Bottaro D, Shepro D, Peterson S, Hechtman H B (1985). Serotonin, histamine, and norepinephrine mediation of endothelial and vascular smooth muscle cell movement. *Am J Physiol* **248**: C252–7.
52. Bell L, Madri J A (1989). Effect of platelet factors on migration of cultured bovine aortic endothelial and smooth muscle cells. *Circ Res* **65**: 1057–65.
53. Lee S L, Wang W W, Moore B J, Fanburg B L (1991). Dual effects of serotonin on growth of bovine pulmonary artery smooth muscle cells in culture. *Circ Res* **68**: 1362–8.
54. Shuey D L, Sadler T W, Lauder J M (1992). Serotonin as a regulator of craniofacial morphogenesis: site specific malformations following exposure to serotonin uptake inhibitors. *Teratology* **46**: 367–78.
55. Yavarone M S, Shuey D L, Tamir H, Sadler T W, Lauder J M (1993). Serotonin and cardiac morphogenesis in the mouse embryo. *Teratology* **47**: 573–84.
56. Moiseiwitch J R D, Lauder J M (1995). Serotonin regulates mouse cranial neural crest migration. *Proc Natl Acad Sci USA* **92**: 7182–6.
57. Moiseiwitsch J R, Lauder J M (1996). Stimulation of murine tooth development in organotypic culture by the neurotransmitter serotonin. *Arch Oral Biol* **41**: 161–5.
58. Moiseiwitsch J R, Lauder J M (1997). Regulation of gene expression in cultured embryonic mouse mandibular mesenchyme by serotonin antagonists. *Anat Embryol* **195**: 71–8.
59. Choi D S, Ward S J, Messaddeq N, Launay J M, Maroteaux L (1997). 5-HT_{2B} receptor-mediated serotonin morphogenetic functions in mouse cranial neural crest and myocardial cells. *Development* **124**: 1745–55.
60. Fanburg B L, Lee S L (1997). A new role for an old molecule: serotonin as a mitogen. *Am J Physiol* **272**: L795–806.
61. Tamura K, Kanzaki T, Saito Y, Otabe M, Saito Y, Morisaki N (1997). Serotonin (5-hydroxytryptamine, 5-HT) enhances migration of rat aortic smooth muscle cells through 5-HT2 receptors. *Atherosclerosis* **132**: 139–43.
62. Lee S L, Wang W W, Finaly G A, Fanburg F L (1999). Serotonin stimulates mitogen-activated protein kinase activity through the formation of superoxide anions. *Am J Physiol* **277**: L282–91.
63. Lee S L, Simon A R, Wang W W, Fanburg B L (2001). H_2O_2 signals 5-HT-induced ERK MAP kinase activation and mitogenesis of smooth muscle cells. *Am J Physiol* **281**: L646–52.

64. Pavone L M, Mithbaokar P, Mastellone V, *et al.* (2007). Fate map of serotonin transporter-expressing cells in developing mouse heart. *Genesis* **45**: 689–95.
65. Nebigil C G, Launay J M, Hickel P, Tournois C, Maroteaux L (2000b). 5-Hydroxytryptamine 2B receptor regulates cell-cycle progression: cross-talk with tyrosine kinase pathways. *Proc Natl Acad Sci USA* **97**: 2591–6.
66. Nebigil C G, Choi D S, Dierich A, *et al.* (2000a). Serotonin 2B receptor is required for heart development. *Proc Natl Acad Sci USA* **97**: 9508–13.
67. Lambert H W, Weiss E R, Lauder J M (2001). Activation of 5-HT receptors that stimulate the adenylyl cyclase pathway positively regulates IGF-I in cultured craniofacial mesenchymal cells. *Dev Neurosci* **23**: 70–7.
68. Azmitia E C (2001). Modern views of an ancient chemical: serotonin effects on cell proliferation, maturation, and apoptosis. *Brain Res Bull* **56**: 413–24.
69. Mukhin Y V, Garnovskaya M N, Collinsworth G, *et al.* (2000). 5-Hydroxytryptamine$_{1A}$ receptor/$G_i\beta\gamma$ stimulates mitogen-activated protein kinase via NAD(P)H oxidase and reactive oxygen species upstream of Src in Chinese hamster ovary fibroblasts. *Biochem J* **347**: 61–7.
70. Choi D S, Kellermann O, Richard J F, *et al.* (1998). Mouse 5-HT$_{2B}$ receptor-mediated serotonin trophic functions. *Ann NY Acad Sci* **861**: 67–73.
71. Adayev T, Ray I, Sondhi R, Sobocki T, Banerjee P (2003). The G protein-coupled 5-HT$_{1A}$ receptor causes suppression of caspase-3 through MAPK and protein kinase Cα. *Biochem Biophys Acta* **1640**: 85–96.
72. Serafeim A, Grafton G, Chamba A, *et al.* (2002). 5-Hydroxytryptamine drives apoptosis in biopsylike Burkitt lymphoma cells: reversal by selective seoronin reuptake inhibitors. *Blood* **99**: 2545–53.
73. Persico A M, Baldi A, Dell'Acqua M L, *et al.* (2003). Reduced programmed cell death in brains of serotonin transporter knockout mice. *NeuroReport* **14**: 341–4.
74. Scharper C, Zhu Y, Kouklei M, Culmsee C, Krieglstein J (2000). Stimulation of 5-HT 1A receptors reduces apoptosis after transient forebrain ischemia in the rat. *Brain Res* **883**: 41–50.
75. Stankovski L, Alvarez C, Ouimet T, *et al.* (2007). Developmental cell death is enhanced in the cerebral cortex of mice lacking the brain vesicular monoamine transporter. *J Neurosci* **27**: 1316–24.
76. Zilkha-Falb R, Ziv I, Nardi N, Offen D, Melamed E, Barzilai A (1997). Monoamine-induced apoptotic neuronal cell death. *Cell Mol Neurobiol* **17**: 101–18.
77. Mathews T A, Fedele D E, Coppelli F M, Avila A M, Murphy D L, Andrews A M (2004). Gene dose-dependent alterations in extraneuronal serotonin but not dopamine in mice with reduced serotonin transporter expression. *J Neurosci Meth* **140**: 169–81.
78. Bengel D, Murphy D L, Andrews A M, *et al.* (1998). Altered brain serotonin homeostasis and locomotor insensitivity to 3,4-methylenedioxymethamphetamine ("Ecstasy") in serotonin transporter-deficient mice. *Mol Pharmacol* **53**: 649–55.
79. Rakic P (1995). Radial versus tangential migration of neuronal clones in the developing cerebral cortex. *Proc Natl Acad Sci USA* **92**: 11 323–7.
80. Levitt P, Eagleson K L, Powell E M (2004). Regulation of neocortical interneuron development and the implications for neurodevelopmental disorders. *Trends Neurosci* **27**: 400–06.
81. Lidov H G, Molliver M E (1982). An immunohistochemical study of serotonin neuron development in the rat: ascending pathways and terminal fields. *Brain Res Bull* **8**: 389–430.
82. Wallace J A, Lauder J M (1983). Development of the serotonergic system in the rat embryo: an immunocytochemical study. *Brain Res Bull* **10**: 459–79.

83. Dori I, Dinopoulos A, Blue M E, Parnavelas J G (1996). Regional differences in the ontogeny of the serotonergic projection to the cerebral cortex. *Exp Neurol* **138**: 1–14.
84. Rice F L (1995). Comparative aspects of barrel structure and development. In Jones E G, Diamond I T, editors. *Cerebral cortex, Vol. 11 – The barrel cortex of rodents*. New York: Plenum Press, pp. 1–76.
85. Erzurumlu R S, Kind P C (2001). Neural activity: sculptor of 'barrels' in the neocortex. *Trends Neurosci* **24**: 589–95.
86. Wong-Riley M T T, Welt C (1980). Histochemical changes in cytochrome oxydase of cortical barrels after vibrissal removal in neonatal and adult mice. *Proc Natl Acad Sci USA* **77**: 2333–7.
87. Woolsey T A, Wann J R (1976). Areal changes in mouse cortical barrels following vibrissal damage at different postnatal ages. *J Comp Neurol* **170**: 53–66.
88. Fuchs J L (1995). Neurotransmitter receptors in developing barrel cortex. In Jones E G, Diamond I T, editors. *Cerebral cortex, Vol. 11 – The barrel cortex of rodents*. New York: Plenum Press, pp. 375–409.
89. Hedreen J C, Bacon S J, Price D L (1985). A modified histochemical technique to visualize acetylcholinesterase-containing axons. *J Histochem Cytochem* **33**: 134–40.
90. Blue M E, Erzurumlu R S, Jhaveri S (1991). A comparison of pattern formation by thalamocortical and serotonergic afferents in the rat barrel field cortex. *Cereb Cortex* **1**: 380–9.
91. Senft S L, Woolsey T A (1991). Growth of thalamic afferents into mouse barrel cortex. *Cereb Cortex* **1**: 308–35.
92. Erzurumlu R S, Jhaveri S (1990). Thalamic axons confer a blueprint of the sensory periphery onto the developing rat somatosensory cortex. *Dev Brain Res* **56**: 229–34.
93. Jhaveri S, Erzurumlu R S, Crossin K (1991). Barrel construction in rodent neocortex: role of thalamic afferents versus extracellular matrix molecules. *Proc Natl Acad Sci USA* **88**: 4489–93.
94. Van der Loos H, Woolsey T A (1973). Somatosensory cortex: structural alterations following early injury to sense organ. *Science* **179**: 395–8.
95. Calia E, Persico A M, Baldi A, Keller F (1998). BDNF and NT-3 applied in the whisker pad reverse cortical changes after peripheral deafferentation in neonatal rats. *Eur J Neurosci* **10**: 3194–200.
96. Baldi A, Calia E, Ciampini A, *et al.* (2000). Deafferentation-induced apoptosis of neurons in thalamic somatosensory nuclei of the newborn rat: critical period and rescue from cell death by peripherally applied neurotrophins. *Eur J Neurosci* **12**: 2281–90.
97. Henderson T A, Woolsey T A, Jacquin M F (1992). Infraorbital nerve blockade from birth does not disrupt central trigeminal pattern formation in the rat. *Dev Brain Res* **66**: 146–52.
98. Diamond M E, Huang W, Ebner F F (1994). Laminar comparison of somatosensory cortical plasticity. *Science* **265**: 1885–8.
99. Wallace H, Fox K (1999). The effect of vibrissa deprivation pattern on the form of plasticity induced in rat barrel cortex. *Somatosens Mot Res* **16**: 122–38.
100. Fujimiya M, Kimura H, Maeda T (1986). Postnatal development of serotonin nerve fibers in the somatosensory cortex of mice studied by immunohistochemistry. *J Comp Neurol* **246**: 191–201.
101. D'Amato R J, Blue M E, Largent B L, *et al.* (1987). Ontogeny of the serotonergic projection to rat neocortex: transient expression of a dense innervation to primary sensory areas. *Proc Natl Acad Sci USA* **84**: 4322–6.

102. Rhoades R W, Mooney R D, Chiaia N L, Bennett-Clarke C A (1990). Development and plasticity of the serotonergic projection to the hamster's superior colliculus. *J Comp Neurol* **299**: 151–66.
103. Bennett-Clarke C A, Mooney R D, Chiaia N L, Rhoades R W (1991). Serotonin immunoreactive neurons are present in the superficial layers of the hamster's, but not the rat's, superior colliculus. *Exp Brain Res* **85**: 587–97.
104. Bennett-Clarke C A, Leslie M J, Lane R D, Rhoades R W (1994). Effect of serotonin depletion on vibrissa-related patterns of thalamic afferents in the rat's somatosensory cortex. *J Neurosci* **14**: 7594–607.
105. Lebrand C, Cases O, Adelbrecht C, *et al.* (1996). Transient uptake and storage of serotonin in developing thalamic neurons. *Neuron* **17**: 823–35.
106. Bennett-Clarke CA, Leslie M J, Chiaia N L, Rhoades R W (1993). Serotonin 1B receptors in the developing somatosensory and visual cortices are located on thalamocortical axons. *Proc Natl Acad Sci USA* **90**: 153–7.
107. Leslie M J, Bennett-Clarke C A, Rhoades R W (1992). Serotonin 1B receptors form a transient vibrissa-related pattern in the primary somatosensory cortex of the developing rat. *Dev Brain Res* **69**: 43–148.
108. Cases O, Seif I, Grimsby J, *et al.* (1995). Aggressive behavior and altered amounts of brain serotonin and norepinephrine in mice lacking MAOA. *Science* **268**: 1763–6.
109. Upton A L, Salichon N, Lebrand C, *et al.* (1999). Excess of serotonin (5-HT) alters the segregation of ispilateral and contralateral retinal projections in monoamine oxidase A knock-out mice: possible role of 5-HT uptake in retinal ganglion cells during development. *J Neurosci* **19**: 7007–24.
110. Vitalis T, Cases O, Callebert J, *et al.* (1998). Effects of monoamine oxidase A inhibition on barrel formation in the mouse somatosensory cortex: determination of a sensitive developmental period. *J Comp Neurol* **393**: 169–84.
111. Rebsam A, Seif I, Gaspar P (2002). Refinement of thalamocortical arbors and emergence of barrel domains in the primary somatosensory cortex: a study of normal and monoamine oxidase A knock-out mice. *J Neurosci* **22**: 8541–52.
112. Burnet H, Bevengut M, Chakri F, *et al.* (2001). Altered respiratory activity and respiratory regulations in adult monoamine oxidase A-deficient mice. *J Neurosci* **21**: 5212–21.
113. Rebsam A, Seif I, Gaspar P (2005). Dissociating barrel development and lesion-induced plasticity in the mouse somatosensory cortex. *J Neurosci* **25**: 706–10.
114. Persico A M, Mengual E, Moessner R, *et al.* (2001). Barrel pattern formation requires serotonin uptake by thalamocortical afferents, and not vesicular monoamine release. *J Neurosci* **21**: 6862–73.
115. Salichon N, Gaspar P, Upton A L, *et al.* (2001). Excessive activation of serotonin (5-HT) 1B receptors disrupts the formation of sensory maps in monoamine oxidase A and 5-HT transporter knock-out mice. *J Neurosci* **21**: 884–96.
116. Altamura C, Dell'Acqua M L, Moessner R, Murphy D L, Lesch K P, Persico A M (2007). Altered neocortical cell density and layer thickness in serotonin transporter knockout mice: a quantitation study. *Cereb Cortex* **17**: 1394–401.
117. Erzurumlu R S, Ebner F F (1988). Maintenance of discrete somatosensory maps in subcortical relay nuclei is dependent on an intact sensory cortex. *Dev Brain Res* **44**: 302–08.
118. Luo X, Persico A M, Lauder J M (2003). Serotonergic regulation of somatosensory cortical development: lessons from genetic mouse models. *Dev Neurosci* **25**: 173–83.
119. Gaspar P, Cases O, Maroteaux L (2003). The developmental role of serotonin: news from mouse molecular genetics. *Nat Rev Neurosci* **4**: 1002–12.

120. Osterheld-Haas M C, Van der Loos H, Hornung J P (1994). Monoaminergic afferents to cortex modulate structural plasticity in the barrelfield of the mouse. *Dev Brain Res* **77**: 189–202.
121. Persico A M, Altamura C, Calia E, *et al.* (2000). Serotonin depletion and barrel cortex development: impact of growth impairment vs 5-HT effects on thalamocortical endings. *Cereb Cortex* **10**: 181–91.
122. Alvarez C, Vitalis T, Fon E A, *et al.* (2002). Effects of genetic depletion of monoamines on somatosensory cortical development. *Neuroscience* **115**: 753–64.
123. Wang Y M, Gainetdinov R R, Fumagalli F, *et al.* (1997). Knockout of the vesicular monoamine transporter 2 gene results in neonatal death and supersensitivity to cocaine and amphetamine. *Neuron* **19**: 1285–96.
124. Whitaker-Azmitia P M, Lauder J M, Shemmer A, Azmitia E C (1987). Postnatal changes in serotonin receptors following prenatal alterations in serotonin levels: further evidence for functional fetal serotonin receptors. *Brain Res* **430**: 285–9.
125. Okado N, Shibanoki S, Ishikawa K, Sako H (1989). Developmental changes in serotonin levels in the chick spinal cord and brain. *Dev Brain Res* **50**: 217–23.
126. Okado N, Cheng L, Tanatsugu Y, Hamada S, Hamaguchi K (1993). Synaptic loss following removal of serotonergic fibers in newly hatched and adult chickens. *J Neurobiol* **24**: 687–98.
127. Chen L, Hamaguchi K, Ogawa M, Hamada S, Okado N (1994). PCPA reduces both monoaminergic afferents and nonmonoaminergic synapses in the cerebral cortex. *Neurosci Res* **19**: 111–5.
128. Niitsu Y, Hamada S, Hamaguchi K, Mikuni M, Okado N (1995). Regulation of synapse density by 5-HT_{2A} receptor agonist and antagonist in the spinal cord of chicken embryo. *Neurosci Lett* **195**: 159–62.
129. Durig J, Hornung J P (2000). Neonatal serotonin depletion affects developing and mature mouse cortical neurons. *Dev Neurosci* **4**: 833–7.
130. Crowley J C, Katz L C (2002). Ocular dominance development revisited. *Curr Opin Neurobiol* **12**: 104–09.
131. Reh T A, Constantine-Paton M (1985). Eye-specific segregation requires neural activity in three-eyed *Rana pipiens*. *J Neurosci* **5**: 1132–43.
132. Stellwagen D, Shatz C J (2002). An instructive role for retinal waves in the development of retinogeniculate connectivity. *Neuron* **33**: 357–67.
133. Kanold P O, Kara P, Reid R C, Shatz C J (2003). Role of subplate neurons in functional maturation of visual cortical columns. *Science* **301**: 521–4.
134. Adams D L, Horton J C (2003). Shadows cast by retinal blood vessels mapped in primary visual cortex. *Science* **298**: 572–6.
135. Iwasato T, Erzurumlu R S, Huerta P T, *et al.* (1997). NMDA receptor-dependent refinement of somatotopic maps. *Neuron* **19**: 1201–10.
136. Iwasato T, Datwani A, Wolf A M, *et al.* (2000). Cortex-restricted disruption of NMDAR1 impairs neuronal patterns in the barrel cortex. *Nature* **406**: 726–31.
137. O'Leary D D M, Nakagawa Y (2002). Patterning centers, regulatory genes and extrinsic mechanisms controlling arealization of the neocortex. *Curr Opin Neurobiol* **12**: 14–25.
138. Agmon A, O'Dowd D K (1992). NMDA receptor-mediated currents are prominent in the thalamocortical synaptic response before maturation of inhibition. *J Neurophysiol* **68**: 345–8.
139. McCandlish C A, Li C X, Waters R S (1993). Early development of the SI cortical barrel field representation in neonatal rats follows a lateral-to-medial gradient: an electrophysiological study. *Exp Brain Res* **92**: 369–74.

140. Melzer P, Welker E, Doerfl J, Van der Loos H (1994). Maturation of the neuronal metabolic response to vibrissae stimulation in the developing whisker-to-barrel pathway of the mouse. *Exp Brain Res* **77**: 227–50.
141. Persico A M, Di Pino G, Levitt P (2006). Multiple receptors mediate the trophic effects of serotonin on ventroposterior thalamic neurons in vitro. *Brain Res* **1095**: 17–25.
142. Young-Davies C L, Bennett-Clarke C A, Lane R D, Rhoades R W (2000). Selective facilitation of the serotonin(1B) receptor causes disorganization of thalamic afferents and barrels in somatosensory cortex of rat. *J Comp Neurol* **425**: 130–8.
143. Laurent A, Goaillard J M, Cases O, Lebrand C, Gaspar P, Ropert N (2002). Activity-dependent presynaptic effect of serotonin 1B receptors on the somatosensory thalamocortical transmission in neonatal mice. *J Neurosci* **22**: 886–900.
144. Berg K A, Clarke W P (2001). Regulation of 5-HT$_{1A}$ and 5-HT$_{1B}$ receptor systems by phospholipid signaling cascades. *Brain Res Bull* **56**: 471–7.
145. Abdel-Majid R M, Leong W L, Schalkwyk L C, *et al.* (1998). Loss of adenylyl cyclase I activity disrupts patterning of mouse somatosensory cortex. *Nat Genet* **19**: 289–91.
146. Lotto B, Upton L, Price D J, Gaspar P (1999). Serotonin receptor activation enhances neurite outgrowth of thalamic neurones in rodents. *Neurosci Lett* **269**: 87–90.
147. Bonnin A, Torii M, Wang L, Rakic P, Levitt P (2007). Serotonin modulates the response of embryonic thalamocortical axons to netrin-1. *Nat Neurosci* **10**: 588–97.
148. Chiaia N L, Fish S E, Bauer W R, Bennett-Clarke C A, Rhoades R W (1992). Postnatal blockade of cortical activity by tetrodoxin does not disrupt the formation of vibrissa-related patterns in the rat's somatosensory cortex. *Dev Brain Res* **66**: 244–50.
149. Rhoades R W, Chiaia N L, Lane R D, Bennett-Clarke C A (1998). Effect of activity blockade on changes in vibrissae-related patterns in rat's primary somatosensory cortex induced by serotonin depletion. *J Comp Neurol* **402**: 276–83.
150. Basu B, Desai R, Balaji J, *et al.* (2008). Serotonin in pre-implantation mouse embryos is localized to the mitochondria and can modulate mitochondrial potential. *Reproduction* **135**: 657–69.
151. Brookes P S, Yoon Y, Robotham J L, Anders M W, Sheu S S (2004). Calcium, ATP, and ROS: a mitochondrial love–hate triangle. *Am J Physiol Cell Physiol* **287**: C817–33.
152. Walther D J, Peter J U, Winter S, *et al.* (2003). Serotonylation of small GTPases is a signal transduction pathway that triggers platelet alpha-granule release. *Cell* **115**: 851–62.
153. Moessner R, Dringen R, Persico A M, *et al.* (2002). Increased hippocampal DNA oxidation in serotonin transporter deficient mice. *J Neural Transm* **109**: 557–65.
154. Bastmeyer M, O'Leary D D M (1996). Dynamics of target recognition by interstitial axon branching along developing cortical axons. *J Neurosci* **16**: 1450–9.
155. Velez Pardo C, Jimenez del Rio M, Pinxteren J, De Potter W, Ebinger G, Vauquelin G (1995). Fe(2+)-mediated binding of serotonin and dopamine to skeletal muscle actin: resemblance to serotonin binding proteins. *Eur J Pharmacol* **288**: 209–18.

156. Betten A, Dahlgren C, Hermodsson S, Hellstrand K (2001). Serotonin protects NK cells against oxidatively induced functional inhibition and apoptosis. *J Leukoc Biol* **70**: 65–72.
157. Hadi N, Singh S, Ahmad A, Zaidi R (2001). Strand scission in DNA induced by 5-hydroxytryptamine (serotonin) in the presence of copper ions. *Neurosci Lett* **308**: 83–6.
158. Park J W, Youn Y C, Kwon O S, Jang Y Y, Han E S, Lee C S (2002). Protective effect of serotonin on 6-hydroxydopamine- and dopamine-induced oxidative damage of brain mitochondria and synaptosomes and PC12 cells. *Neurochem Int* **40**: 23–33.
159. Velez Pardo C, Jimenez del Rio M, Ebinger G, Vauquelin G (1996). Redox cycling activity of monoamine-serotonin binding protein conjugates. *Biochem Pharmacol* **51**: 1521–5.
160. Roerig B, Sutor B (1996). Serotonin regulates gap junction coupling in the developing rat somatosensory cortex. *Eur J Neurosci* **8**: 1685–95.
161. Bauman A L, Apparsundaram S, Ramamoorthy S, Wadzinski B E, Vaughan R A, Blakely R D (2000). Cocaine and antidepressant-sensitive biogenic amine transporters exist in regulated complexes with protein phosphatase 2A. *J Neurosci* **20**: 7571–8.
162. Ramamoorthy S, Blakely R D (1999). Phosphorylation and sequenstration of serotonin transporters differentially modulated by psychostimulants. *Science* **285**: 763–6.
163. Carneiro A M, Cook E H, Murphy D L, Blakely R D (2008). Interactions between integrin alphaIIbbeta3 and the serotonin transporter regulate serotonin transport and platelet aggregation in mice and humans. *J Clin Invest* **118**: 1544–52.
164. Brunner H G, Nelen M, Breakfield X O, Ropers H H, Van Oost B A (1993). Abnormal behavior associated with a point mutation in the structural gene for monoamine oxidase A. *Science* **262**: 578–80.
165. Orr S T, Miller C A (1995). Maternal depressive symptoms and the risk of poor pregnancy outcome. Review of the literature and preliminary findings. *Epidemiol Rev* **17**: 165–71.
166. Misri S, Kostaras D, Kostaras X (2000). The use of selective serotonin reuptake inhibitors during pregnancy and lactation: current knowledge. *Can J Psychiatry* **45**: 285–7.
167. Jensen P N, Olesen O V, Bertelsen A, Linnet K (1997). Citalopram and desmethylcitalopram concentrations in breast milk and in serum of mother and infant. *Ther Drug Monit* **19**: 236–9.
168. Kulin N A, Pastuszak A, Sage S R, *et al.* (1998). Pregnancy outcome following maternal use of the new selective serotonin reuptake inhibitors – a prospective controlled multicenter study. *JAMA* **279**: 609–10.
169. Ericson A, Kallen B, Wiholm B (1999). Delivery outcome after the use of antidepressants in early pregnancy. *Eur J Clin Pharmacol* **55**: 503–08.
170. Einarson A, Fatoye B, Sarkar M, *et al.* (2001). Pregnancy outcome following gestational exposure to venlafaxine: a multicenter prospective controlled study. *Am J Psychiatry* **158**: 1728–30.
171. Hendrick V, Smith L M, Suri R, Hwang S, Haynes D, Altshuler L (2003). Birth outcomes after prenatal exposure to antidepresant medication. *Am J Obstet Gynecol* **188**: 812–5.
172. Nulman I, Rovet J, Stewart D E, *et al.* (1997). Neurodevelopment of children exposed in utero to antidepressant drugs. *N Engl J Med* **336**: 258–62.
173. Chambers C D, Johnson K A, Dick L M, Felix R J, Jones K L (1996). Birth outcomes in pregnant women taking fluoxetine. *N Engl J Med* **335**: 1010–15.

174. Morrison J L, Riggs K W, Rurak D W (2005). Fluoxetine during pregnancy: impact on fetal development. *Reprod Fertil Dev* **17**: 641–50.
175. Casper C R, Fleiscer B E, Ancajas J C L, *et al.* (2003). Follow up of children of depressed mothers exposed or not exposed to antidepressant drugs during pregnancy. *J Pediatr* **142**: 402–08.
176. Oberlander T F, Eckstein Grunau R, Fitzgerald C, *et al.* (2002). Prolonged prenatal psychotropic medication exposure alters neonatal acute pain response. *Pediatr Res* **51**: 443–53.
177. Koren G (2002). SSRIs in pregnancy – are they safe? *Pediatr Res* **51**: 424–5.
178. Chubakov A R, Gromova E A, Konovalov G V, Sarkisova E F, Chumasov E I (1986). The effects of serotonin on the morpho-functional development of rat cerebral neocortex in tissue culture. *Brain Res* **369**: 285–97.
179. Lieske V, Bennett-Clarke C A, Rhoades R W (1999). Effects of serotonin on neurite outgrowth from thalamic neurons in vitro. *Neuroscience* **90**: 967–74.
180. Rhoades R W, Bennett-Clarke C A, Shi M Y, Mooney R D (1994). Effects of 5-HT on thalamocortical synaptic transmission in the developing rat. *J Neurophysiol* **72**: 2438–50.
181. Sikich L, Hickok J M, Todd R D (1990). $5HT_{1A}$ receptors control neurite branching during development. *Dev Brain Res* **56**: 269–74.

ADAM TRIPP AND ETIENNE SIBILLE

4

SERT models of emotional dysregulation

ABSTRACT

The serotonin system plays a key modulatory role in central nervous system processes that appear to be dysregulated in psychiatric disorders. Specifically, the serotonin transporter (SERT) is thought to be critical to many aspects of emotional dysregulation and has been a successful target for medications that treat several psychiatric disorders. Here, we narrowly focused on two psychiatric conditions; anxiety and depression, for which mice with SERT genetic manipulations have provided insight. Specifically, we suggest that dissecting syndromes according to a trait and state perspective may help us understand the complex and at times contradictory rodent results. The most compelling reason for this approach is provided by human studies, in which increased trait-neuroticism and stress-mediated vulnerability to develop depression were reported for subjects carrying the 5-HTTLPR *s/s* allele of the SERT gene, and thus placing the contribution of SERT to mood disorders in a gene × environment and trait/state context. Accordingly, current behavioral results in SERT knock-out (KO) mice are consistent with both increased trait and state anxiety-like behaviors, while evidence in support of a trait-based model of depression in SERT KO mice are inconsistent and mostly based on tests with limited relevance to human depression. However, comorbid symptoms associated with a wider definition of depression, such as altered gastrointestinal functions, lower pain threshold, and greater sensitivity to stress, have been reported in SERT KO mice, suggesting the presence of a pro-depressive state resulting from low SERT. SERT KO mice as a putative genetic model of

Experimental Models in Serotonin Transporter Research, eds. A. V. Kalueff and J. L. LaPorte. Published by Cambridge University Press.

increased vulnerability to develop a depressive state in response to chronic challenges (i.e. paralleling the *s*-allele mediated vulnerability in humans) has only begun to be investigated. Finally, studies will need to integrate trait/state features and with gender-specific approaches to fully recapitulate the risk factors that are known to influence the vulnerability to develop altered mood regulation in human subjects, namely genetic load, sex, and environment. To this end, SERT mutant mice can provide a critical window into mechanisms leading to increased risk for mood disorders, with the potential to reveal new targets for antidepressant drug development.

INTRODUCTION

The serotonin (5-hydroxytryptamine, 5-HT) system plays a key modulatory role in central nervous system processes that appear to be dysregulated in many psychiatric disorders. These processes include: internal affective states such as anxiety, fear, depression, and aggression; control of sleep; modulation of digestive behaviors; and influence on reward circuits that mediate motivation, hedonic states, and the appetitive properties of drugs of abuse (LeMarquand *et al.*, 1994; Linnoila and Virkkunen, 1992; Murphy and Lesch, 2008; Nestler *et al.*, 2002; Spiller, 2007). The serotonin (5-HT) system has been a successful target for medications that treat many psychiatric disorders (Nemeroff and Owens, 2002). The serotonin transporter (*SLC6A4* gene; protein also characterized as 5-HTT or SERT) is thought to be critical to many aspects of emotional dysregulation in neuropsychiatric disorders in which serotonin is a key modulator. In addition to the comorbid psychiatric symptoms, there are multiple neurological and physiological dysfunctions that are also comorbid with affective disorders, such as multiple sclerosis, dementia, epilepsy, gastrointestinal troubles, and altered pain sensation (Esch *et al.*, 2002; Ghaffar and Feinstein, 2007; Ishihara and Brayne, 2006; Kanner, 2007; O'Brien, 2005). As the scientific literature for all of these conditions is vast, we will be narrowly focusing on two psychiatric conditions within the larger panoply of SERT-related emotional dysregulation, anxiety and depression, for which mice with SERT genetic manipulations have provided insight (Murphy and Lesch, 2008). Focusing on these two affective disorders will illustrate in greater detail the important role, and possible mechanisms, of serotonin and SERT in emotional dysregulation.

Anxiety represents a serious and disabling psychiatric spectrum of disorders, including panic disorder and general anxiety disorder, with multiple comorbidities such as post-traumatic stress disorder (PTSD) and depression. The greatest determinants of the development of anxiety disorders lie in individual environmental factors, although the genetic heritability of anxiety is estimated at 30–40% (Hettema *et al.*, 2001). The rate of suicide with anxiety disorders is increased from the general population, by approximately 18-fold in panic disorder, and significantly increased with comorbid general anxiety disorder (GAD) and depressive symptoms (Weissman *et al.*, 1989). Selective serotonin reuptake inhibitors (SSRIs) are an effective treatment for anxiety-related disorders. The major target of SSRIs is SERT, and blockade of SERT is the mechanism by which excess anxiety or panic is relieved (Nemeroff and Owens 2002). Therefore, a better characterization of the role of key players in the serotonin system throughout life is crucial to the investigation of the neurobiology of anxiety as well as to identify new therapeutic targets for the treatment of this disabling psychiatric disorder.

Blockade of SERT function results in an anxiolytic effect in adult and adolescent patients. This pharmacologic anxiolytic response occurs with prolonged neurotransmission of serotonin by chronic SSRI block of its reuptake from the synaptic cleft. Intuitively one would guess that constitutive genetic downregulation of SERT expression would result in a non-anxious phenotype throughout the life of the individual. However, depending on its timing, a SERT blockade can have opposite and paradoxical behavioral outcomes. This paradox is illustrated in the context of a common promoter polymorphism of the human SERT gene (SERT gene-linked polymorphic region, 5-HTTLPR). The 5-HTTLPR polymorphism occurs in short (*s*) and long (*l*) allelic variants and has demonstrable effects on lymphoblast SERT messenger RNA (mRNA) and binding, and platelet serotonin reuptake; the (*s*) variant is a common 44-base pair insertion/deletion polymorphism associated with lower levels of SERT transcription, expression, function, and increased serotonin in the extracellular space in cell lines (Lesch *et al.*, 1996). However, associations with reduced RNA or binding levels in the adult brain have been more difficult to establish (Lim *et al.*, 2006; Mann *et al.*, 2000; Parsey *et al.*, 2006; Shioe *et al.*, 2003), likely reflecting the presence of additional factors contributing to SERT regulation (Serretti *et al.*, 2006).

Contrary to the effects seen with SERT blockade in patients on SSRI antidepressant treatment, the *s*/*s* polymorphism is associated with increased neuroticism and anxiety, and with increased vulnerability to affective disorders in concert with increased childhood stressful life events (Caspi *et al.*, 2003; Collier *et al.*, 1996; Gutierrez *et al.*, 1998;

Kendler *et al.*, 2005; Lesch *et al.*, 1996; Mazzanti *et al.*, 1998). These contrasting reports highlight the complexity of the role of serotonin in mood regulation and emphasize the need to investigate putative neurobiological and neurodevelopmental mechanisms by which serotonin, SERT, and the 5-HTTLPR *s/s* polymorphism influences the vulnerability to develop anxiety-related and depressive states.

Several imaging studies have identified neural networks involved in anxious phenotypes that are influenced by the *s/s* 5-HTTLPR polymorphism. Hariri *et al.* (2002) report that individuals with one or two copies of the short allele of the serotonin transporter (5-HTT) promoter polymorphism exhibited greater amygdala neuronal activity, as assessed by blood oxygenation level-dependent (BOLD) functional magnetic resonance imaging (fMRI), in response to fearful stimuli compared with individuals homozygous for the long allele. BOLD fMRI identifies "active brain areas" through a process called the hemodynamic response: blood releases oxygen to metabolically active neurons at a greater rate than to inactive neurons, and the difference in magnetic susceptibility between oxyhemoglobin and deoxyhemoglobin and thus oxygenated or deoxygenated blood leads to magnetic signal variation, which can be detected using an MRI scanner. This study was independently confirmed, further implicating the amygdala, SERT, and the pathways that may inhibit or activate under fearful or depressive stimuli (Heinz *et al.*, 2005). Pezawas *et al.* have also reported functional consequences of the presence of the *s*-allele on the structure, function, and functional coupling of the perigenual cingulate cortex (rACC) and amygdala (Pezawas *et al.*, 2005). The variance associated with the *s/l* polymorphism in amygdala–rACC functional connectivity was responsible for 30% of temperament variance in harm-reduction subscale scores from the Tridimensional Personality Questionnaire. Moreover, the presentation of fearful stimuli revealed an uncoupling of the functional interaction of this regulatory circuit in *s/s* patients. Together, this study provided a rationale for the amygdala–rACC coupling as a feedback mechanism for amygdala regulation and a putative mechanism by which the 5-HTTLPR *s/s* carrier was associated with a more neurotic and anxious phenotype.

Major depressive disorder is a significant psychiatric illness, contributing to death by suicide, as well as the fourth most common cause of disability per the World Health Organization (WHO) (Murray, 1996). The lifetime prevalence for suicide attempts in individuals with unipolar depression is ~16%, about half the rate of those with bipolar disorder, and four times greater than those with any other Axis I disorder (Chen and Dilsaver, 1996). Significant clinical symptoms include sleep disturbances, anergia, anhedonia, changes in appetite, poor concentration, and the appearance of suicidal ideation. Lifetime incidence reaches 20% and is often found comorbid with PTSD, anxiety, and alcohol and substance use disorders. PTSD is characterized as development of characteristic symptoms following exposure to an extreme traumatic stressor involving direct personal experience of an event. This exposure results in intense fear and/or helplessness, persistent re-experiencing of the traumatic event, persistent avoidance of stimuli associated with the trauma, and numbing of general responsiveness, and persistent symptoms of increased arousal, that cause significant interference with normal daily social and psychological functioning. Multiple environmental and genetic factors act additively or synergistically to produce a depressive phenotype, with no one environmental or genetic factor contributing more than 5% of the variance between normal subjects and depressed subjects (Leonardo and Hen, 2006; Mann and Currier, 2006; Nestler *et al.*, 2002). Depression is also a significant contributor to systemic organ diseases (Murray and Lopez, 1996), including potential shared etiology for numerous comorbid symptoms and diseases, such as anxiety, increased pain sensitivity, irritable bowel syndrome (IBS), and overactive bladder. SSRIs were originally used as antidepressants, and blockade of SERT is the mechanism by which the cluster of depressive symptoms is relieved (Nemeroff and Owens, 2002). Similar to studies examining anxiety, the 5-HTTLPR *s/s* polymorphism has both provided answers and raised many additional questions regarding the role of SERT and serotonin in depression.

In a seminal study, Caspi *et al.* identified reduced resilience for stressful life events in *s/s* carriers compared to *l/l* carriers, a strong clinically relevant and statistically significant direct correlation between number of stressful life events and depressive symptoms in *s/s* carriers, and an increased likelihood of suicide attempts or ideation with increased stressful life events (Caspi *et al.*, 2003). The authors have speculated that 5-HTTLPR *s/s* is a factor that predisposes individuals towards PTSD or depression through gene × environment interaction rather than being a direct correlate of depression. This group also alluded to the gene × gene interaction that may work additively or synergistically to create depressive phenotypes. These findings have been replicated in some studies (Kendler *et al.*, 2005), but not all (Gillespie *et al.*, 2005). Nevertheless, these results are difficult to reconcile with the general assumption that depression is associated with decreased central serotonin levels, and anxiety with increased central serotonin levels (Lowry *et al.*, 2005). How can it be that the *s/s* genotype is linked to both anxiety and depression? A potential explanation, which is partially supported by current pharmacological and genetic studies in mice (Ansorge *et al.*, 2004), could be that the acute consequence of the *s*-allele on the serotonin system may regulate anxiety levels, while changes in adult systems that are secondary to altered developmental events related to SERT genetic variations place the system at risk for developing depression (Sibille and Lewis, 2006). These observations illustrate the need for more tractable models to investigate mechanisms that are downstream from SERT function, and that can investigate additional gene × gene or environment × gene interactions, in order to provide a better understanding of the complexity of the genetics of depression (Gillespie *et al.*, 2005). Indeed, while 5-HTTLPR studies have shed some light on the differential role of SERT in the neurobiology of anxiety and depression, there is a need for animal models, where experimental manipulation of SERT expression (such as transgenic and SERT KO rodents) can establish causality relationships and set the stage to investigate cellular and molecular mechanisms by which changes in SERT affect brain function, emotional regulation, and symptoms of neuropsychiatric disorders.

SERT MUTANT MICE

SERT knock-out (KO) mice (Bengel *et al.*, 1998; Lira *et al.*, 2003), and recently rats (Homberg *et al.*, 2007), have provided useful models to investigate mechanisms by which SERT may regulate emotional behavior. SERT KO mice were derived by different groups independently (Ansorge *et al.*, 2004; Bengel *et al.*, 1998; Homberg *et al.*, 2007). The first SERT KO mouse was generated via homologous recombination by replacing the second exon of the SERT gene with a neomycin cassette (Bengel *et al.*, 1998). This alteration leads to a loss of the full-length, functional SERT protein in the brain (Bengel *et al.*, 1998). This mouse was back-crossed onto the C57BL/J6 (B6) strain. Mice homozygous for the null mutation (SERT−/− or KO) exhibit an absence of serotonin reuptake, resulting in a decreased rate of synaptic serotonin clearance and a 6–10-fold increase in basal levels of forebrain extracellular serotonin, and a compensatory 60–80% reduction in tissue levels of serotonin (Mathews *et al.*, 2004; Montanez *et al.*, 2003). Heterozygous (HZ) mutant mice lacking one SERT allele (SERT HZ) show a deficiency in serotonin reuptake and clearance that is intermediate between that observed in SERT KO mice and wildtype (WT) controls (Mathews *et al.*, 2004; Montanez *et al.*, 2003). However, despite the 50% reduction in SERT expression, SERT

HZ mice do not show the low locomotor activity phenotype that is characteristic of KO mice (Holmes *et al.*, 2002b; Kalueff *et al.*, 2007b), and exhibit either more subtle behavioral differences compared to KO or, in the majority of studies, no differences in testing compared to their WT controls (Bengel *et al.*, 1998; Kalueff *et al.*, 2007b; Li *et al.*, 1999). These results were confirmed in an independently derived SERT mutant line where the first exon of SERT was replaced with a neomycin cassette (Lira *et al.*, 2003). This line has been mostly maintained on the 129S6/SvEv (S6) genetic background (Lira *et al.*, 2003). Other SERT genetic manipulations have included the use of siRNA to downregulate SERT in adult male BALB/c mice, which resulted in a phenocopy of adult SSRI treatment in WT mice (Thakker *et al.*, 2005). Finally, Zhao *et al.* (2006) have recently trapped exon 14 of SERT, creating a nonfunctional truncated SERT protein at the C-terminus, rather than the N-terminus for the other two groups, with a phenotype similar to the other SERT KO strains (Bengel *et al.*, 1998; Holmes *et al.*, 2003a; Lira *et al.*, 2003).

A recent study investigated the neurochemical and behavioral effects of increased SERT expression by generating a novel transgenic mouse model that expresses huSERT from a yeast artificial chromosome construct (El Yacoubi and Vaugeois, 2007) in addition to endogenous murine SERT (Jennings *et al.*, 2006). huSERT consists of the human 5-HTT (h5-HTT) gene flanked by 150 kb of 5′ and 300 kb of 3′ sequences with the "short" allele of the 5-HTTLPR in the promoter region and the 10-repeat allele of the variable number tandem repeat in intron 2 inserted into the yeast artificial chromosome (YAC) construct, that was ultimately injected into fertilized eggs. These transgenic mice showed reduced tissue levels (~15–35%) of serotonin in the hippocampus, frontal cortex, hypothalamus, brain stem, and midbrain compared with wildtype animals. However, in microdialysis experiments, SERT over-expressing mice demonstrated constantly lower (50–60%) basal extracellular levels of serotonin in both the prefrontal cortex and hippocampus compared with wildtype mice. This difference was stable and maintained over 3–4 h of baseline sampling. Also, in both regions, the increase in serotonin evoked by local application of high potassium was significantly less (40–80%) in the transgenic mice compared with wildtype. Separate experiments showed that the low levels of extracellular serotonin in the prefrontal cortex of SERT over-expressing mice could be reversed and normalized by local application of 1 μM paroxetine. While the genetic mutation is in some ways opposite to that in SERT KO mice, the two lines share some unexpected similarities, such as reduced tissue levels of serotonin, thus prompting additional questions on the neurobiology of SERT expression in the brain, and suggesting differential possibilities for compensatory mechanisms following dysregulated SERT function (see the section on anxiety behavior later).

Studies in SERT mutants have also reported crucial adaptive mechanisms and compensations resulting from decreased or absent SERT function. SERT KO mice, and to a lesser extent HZ mice, displayed reduced dorsal raphe serotonergic neuronal firing, a reduction in serotonin neurons, and a desensitization and downregulation of somatodendritic 5-HT1A autoreceptors (Gobbi *et al.*, 2001; Li *et al.*, 2000; Lira *et al.*, 2003; Mannoury la Cour *et al.*, 2001). Binding density reductions of postsynaptic 5-HT1A receptors are seen in SERT KO mice in the frontal cortex, amygdala, septum, and hypothalamus, but not the hippocampus (Li *et al.*, 2000; Mannoury la Cour *et al.*, 2001). Changes in the expression of other serotonin receptor subtypes appear to be less profound and more region-specific. SERT KO mice show reduced 5-HT1B receptor binding density in the substantia nigra but not other brain regions (Fabre *et al.*, 2000), and fail to respond to the locomotor-stimulating effects of 5-HT1B receptor activation (Holmes *et al.*, 2002b). The binding density of 5-HT2A and 5-HT2C receptors is increased in the hypothalamus and amygdala, respectively (Li *et al.*, 2003), while 5-HT3 mRNA levels are reduced in the enteric nervous system of SERT KO mice (Liu *et al.*, 2002). In SERT KO mice, modest residual serotonin reuptake into axons is accomplished by dopamine or norepinephrine transporter function (Montanez *et al.*, 2003; Murphy *et al.*, 2001) and by compensatory upregulation of the OCT3 transporter (Schmitt *et al.*, 2003), although not as efficiently (Daws *et al.*, 2006; Holmes *et al.*, 2002b; Mathews *et al.*, 2004; Schmitt *et al.*, 2003). Together, these neurochemical characterizations revealed significant downstream compensations due to altered expression of functional SERT, and highlight the complexity of changes and putative confounding effects that will need to be taken into consideration when investigating the contribution of SERT and SERT mutant models in anxiety and depressive disorders.

ANXIETY

The constitutive silencing of SERT expression results in elevated anxiety-like behavior in adult mice (Holmes *et al.*, 2003b). These findings were replicated in different KO variants in mice (Lira *et al.*, 2003) and rats (Olivier *et al.*, 2008), but also appeared to be modulated by differences in genetic background (Holmes *et al.*, 2002b). Early blockade of SERT by chronic SSRI treatment recreates the adult SERT KO phenotype

(Ansorge *et al.*, 2004). Finally, SERT over-expression resulted in the opposite phenotype, a low anxiety- or anxiety-resistant phenotype (Jennings *et al.*, 2006).

Holmes *et al.* examined anxiety-related behaviors in SERT KO and HZ mice using the original strain of SERT KO mice on the C57B6 genetic background in the light–dark exploration, emergence, open field, and elevated plus maze tests (Bengel *et al.*, 1998; Holmes *et al.*, 2002b). SERT KO mice spent less time in the aversive, open arms of the elevated plus-maze and made fewer entries into the open arm, thus exhibiting more inhibited, less explorative anxiety-like behavior compared to WT controls. Knock-out mice showed less exploration of brightly lit areas in both the light–dark exploration and emergence tests, ~50–75% less time compared to WT controls. Knock-out mice also showed a general reduction in exploratory locomotion and greater "wall-hugging" in a brightly lit open field arena. These findings suggest a robust increase in anxiety-like behavior in SERT KO mice. Interestingly, despite exhibiting a gene-dosage dependent alteration in serotonin neurotransmission (e.g. partially elevated basal synaptic serotonin), SERT HZ mice fail to exhibit clear behavioral abnormalities in these tests. No robust gender-linked differences were observed. Together, SERT KO mice on the C57B6 genetic background were uniformly more anxious than their WT controls (Holmes *et al.*, 2002b).

In contrast, phenotypic abnormalities were not observed in SERT KOs that were bred onto a congenic 129S6 background (Holmes *et al.*, 2002b; Holmes *et al.*, 2003a), as measured in the elevated plus maze and light–dark exploratory tests. A possible explanation for these findings is that the naturally elevated anxiety-related behavioral baseline of 129S6 WT controls precluded the detection of further anxiety-like abnormalities caused by the SERT KO mutation, especially in tests that rely on locomotor activity and that suffer from known floor effects in high-anxiety groups. This is especially relevant since SERT KO mice exhibit a hypoactive locomotor phenotype in a home cage environment (Holmes *et al.*, 2002b), which may have contributed to the lack of detectable abnormal behavior in exploration-based tests for anxiety-like behavior (Holmes, 2001).

The absence of an increased anxiety-related phenotype in SERT KO mice on the 129S6 genetic background appeared to be confirmed in a separate line of SERT mutant mice (Lira *et al.*, 2003). These mice exhibited no behavioral phenotypic differences related to anxiety measurements in the open field and elevated plus maze tests. In the elevated plus maze test, Lira *et al.* observed no gender or genotypic differences in time spent or percent of entries to the open and closed arms; however, activity differed between the genotypes, with SERT KO mice showing less total arm entries and fewer head dips than their WT controls by ~25%. This is in contrast to the findings of Holmes *et al.*, which did not find activity-related differences in elevated plus maze testing, but consistent with prior reports of lower activity of SERT KO mice in open field (Holmes *et al.*, 2002b). More subtle behavioral differences have suggested differences in anxiety-like behavior in SERT KO mice on the 129S6 genetic background as well. Indeed, Ansorge *et al.* (2004) reported no difference in the percentage of entries or time spent in the open arms of the elevated plus maze, as well as no difference in the percentage of time in the center of the test chamber using the open field test. However, SERT KO mice displayed significant reductions, by ~33–50% depending on the test, in the total arm entries, total ambulatory time, as well as total vertical activity counts, which was interpreted by the authors as anxiety-like behavior, and not simply a matter of baseline reduced locomotor activity, since no differences in home cage activity were observed between KO and WT control mice.

A more compelling argument for elevated anxiety-like behaviors for SERT KO mice on the 129S6 background may actually be provided by results from the same group in the novelty suppressed feeding (NSF) test. Although the NSF has been used recently to investigate the long-term behavioral response to chronic antidepressant activity (Santarelli *et al.*, 2003), the latency to feed in a threatening novel environment of the NSF chamber correlates with fearfulness and decreases after acute treatment with both anxiolytic drugs (Bodnoff *et al.*, 1988) or chronic antidepressant exposure (Santarelli *et al.*, 2003). This pharmacological response suggests that mechanisms underlying changes in the latency to start feeding involve both anxiety-like and antidepressant-like processes. Moreover, this test is mostly activity-independent, and thus less likely to be confounded by the low locomotor activity of SERT KO mice. In this test, 129S6 SERT KO mice displayed a significant increase in the latency to start eating (Ansorge *et al.*, 2004), thus providing supporting evidence for an anxiety-related phenotype on that genetic background as well, which the authors characterized as "emotional" behavior. Alternatively, background genetic differences present in one strain (129S6), but not another, might partially protect against the anxiety-promoting effects of the SERT KO mutation. It is also worth noting that there were no appreciable sex differences in C57B6 or 129S6 WT, HZ, or KO mice on anxiety-related behavioral testing, in contrast to the known sex differences in mood disorders observed in human subjects. Taken together, these findings underscore the utility of assessing mutants on multiple genetic backgrounds, and in using multiple tests that do not all rely on behavioral inhibition.

In a follow up study, Ansorge *et al.* (2004) determined that early postnatal blockade of SERT in WT mice with fluoxetine and then normalization in adulthood mimicked the elevated emotional phenotype of constitutive SERT KO mice. They pinpointed the necessary period of SERT blockade for the emotional phenotype by parallel testing of KO mice and chronic early treatment of WT mice with fluoxetine. No differences were observed in the percentage of entries into the open arms or time spent in open arms, as well as no difference in the percentage of time in the center of the test chamber using the open field test. However, SERT KO mice and postnatally fluoxetine-treated mice showed significant reductions in total arm entries, total ambulatory time, and total vertical activity counts. The developmental origin of the adult "emotional" phenotype was clearly demonstrated in the NSF test as WT mice treated with fluoxetine between postnatal days 4–21 pheno-copied the increased latency to start feeding in the NSF test of SERT KO mice. The authors have recently replicated their findings and showed that this effect was specific to SERT compared to postnatal blockade of the norepinehrine transporter (Ansorge *et al.*, 2008). In summary, these studies demonstrated that early disruption of normal SERT function can result in a trait-based emotional phenotype, which may be relevant to anxiety-like but also to a pro-depressive behavior due to the pharmacological validations of the NSF test by both anxiolytic and antidepressant drugs.

By shifting the time frame to earlier developmental events, these rodent studies may shed light on the apparent discrepancies between the similar biological effects of the 5-HTTLPR *s*-allele and SSRI treatment in human subjects (decreased serotonin uptake through either reduced SERT expression or pharmacological blockade, respectively) and the opposite clinical outcomes (greater risk for depression with the *s*-allele versus therapeutic improvement with SSRIs). Specifically, these studies suggest that serotonin, as a trophic factor, can influence the development and establishment of neural networks that participate in mood regulation later in life (Sibille and Lewis, 2006). Accordingly, once established, these altered neural networks may mediate the increased vulnerability to depression in adulthood, independent of the current state of serotonin function.

Finally, additional evidence for a causal role for SERT in modulating anxiety-like behavior was provided by Jennings *et al.* (2006) using a line of SERT over-expressing mice. C57B6-transgenic SERT over-expressor mice expressed a more resilient and low anxiety phenotype compared to normal controls. Specifically, they displayed increased entries (two-fold) and a decreased latency (~50% reduction) to enter the open arms of the elevated plus maze, as well as a significant reduction in latency to eat in the NSF test (Jennings *et al.*, 2006), contrasting with the increased latency observed in SERT KO mice (Ansorge *et al.*, 2004). Interestingly, paroxetine treatment of SERT over-expressing mice reversed the low-anxiety phenotype in the elevated plus maze test, suggesting that mechanisms responsible for the decreased anxiety-like phenotype were directly related to increased SERT function.

The study of Jennings *et al.* dovetailed with SERT KO mice studies, showing that constitutive lack of SERT expression, or early SERT blockade during development, resulted in increased anxiety phenotype, suggesting altogether that SERT expression may act like a "temperamental thermostat," with more SERT resulting in less anxiety, and vice versa. Thus SERT genetic murine studies support the idea of serotonin as a temperamental thermostat, where an increased amount of serotonin in synaptosomes early in development results in adult animals that are more prone to affective extremes of anxiety and depression, and less able to modulate their affective state, compared to mice with normal or increased levels of SERT expression displaying normal or low anxiety levels. The importance of the time window of SERT downregulation (i.e. developmental versus constitutive blockade) and of multiple compensatory mechanisms in SERT KO mice also suggest that mechanisms supporting the increased anxiety phenotype may be remote from the original SERT disruption in some cases. Specifically, changes in SERT activity early in development suggest developmental adaptations that in turn may disrupt the formation of neural networks that are critical for normal adult functions.

Nevertheless, potential discrepancies in anxiety-related phenotypes in SERT KO mice suggest the following question: Would an anxiety-like abnormality in SERT KO mice clearly manifest under high or chronic stress conditions? This would test for potential differences between an anxiety-like "state" rather than "trait" phenotype in SERT KO mice. Testing this hypothesis is only beginning in SERT KO mice. In a recent study, male SERT KO mice on the C57B6 background, but not HZ, were more susceptible to mild stress (cat odor), as measured by increased anxiety-like behavior in open arm entries in elevated plus maze testing and dark–light box testing (Adamec *et al.*, 2006b). Interestingly, the more handled the mice were, the less their basal differences were apparent (i.e. nurtured/handled SERT KO mice seem to be less anxious than naïve SERT-KO mice). These results parallel the effects of nurturing on the impact of the 5-HTTLPR *s/s* polymorphism in non-human primates and humans (Bennett *et al.*, 2002; Caspi *et al.*, 2003; Champoux *et al.*, 2002; Kendler *et al.*, 2005). In this particular study, an anxious predisposition was unmasked in SERT KO mice with repeat exposure to stress, echoing a variety of mammalian models demonstrating the important interaction of gene and environment in the resiliency, or lack thereof, to neuropsychiatric disorders under different environmental conditions (Bennett *et al.*, 2002; Champoux *et al.*, 2002; Wellman *et al.*, 2007). Adamec *et al.* (2006b) previously demonstrated that female C57/B6 WT mice, but not male mice, showed an increased susceptibility to stress and anxiety after being exposed to cat odor. Thus, they postulated that they partially recreated a "female-like" susceptibility to anxiety and stress in male SERT KO mice by subcutaneous implantation of estradiol-β releasing pellets, and that resultant downstream changes in 5-HT1A and 5-HT2A binding may have played a role in these adaptive differences in anxiety-like behavioral outcomes (Ren-Patterson *et al.*, 2006). This study helps to define similarities and differences in state versus trait testing of anxiety, in addition to testing the role of critical factors in the expression of anxiety-related phenotypes, including differences based on the extent of nurturing and gender.

Neurotrophic factors such as brain-derived neurotrophic factor (BDNF) can interact with SERT to affect the levels of serotonin in extraneuronal space as well as modulate anxiety-like behavior. Interestingly, SERT/BDNF double KO mice display gender differences in which females, perhaps through estrogen expression, are more resilient to the effects of increased serotonin in the extraneuronal space in behavioral testing (Ren-Patterson *et al.*, 2006). Female SERT−/− × BDNF+/− mice showed a protective effect, through increased TrKB receptor expression, and BDNF modulation (Ren-Patterson *et al.*, 2006), in that significantly fewer reductions in serotonin concentrations were observed in hypothalamus and other brain regions than males, relative to controls. Likewise, in the elevated plus maze, female SERT−/− × BDNF+/− deficient mice also demonstrated no increases in the anxiety-like behaviors previously found in males SERT−/− × BDNF+/−. Female SERT−/− × BDNF+/− mice did not manifest the ~40% reduction in the expression of TrkB receptors or the ~30% reductions in dopamine and its metabolites that male SERT−/− × BDNF+/− did. After estradiol implantation in male SERT−/− × BDNF+/− mice, hypothalamic serotonin was significantly increased compared to vehicle-implanted mice. These findings support the hypothesis that estrogen may enhance BDNF function via its TrkB receptor, leading to alterations in the serotonin circuits which modulate anxiety-like behaviors. Together, the sex effects were reversed by estrogen implants in males or ovarectomy in females, identifying estrogen as a potential important modulator in the behavioral outcomes and altered serotonin levels in extraneuronal spaces.

In short, SERT KO mice exhibit a robust baseline difference in anxiety-like behaviors, although modified by the background strain of the KO mice, suggesting the presence of modifier genes interacting with SERT function. These findings parallel human studies with the 5-HTTLPR polymorphism, in which the *s/s* allele can make individuals more susceptible to anxiety disorders, but anxiety disorders are still multifactorial, and not solely due to disruption of one gene. Comparisons between constitutive deletion and pharmacological manipulations have been instrumental in determining the critical developmental time window for the long-lasting effects of the lack of SERT expression on adult anxiety-like behavior. Studies in SERT/BDNF double KO have started to investigate interactions of SERT with other key genetic (BDNF) or neuroendocrine (estrogen) modulators that act in concert with SERT to establish levels of anxiety-like behaviors. Together, the somewhat conflicting results in gender and strain differences illustrate the complex nature of gene and environment interactions even for a "pure" affect-related syndrome such as anxiety, in contrast to depression, which is characterized by clusters of symptoms, each of those potentially supported by different neurobiological systems and potentially acting with relative autonomy.

DEPRESSION

SERT plays an important role both in putative mechanisms underlying the pathophysiology of depression, as well as in its pharmacological treatment. Interestingly, current studies suggest that the constitutive lack of SERT expression may result in some depression-like behaviors. Since SERT pharmacological blockade relieves depression, these results are in contrast to what was hypothesized initially, which was that the lack of serotonin reuptake would result in a mouse that, if anything, would be more resistant to developing depression-like behavior. Remarkably, behavioral studies in SERT KO mice suggest just the opposite phenotype, with more anxiety-like behavior and potential increased susceptibility to stress and depression.

However, numerous limitations to modeling a depressive syndrome may mitigate these conclusions and must be addressed first. The difficulties associated with studying depression in rodents could be framed by the following facts: (1) the lack of a model to induce a validated depressive pathology; (2) an almost exclusive focus on tests for antidepressant mechanisms, rather than on the primary pathology of the disorder; and (3) the heterogeneity of a disorder with multiple symptom dimensions. Thus, to establish a rodent model of depression, as a cluster-based syndrome (i.e. paralleling the definition of the human syndrome in DSM-IV and ICD-10), several criteria would need to be fulfilled, including: (1) good face validity (close ethological counterpart for emotion-related and anhedonia-like behaviors); (2) good construct validity (for instance, unpredictable psycho-social stress mimics real-life stress etiology and recruits equivalent neuroendocrine and biological systems); and (3) good predictive validity (antidepressant reversal respects the time courses for mechanisms of disease and drug reversal).

It is important to note that the majority of paradigms that are frequently used either to induce or characterize depressive-like states (social defeat, learned helplessness), or to predict antidepressant activities (forced swim and tail suspension tests), follow at best one or two of these criteria or do not model epidemiological characteristics of human depression and neurobiological mechanisms. Thus, conclusions drawn from these tests have only limited relevance to the human depressive syndrome. In this section, we first review results from some of these behavioral tests, which have been used mostly for predictive values of antidepressant effects. Then, in the absence of a current validated model with good face and construct validities for the full depressive syndrome, we argue that reviewing sets of symptoms that are commonly found comorbid with depression and that are affected by the lack of SERT would in the meantime contribute to our understanding of the role of SERT in depression. Indeed, some or all of the following overlapping symptoms may be found along with depressive-like behavior, and are believed to share some genetic and environmental components: (i) increased alcohol and/or substance use, (ii) anxiety, (iii) increased or decreased aggression, and (iv) additional physiological symptoms – potentially mediated by peripheral serotonin and SERT – such as IBS and/or chronic pain (Cryan and Holmes, 2005; Gross and Hen, 2004; Hariri and Holmes, 2006; Jann and Slade, 2007; Leonardo and Hen, 2006; Nestler *et al.*, 2002). In other words, the goal is to assess multiple features of a depressive-like phenotype in SERT KO mice, as a means to help us understand the overall role of SERT in this syndrome.

Holmes *et al.* (2002b) assessed the presence of a depressive-like phenotype in SERT KO mice through forced swim test (FST) and tail suspension test (TST) for inescapable stress-related behavior. In the FST, SERT KO mice back-crossed onto a 129S6 genetic background spent significantly more time in passive immobility than WT controls. Because reduced immobility in this test is opposite to the effects of antidepressants, such a profile could be indirectly interpreted as a "depression-like" response to inescapable stress. However, SERT KO mice on the C57B6 background did not show any differences in FST or TST testing (Holmes *et al.*, 2002b) while reduced immobility in TST testing for 129S6 SERT KO strain was reported in the same study, just the opposite of what would be expected for a "depressive" phenotype. Limitations of the TST and FST tests and present results at addressing potential molecular or cellular mechanisms of depression include paradoxical responses in the two tests, and, importantly, a time course for pharmacological validation of these tests that rely on minutes, rather than weeks, as observed in depression. Therefore, these studies provide only weak, and contentious, evidence for a putative trait-based depression-like phenotype (Holmes *et al.*, 2002b).

As mentioned above, Ansorge *et al.*, using the 129S6 SERT KO strain, reported heightened "emotional" behavior in the activity-independent NSF test. SERT KO mice and postnatally fluoxetine-treated WT mice both showed increased latency to feed in the NSF test compared to HZ and WT control mice. Again, the pharmacological validation of this test by chronic exposure to antidepressants (Santarelli *et al.*, 2003) suggests that increased latency in that test may also be consistent with a depressive-like phenotype. Similar results were reported with the foot shock avoidance test, where both fluoxetine-treated mice and constitutive SERT KO mice showed an increased latency to avoiding shock, considered "learned helplessness" behavior. Activity was controlled for by observing intershock activity and did not differ across groups. Together, these studies suggest evidence for trait-based depressive-like behavior in SERT KO mice, although they highlight the difficulty of clearly separating depressive-like from anxiety-like behaviors. Alternatively, these tests may be viewed as assessing an emotional dimension of behavior that is present in both syndromes, and that should be interpreted in the context of additional behavioral dimensions for conclusive evidence supporting a depressive-like phenotype. Importantly, these studies only assessed trait-like behaviors and did not address the possibility of SERT KO mice state-based depressive behavior, as induced by interactions with the environment. Stress has been most often used to induce higher emotion-related states. Here, in support of impaired stress responses resulting from the lack of functional SERT, SERT KO mice show exaggerated plasma adrenocorticotropin and catecholamine responses to 15 min of immobilization or saline injection (Li *et al.*, 1999; Tjurmina *et al.*, 2002), deficits on active avoidance in the shock avoidance test (Lira *et al.*, 2003).

In the face of these conflicting results and lack of all-encompassing tests for depression, how then should SERT KO mice be evaluated as a potential animal model of depression? What additional evidence has been provided by studies performed in SERT KO with regard to other putative comorbid "symptoms"? We suggest that the presence of these symptoms (i.e. including aggression, chronic pain, IBS, and fear conditioning) should be included and considered in a wider definition of a depressive syndrome, and that they should help us define the role of SERT in potentially modulating multiple symptom dimensions that are either comorbid or interactive with depression. We suggest that the overall pattern of changes observed reflects a potential trait-like pro-depressive and cluster-based behavioral phenotype in SERT KO mice, and suggests that induced state-based behavioral paradigms should be investigated.

Changes in *aggression* levels and *agonistic behaviors* are often comorbid with human depression. Holmes *et al.* (2002a) have reported reduced aggression levels in SERT KO mice (C57B6 background) using the resident-intruder test. SERT KO mice took longer to initiate the first attack and, generally, attacked less frequently and less intensely than WT controls. In a rare example of intermediate phenotype, SERT HZ mice showed an intermediate aggressive phenotype, attacking as quickly as WT controls but generally with lower frequency. To test whether aggression in SERT KO mice would emerge under further provocation, mice were exposed to an intruder for a second time. Repeated testing increased aggression in SERT HZ and WT control mice, while aggressive behavior in SERT KO mice remained low. The amount of time SERT mutant mice spent in non-aggressive, social investigative behavior was similar to that of the other genotypes, thus suggesting a specific inhibition of aggressive responses, rather than a more general social deficit, in SERT KO mice. However, some recent studies have shown global social deficits in SERT KO mice (Kalueff, 2007; Kalueff *et al.*, 2007a, 2007b). This decreased aggression phenotype in SERT KO parallels clinical findings in some studies in human depression (Holmes *et al.*, 2002a; Linnoila and Virkkunen, 1992). Interestingly, this study not only evaluated aggression as a baseline trait, but also as an induced state over time. With increasing exposure to intruders, SERT KO mice remained more docile, thus displaying a consistent trait and state-decreased aggressive behavior phenotype.

Chronic pain is often comorbid in individuals experiencing depression. In a recent study, Vogel *et al.* (2003) examined changes in pain perception in SERT KO mice. In these mice, reduced serotonin levels in the injured peripheral nerves correlate with diminished behavioral signs of thermal hyperalgesia, a pain-related symptom caused by peripheral sensitization. In contrast, bilateral mechanical allodynia ("other pain": pain from stimuli which are not normally painful), a centrally mediated phenomenon, was associated with decreased spinal serotonin concentrations in SERT KO mice and may possibly be caused by a lack of spinal inhibition. In short, lack of serotonin does not activate heat hyperalgesia at local site, but lack of serotonin causes a lack of central inhibition in the spine and an increase in mechanical pain, making it bilateral rather than remaining unilateral, through a lack of 5-HT2A and 5-HT3 activation or downregulation of these receptors. This study finds increased pain in SERT KO mice to stimuli that otherwise do not elicit pain, demonstrating the presence of another analogous pro-depressive characteristic of trait-based depression, paralleling observations in some depressed human subjects (Jann and Slade, 2007).

Other comorbid peripheral conditions often observed in depressive disorders include IBS and overactive bladder (Chen *et al.*, 2001; Cornelissen *et al.*, 2005). Gastrointestinal and bladder functions are mediated by peripheral serotonin that is synthesized in the gastrointestinal tract and transported back into the cell by SERT as well. Gastrointestinal and bladder dysfunction were reported in SERT KO mice (Chen *et al.*, 2001; Cornelissen *et al.*, 2005). Stool water and colon motility were increased in most SERT KO animals; however, the increase in motility (diarrhea) occasionally alternated irregularly with decreased motility (constipation) (Chen *et al.*, 2001). The watery diarrhea is probably attributable to the potentiation of serotonergic signaling in SERT KO mice, whereas the transient constipation may be caused by episodes of enhanced serotonin release leading to serotonin receptor desensitization. Cornelissen *et al.* (2005) found this attribute more robust in female mice, leading to a clinical correlation mimicking the comorbidities found in human subjects with depression, bladder dysfunction, and IBS. These studies were performed in SERT KO mice back-crossed on a C57B6 background strain.

Importantly, these studies did not evaluate depressive behavior directly, but rather addressed comorbid conditions associated with depression observed in human studies, providing additional evidence for potential links between central and peripheral symptoms related to a more encompassing definition of a depressive syndrome, and which may help our overall understanding of depression (Zorn *et al.*, 1999). This study illustrates peripheral mechanisms of serotonin dysregulation, increased serotonin release resulting in alternate diarrhea and transient constipation, similar to human IBS, in which SSRI treatment improves global quality of life by acting on central CNS targets, but does not affect peripheral serotonin receptor activation, or improve gut pathophysiology (North *et al.*, 2007).

Human imaging studies have reported and characterized a link between the *s/s* 5-HTTLPR polymorphism, rACC–amygdala coupling and increased avoidance, and amygdala activation with fearful stimuli (Hariri *et al.*, 2002; Pezawas *et al.*, 2005). These results provide network-based evidence for a role of SERT in emotional regulation, and additional evidence in support of the link between fear, depression, and SERT function. One recent study has evaluated the effects of fear conditioning and repeated exposure to FST on fear extinction and depressive-like behavior (FST) resulting from stress exposure, a potential model of "state-based" depressive behavior in mice (Wellman *et al.*, 2007). The fear memory was then extinguished by repeatedly presenting the fear-associated stimulus in the absence of aversive outcome. During the first session of extinction learning, SERT KO and WT mice exhibited similar progressive reductions in conditioned freezing. In contrast, whereas both genotypes showed an expected spontaneous recovery of the fear response when tested for recall of the extinction memory 24 h later, the response was markedly higher in SERT KO mice than in WT mice. SERT KO mice were subsequently able to (re)extinguish to WT levels with additional repeated exposure to the conditioned stimulus. This has parallels with individuals with PTSD, as well as depressed individuals with the 5-HTTLPR *s/s* polymorphism (Caspi *et al.*, 2003; Kendler *et al.*, 2005; Lee *et al.*, 2005).

The results of this study identified stronger spontaneous recovery of the fear response to the conditioned stimulus, a PTSD-like behavior, in SERT KO mice, supporting the potential use of this model to investigate neuropsychiatric disorders, such as PTSD, in addition to anxiety and depression. One of the limitations of this mouse study is that only male mice were used, and that sex differences were not assessed. Again, the use of the FST as a test of depressive-like behavior, rather than antidepressant predictability, has been questioned (Cryan and Holmes, 2005; Kalueff *et al.*, 2007a; Lucki, 2001; Mayorga and Lucki, 2001), and another test such as the sucrose preference test or NSF may have strengthened the results.

A recent study by Carola *et al.* (2008) has investigated the role of SERT in gene × environment interaction using SERT HZ mice under different maternal care conditions, using C57B6/BALBc crossed mice that differ in terms of nurturing and grooming time. In mice with high maternal care, there were no differences in testing for anxiety-like behavior (open field test, elevated plus maze) or depression-like behavior (TST) between HZ SERT mice or WT controls. However, HZ mice exposed to low maternal care consistently showed increased anxiety- and depression-like behaviors. This phenotype was observed only in mice with normal serotonin turnover, while lower serotonin turnover associated with the tryptophan hydroxylase (TPH-2)$^{P/R}$ polymorphism negated the expressivity of the low maternal care/SERT HZ phenotype, at least for anxiety-like behavior. Thus, this study highlighted a SERT by environmental factors interaction in behavioral phenotypes that paralleled results in human and nonhuman primate studies (Caspi *et al.*, 2003; Champoux *et al.*, 2002). Together, these last two reports are the first studies to address "state-based" or evoked depressive-like behavior in SERT KO mice after exposure to repeated environmental stress or early life stress, therefore providing insight into more clinically relevant scenarios of rodent models for anxiety, depression, and PTSD. Similar studies will need to be performed to examine trajectories and dynamics that are involved in these behavioral, genetic, and state/trait interactions.

In summary, we postulate that unlike anxiety, and similar to the way it is diagnosed in a human population, investigating "depression" in rodents may benefit from the inclusion of a "cluster of symptoms" (Figure 4.1) rather than a more limited focus on affect-related behaviors. Numerous studies have addressed components of this cluster. In some cases (i.e. depressive-like behavior), the results have been conflicting, while for other symptoms or comorbid conditions (i.e. anxiety and IBS), the effects of SERT KO are more robust. Although it is far from conclusive at this point, taken together, these studies provide some level of evidence suggesting the presence of a "trait-based" depressive phenotype in SERT KO mice, as manifested by elevated anxiety, altered agonistic behavior, higher susceptibility to stress, decrease in fear extinction, IBS and overactive bladder, and increase in pain experience. Also, few studies (Avgustinovich *et al.*, 2005; Kudryavtseva *et al.*, 1991; Mineur *et al.*, 2006; Wellman *et al.*, 2007; Willner *et al.*, 1992) have examined a "state-based" model of depression, evoking depressive-like behavior after exposure to environmental stressors. Here, one study suggests that SERT KO mice may be useful as a potential state-based model of depression

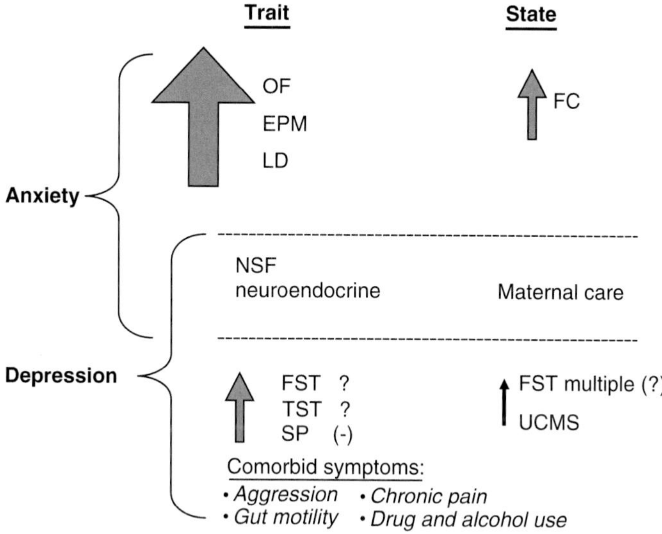

Figure 4.1. Developmental view of cortical serotoninergic and thalamocortical afferents. Serotonergic neurons synthesize 5-HT (*black dots*) from tryptophan (Trp) through the rate limiting enzyme tryptophan hydroxylase 2 and an amino acid decarboxylase, which generate 5-hydroxytryptophan (5-OHTrp) and 5-HT, respectively; 5-HT is then either transported into vesicles by VMAT-2 (*gray triangles*) to eventually undergo Ca^{2+}-mediated release, or it is metabolized through deamination by MAO-A, located on the outer mitochondrial membrane, followed by further oxidation to 5-HIAA (*gray dots*) by an aldehyde dehydrogenase (Ald DH). Neurochemical and paracrine extracellular 5-HT activity is terminated by the SERT (*black triangles*), which under certain conditions can also reverse its direction and mediate vesicle-independent neurotransmitter release. In the somatosensory cortex of neonatal rodents, the transient barrel-like 5-HT pattern visible in layer IV is due to 5-HT uptake and vesicular storage in thalamocortical neurons, devoid of 5-HT-synthesizing enzymes but transiently expressing both SERT and VMAT-2.

(Wellman *et al.*, 2007), although little is currently known about state-based changes in depressive behavior in SERT KO mice.

LIMITATIONS/FUTURE DIRECTIONS

The limitations of current studies using SERT KO mice at addressing potential mechanisms involved in the neurobiology of depression and anxiety can be summarized along four general lines.

The first limitation is inherent to the constitutive nature of the genetic manipulation, in that SERT KO mice are an artificial construct, where lifelong constitutive lack of functional SERT expression has no parallel with depressed or anxious patients. Depression and anxiety are complex diseases, and most likely involve a complex series of mild genetic alterations that contribute to these conditions, thus SERT HZ may be more valuable as a putative and clinically relevant research model (Kalueff *et al.*, 2007b). It is also important to note that the current studies do not directly model the role of the commonly investigated *s/l* SERT polymorphisms in human anxiety and depression, as SERT levels do not necessarily correlate with *s/l* polymorphism in the adult human brain (Lim *et al.*, 2006; Mann *et al.*, 2000; Parsey *et al.*, 2006; Shioe *et al.*, 2003), rather these studies are investigating the impact of variable SERT levels to anxiety-like and depression-related behaviors. In view of the critical role of low SERT during development (Ansorge *et al.*, 2007), it will be essential to develop new lines of mutant mice with better temporal control of SERT expression in order to confirm genetically and further investigate early time windows of selective vulnerability in establishing neural networks that regulate emotion-related behaviors later in life. That adult knock-down of SERT recapitulates the pharmacological blockade of SERT (Thakker *et al.*, 2005), and not the KO or HZ phenotype, and that SSRIs reduce the low anxiety phenotype of SERT-over-expressing mice (Jennings *et al.*, 2006), further emphasizes this latter point. In view of the considerable biological adaptations and developmental compensations that take place in constitutive SERT KO mice, further such fine-tuned genetic manipulations will be valuable in identifying changes that are critical to mood regulation and to segregate relevant biological events from epiphenomena.

The second categorical limitation relates to background strain variance and limitations of tests at assessing depression-related mechanisms. Indeed, variable anxiety- and depression-related results were obtained depending on the behavioral tests and genetic background of SERT KO mice (Holmes *et al.*, 2002b). In addition to a reduced locomotor activity phenotype in SERT-KO mice (Holmes *et al.*, 2002b), the 129S6 strain itself is hypoactive, together leading to potentially false positive results on locomotion-based tests for anxiety measurements, such as the elevated plus maze and open field, and on depression-like behavioral tests, such as the FST and TST. Moreover, while these latter behavioral tasks demonstrate good predictive validity for the acute effects of antidepressants, it is unclear how they relate to the complex neurobiology of human depression (Cryan and Holmes, 2005). Thus in view of behavioral differences due to genetic background variability, and due to inconsistent results in SERT KO mice in tests that are similar in construct (FST and TST) but that are more limited in face validity for putative implication on depression mechanisms, caution is needed when interpreting data on altered depression-like behavior in SERT KO mice.

Taken together, this suggests that a depression phenotype in SERT KO mice cannot be established only by "despair" tests such as the FST and TST, and would benefit from re-evaluation using other depression paradigms. Accordingly, the absence of difference between WT, HZ, and KO mice in the activity-independent sucrose preference test (Kalueff *et al.*, 2006), a model for anhedonia that has better face and construct validities for studying depressive characteristics, further suggests that SERT KO mice may not be "depressed" (Kalueff *et al.*, 2007b), or at least do not display trait-based depression-like behaviors. These conclusions are only mitigated at this point by the results from Ansorge *et al.* (2004) in the NSF test, due to the dual assessment of depressive- and anxiety-like features of this test, and by the presence of several additional related symptoms that are often comorbid, and potentially related to a depressive phenotype, as described earlier.

The third major limitation relates to the lack of in-depth assessment of sex differences. Indeed, in view of the well-characterized increased prevalence of mood disorders in female subjects, it is surprising that sex differences in behavioral assays have not been more systematically investigated in SERT KO mice. Some sex-specific effects have been identified, female BDNF+/−/SERT−/− (sb) appear to be more adaptive to a lack of SERT expression, having significantly diminished reductions in serotonin concentrations in hypothalamus and other brain regions compared to males (Ren-Patterson *et al.*, 2006). Likewise, in the elevated plus maze, female sb mice demonstrated no increase in anxiety-like behaviors and did not manifest the ~40% reduction in the expression of TrkB receptor observed in male sb mice. The authors suggest that estrogen may exert a protective and moderating effect on compensatory changes occurring in SERT KO mice (Ren-Patterson *et al.*, 2006). Together, these studies represent only the beginning of investigations aimed at understanding and identifying the potential biological substrates of sex by serotonin interactions in mood regulation.

Finally, the last major limitation of the current studies is the lack of evocative testing and modeling, or lack of comparisons between trait- and state-based models of anxiety and depression in SERT KO mice. The most compelling reason suggesting that such studies are needed is provided by studies in human subjects carrying the 5-HTTLPR *s/s* polymorphism, where prior exposure to some form of stress is necessary to reveal the genetic contribution of SERT to the development of depressive episodes, thus clearly identifying a gene × environment interaction (Caspi *et al.*, 2003; Hariri and Holmes, 2006; Kendler *et al.*, 2005). Also, there is significant comorbidity of affective disorders, with other disorders affected by stress, including PTSD, multiple sclerosis, chronic pain, and fibromyalgia (Buskila and Cohen, 2007; Esch *et al.*, 2002; Fietta *et al.*, 2007; Ghaffar and Feinstein, 2007; Lee *et al.*, 2005). Thus, projecting back to rodent models, how would SERT KO and HZ respond to unpredictable chronic mild stress or to a social defeat paradigm, two models used to induce depressive-like states?

Trait-based studies in SERT KO mice on one hand, and evoked or state-based studies in normal WT mice on the other, have been missing out on important factors in the gene × environment model of depression. In other words, while SERT KO mice may represent, at best, a poor model of trait-based depression, does the lack of SERT function result in an increased vulnerability to develop a depressive-like state? Studies using fear conditioning and repeated exposure to stressful stimuli (Wellman *et al.*, 2007) have suggested increased stress reactivity and impaired fear extinction, thus representing first attempts at investigating evoked states in SERT KO mice. Also, the recent study examining the interaction between maternal care and HZ SERT mice illustrates not only the synergistic effects, but also other related genes that modulate the affective phenotype, such as TPH-2 (Carola *et al.*, 2008). Preliminary studies from our lab indicate that unpredictable chronic mild stress induces robust increases in emotional behavior in the NSF test in all genotype groups (WT, HZ, and KO; C57B6 background) and that maximal evoked behaviors are achieved in SERT KO mice, with female SERT KO mice displaying highest emotional behavior compared to all other groups (Edgar *et al.*, 2007), thus suggesting the presence of an increased vulnerability to develop elevated emotional behavior in SERT KO mice, and mimicking the increased prevalence of mood disorders in female subjects. Together, these preliminary results suggest that SERT KO mice may not yet be ruled out as a model, if not of trait depression, then of increased vulnerability to develop depressive states.

SUMMARY

Now that we have briefly addressed the limitations of knocking down, out and over-expressing SERT in modeling aspects of anxiety-like and depression-related behaviors, what can we say about SERT and emotional dysregulation? In short, SERT KO may represent a good model of trait anxiety, a poor model of trait depression, and putatively a better model for evoking state depression. However, much work remains to be done to assert these conclusions, especially with regards to evoked anxiety-like and depression-related states. Studies on gene × gene and gene × environment interactions have only just begun, and will need to be integrated with trait/state and gender-specific studies to fully recapitulate risk factors that are known to influence the vulnerability to develop altered mood regulation, namely genetic load, sex, and environment (especially early-life and chronic stress). These new studies will benefit from completing the baseline and evoked characterization of constitutive SERT mutants. If an HZ–SERT mutant ended up representing an intermediate phenotype in evoked states, as suggested by few studies performed to date (Kalueff *et al.*, 2007b), this would validate the use of SERT KO mice to investigate relevant changes in neural networks, as an extreme phenotype, yet still relevant to mechanisms of altered mood regulation.

So how will SERT mutant models help us in identifying cellular and molecular mechanisms that are proximal to an altered mood phenotype? Could a SERT mutant be useful in identifying true new pharmacological targets, beyond the monoamine neurotransmitter systems? Interestingly, adult SERT downregulation from normal or artificially elevated levels has so far suggested a lack of compensatory mechanisms beyond SERT, as RNAi mimicked SSRI application (Thakker *et al.*, 2005) and SSRI reversed the low-anxiety phenotype of SERT over-expressors (Jennings *et al.*, 2006). On the other hand, early SERT blockade has clearly identified a postnatal developmental window that appears to be critical for establishing emotion-related behavior in adulthood (Ansorge *et al.*, 2004). Together, these observations point to two potential directions to focus on: first, identifying developmental switches affected by changes in SERT function; and second, since early developmental periods are unlikely to be realistically targeted for the prevention of mood disorders, identifying the molecular, cellular, and circuitry changes in adult systems that are secondary to altered developmental events related to SERT and that place the system at risk for developing mood disorders (in concert and in addition to already characterized compensations in monoamine systems). To this end, SERT mutant mice provide a critical window into mechanisms leading to increased risk for mood disorders. In turn, this latter set of studies has the potential to reveal new targets for antidepressant drug development. Moreover, it is likely that identified mechanisms underlying adult vulnerability to mood disorders will be subject to modulation from other etiological pathways and may thus represent "common" mechanisms conferring risk for anxiety and depressive disorders.

REFERENCES

Adamec R, Burton P, Blundell J, Murphy D L, Holmes A (2006a). Vulnerability to mild predator stress in serotonin transporter knockout mice. *Behav Brain Res* **170**: 126–40.

Adamec R, Head D, Blundell J, Burton P, Berton O (2006b). Lasting anxiogenic effects of feline predator stress in mice: sex differences in vulnerability to stress and predicting severity of anxiogenic response from the stress experience. *Physiol Behav* **88**: 12–29.

Ansorge M S, Hen R, Gingrich J A (2007). Neurodevelopmental origins of depressive disorders. *Curr Opin Pharmacol* **7**: 8–17.

Ansorge M S, Morelli E, Gingrich J A (2008). Inhibition of serotonin but not norepinephrine transport during development produces delayed, persistent perturbations of emotional behaviors in mice. *J Neurosci* **28**: 199–207.

Ansorge M S, Zhou M, Lira A, Hen R, Gingrich J A (2004). Early-life blockade of the 5-HT transporter alters emotional behavior in adult mice. *Science* **306**: 879–81.

Avgustinovich D F, Kovalenko I L, Kudryavtseva N N (2005). A model of anxious depression: persistence of behavioral pathology. *Neurosci Behav Physiol* **35**: 917–24.

Bengel D, Murphy D L, Andrews A M, *et al.* (1998). Altered brain serotonin homeostasis and locomotor insensitivity to 3,4-methylenedioxymethamphetamine ("Ecstasy") in serotonin transporter-deficient mice. *Mol Pharmacol* **53**: 649–55.

Bennett A J, Lesch K P, Heils A, *et al.* (2002). Early experience and serotonin transporter gene variation interact to influence primate CNS function. *Mol Psychiatry* **7**: 118–22.

Bodnoff SR, Suranyi-Cadotte B, Aitken D H, Quirion R, Meaney M J (1988). The effects of chronic antidepressant treatment in an animal model of anxiety. *Psychopharmacology (Berl)* **95**: 298–302.

Buskila D, Cohen H (2007). Comorbidity of fibromyalgia and psychiatric disorders. *Curr Pain Headache Rep* **11**: 333–8.

Carola V, Frazzetto G, Pascucci T, *et al.* (2008). Identifying molecular substrates in a mouse model of the serotonin transporter × environment risk factor for anxiety and depression. *Biol Psychiatry* **63**: 840–6.

Caspi A, Sugden K, Moffitt T E, *et al.* (2003). Influence of life stress on depression: moderation by a polymorphism in the 5-HTT gene. *Science* **301**: 386–9.

Champoux M, Bennett A, Shannon C, Higley J D, Lesch K P, Suomi S J (2002). Serotonin transporter gene polymorphism, differential early rearing, and behavior in rhesus monkey neonates. *Mol Psychiatry* **7**: 1058–63.

Chen J J, Li Z, Pan H, *et al.* (2001). Maintenance of serotonin in the intestinal mucosa and ganglia of mice that lack the high-affinity serotonin transporter: abnormal intestinal motility and the expression of cation transporters. *J Neurosci* **21**: 6348–61.

Chen Y W, Dilsaver S C (1996). Lifetime rates of suicide attempts among subjects with bipolar and unipolar disorders relative to subjects with other Axis I disorders. *Biol Psychiatry* **39**: 896–9.

Collier D A, Stober G, Li T, *et al.* (1996). A novel functional polymorphism within the promoter of the serotonin transporter gene: possible role in susceptibility to affective disorders. *Mol Psychiatry* **1**: 453–60.

Cornelissen L L, Brooks D P, Wibberley A (2005). Female, but not male, serotonin reuptake transporter (5-HTT) knockout mice exhibit bladder instability. *Auton Neurosci* **122**: 107–10.

Cryan J F, Holmes A (2005). The ascent of mouse: advances in modelling human depression and anxiety. *Nat Rev Drug Discov* **4**: 775–90.

Daws L C, Montanez S, Munn J L, *et al.* (2006). Ethanol inhibits clearance of brain serotonin by a serotonin transporter-independent mechanism. *J Neurosci* **26**: 6431–8.

Edgar N, Joeyen-Waldorf J, Sibille E (2007). Sex and serotonin transporter interactions in pathways to depression. *Poster presented at Society for Neuroscience Meeting*, San Diego, CA.

El Yacoubi M, Vaugeois J M (2007). Genetic rodent models of depression. *Curr Opin Pharmacol* **7**: 3–7.

Esch T, Stefano G B, Fricchione G L, Benson H (2002). The role of stress in neurodegenerative diseases and mental disorders. *Neuro Endocrinol Lett* **23**: 199–208.

Fabre V, Beaufour C, Evrard A, *et al.* (2000). Altered expression and functions of serotonin 5-HT1A and 5-HT1B receptors in knock-out mice lacking the 5-HT transporter. *Eur J Neurosci* **12**: 2299–310.

Fietta P, Fietta P, Manganelli P (2007). Fibromyalgia and psychiatric disorders. *Acta Biomed* **78**: 88–95.

Ghaffar O, Feinstein A (2007). The neuropsychiatry of multiple sclerosis: a review of recent developments. *Curr Opin Psychiatry* **20**: 278–85.

Gillespie N A, Whitfield J B, Williams B, Heath A C, Martin NG (2005). The relationship between stressful life events, the serotonin transporter (5-HTTLPR) genotype and major depression. *Psychol Med* **35**: 101–11.

Gobbi G, Murphy D L, Lesch K, Blier P (2001). Modifications of the serotonergic system in mice lacking serotonin transporters: an in vivo electrophysiological study. *J Pharmacol Exp Ther* **296**: 987–95.

Gross C, Hen R (2004). The developmental origins of anxiety. *Nat Rev Neurosci* **5**: 545–52.

Gutierrez B, Pintor L, Gasto C, *et al.* (1998). Variability in the serotonin transporter gene and increased risk for major depression with melancholia. *Hum Genet* **103**: 319–22.

Hariri A R, Holmes A (2006). Genetics of emotional regulation: the role of the serotonin transporter in neural function. *Trends Cogn Sci* **10**: 182–91.

Hariri A R, Mattay V S, Tessitore A, *et al.* (2002). Serotonin transporter genetic variation and the response of the human amygdala. *Science* **297**: 400–03.

Heinz A, Braus D F, Smolka M N, *et al.* (2005). Amygdala–prefrontal coupling depends on a genetic variation of the serotonin transporter. *Nat Neurosci* **8**: 20–1.

Hettema J M, Neale M C, Kendler K S (2001). A review and meta-analysis of the genetic epidemiology of anxiety disorders. *Am J Psychiatry* **158**: 1568–78.

Holmes A (2001). Targeted gene mutation approaches to the study of anxiety-like behavior in mice. *Neurosci Biobehav Rev* **25**: 261–73.

Holmes A, Lit Q, Murphy D L, Gold E, Crawley J N (2003a). Abnormal anxiety-related behavior in serotonin transporter null mutant mice: the influence of genetic background. *Genes Brain Behav* **2**: 365–80.

Holmes A, Murphy D L, Crawley J N (2002a). Reduced aggression in mice lacking the serotonin transporter. *Psychopharmacology (Berl)* **161**: 160–7.

Holmes A, Murphy D L, Crawley J N (2003b). Abnormal behavioral phenotypes of serotonin transporter knockout mice: parallels with human anxiety and depression. *Biol Psychiatry* **54**: 953–9.

Holmes A, Yang R J, Murphy D L, Crawley J N (2002b). Evaluation of antidepressant-related behavioral responses in mice lacking the serotonin transporter. *Neuropsychopharmacology* **27**: 914–23.

Homberg J R, Olivier J D, Smits B M, *et al.* (2007). Characterization of the serotonin transporter knockout rat: a selective change in the functioning of the serotonergic system. *Neuroscience* **146**: 1662–76.

Ishihara L, Brayne C (2006). A systematic review of depression and mental illness preceding Parkinson's disease. *Acta Neurol Scand* **113**: 211–20.

Jann M W, Slade J H (2007). Antidepressant agents for the treatment of chronic pain and depression. *Pharmacotherapy* **27**: 1571–87.

Jennings K A, Loder M K, Sheward W J, *et al.* (2006). Increased expression of the 5-HT transporter confers a low-anxiety phenotype linked to decreased 5-HT transmission. *J Neurosci* **26**: 8955–64.

Kalueff A V (2007). Neurobiology of memory and anxiety: from genes to behavior. *Neural Plast* **28**: 78 171.

Kalueff A V, Fox M A, Gallagher P S, Murphy D L (2007a). Hypolocomotion, anxiety and serotonin syndrome-like behavior contribute to the complex phenotype of serotonin transporter knockout mice. *Genes Brain Behav* **6**: 389–400.

Kalueff A V, Gallagher P S, Murphy D L (2006). Are serotonin transporter knockout mice 'depressed'? Hypoactivity but no anhedonia. *Neuroreport* **17**: 1347–51.

Kalueff A V, Ren-Patterson R F, Murphy D L (2007b). The developing use of heterozygous mutant mouse models in brain monoamine transporter research. *Trends Pharmacol Sci* **28**: 122–7.

Kanner A M (2007). Epilepsy and mood disorders. *Epilepsia* **48** (Suppl 9): 20–2.

Kendler K S, Kuhn J W, Vittum J, Prescott C A, Riley B (2005). The interaction of stressful life events and a serotonin transporter polymorphism in the prediction of episodes of major depression: a replication. *Arch Gen Psychiatry* **62**: 529–35.

Kudryavtseva N N, Bakshtanovskaya I V, Koryakina L A (1991). Social model of depression in mice of C57BL/6J strain. *Pharmacol Biochem Behav* **38**: 315–20.

Lee H J, Lee M S, Kang R H, *et al.* (2005). Influence of the serotonin transporter promoter gene polymorphism on susceptibility to posttraumatic stress disorder. *Depress Anxiety* **21**: 135–9.

LeMarquand D, Pihl R O, Benkelfat C (1994). Serotonin and alcohol intake, abuse, and dependence: clinical evidence. *Biol Psychiatry* **36**: 326–37.

Leonardo E D, Hen R (2006). Genetics of affective and anxiety disorders. *Annu Rev Psychol* **57**: 117–37.

Lesch K P, Bengel D, Heils A, *et al.* (1996). Association of anxiety-related traits with a polymorphism in the serotonin transporter gene regulatory region. *Science* **274**: 1527–31.

Li Q, Wichems C, Heils A, Lesch K P, Murphy D L (2000). Reduction in the density and expression, but not G-protein coupling, of serotonin receptors (5-HT1A) in 5-HT transporter knock-out mice: gender and brain region differences. *J Neurosci* **20**: 7888–95.

Li Q, Wichems C, Heils A, Van De Kar L D, Lesch K P, Murphy D L (1999). Reduction of 5-hydroxytryptamine (5-HT)(1A)-mediated temperature and neuroendocrine responses and 5-HT(1A) binding sites in 5-HT transporter knockout mice. *J Pharmacol Exp Ther* **291**: 999–1007.

Li Q, Wichems C H, Ma L, Van de Kar L D, Garcia F, Murphy D L (2003). Brain region-specific alterations of 5-HT2A and 5-HT2C receptors in serotonin transporter knockout mice. *J Neurochem* **84**: 1256–65.

Lim J E, Papp A, Pinsonneault J, Sadee W, Saffen D (2006). Allelic expression of serotonin transporter (SERT) mRNA in human pons: lack of correlation with the polymorphism SERTLPR. *Mol Psychiatry* **11**: 649–62.

Linnoila M, Virkkunen M (1992). Biologic correlates of suicidal risk and aggressive behavioral traits. *J Clin Psychopharmacol* **12**: 19S–20S.

Lira A, Zhou M, Castanon N, *et al.* (2003). Altered depression-related behaviors and functional changes in the dorsal raphe nucleus of serotonin transporter-deficient mice. *Biol Psychiatry* **54**: 960–71.

Liu M T, Rayport S, Jiang Y, Murphy D L, Gershon M D (2002). Expression and function of 5-HT3 receptors in the enteric neurons of mice lacking the serotonin transporter. *Am J Physiol Gastrointest Liver Physiol* **283**: G1398–411.

Lowry C A, Johnson P L, Hay-Schmidt A, Mikkelsen J, Shekhar A (2005). Modulation of anxiety circuits by serotonergic systems. *Stress* **8**: 233–46.

Lucki I (2001). A prescription to resist proscriptions for murine models of depression. *Psychopharmacology (Berl)* **153**: 395–8.

Mann J J, Currier D (2006). Effects of genes and stress on the neurobiology of depression. *Int Rev Neurobiol* **73**: 153–89.

Mann J J, Huang Y Y, Underwood M D, *et al.* (2000). A serotonin transporter gene promoter polymorphism (5-HTTLPR) and prefrontal cortical binding in major depression and suicide. *Arch Gen Psychiatry* **57**: 729–38.

Mannoury la Cour C, Boni C, Hanoun N, Lesch K P, Hamon M, Lanfumey L (2001). Functional consequences of 5-HT transporter gene disruption on 5-HT(1a) receptor-mediated regulation of dorsal raphe and hippocampal cell activity. *J Neurosci* **21**: 2178–85.

Mathews T A, Fedele D E, Coppelli F M, Avila A M, Murphy D L, Andrews A M (2004). Gene dose-dependent alterations in extraneuronal serotonin but not dopamine in mice with reduced serotonin transporter expression. *J Neurosci Methods* **140**: 169–81.

Mayorga A J, Lucki I (2001). Limitations on the use of the C57BL/6 mouse in the tail suspension test. *Psychopharmacology (Berl)* **155**: 110–2.

Mazzanti C M, Lappalainen J, Long J C, *et al.* (1998). Role of the serotonin transporter promoter polymorphism in anxiety-related traits. *Arch Gen Psychiatry* **55**: 936–40.

Mineur Y S, Belzung C, Crusio W E (2006). Effects of unpredictable chronic mild stress on anxiety and depression-like behavior in mice. *Behav Brain Res* **175**: 43–50.

Montanez S, Owens W A, Gould G G, Murphy D L, Daws L C (2003). Exaggerated effect of fluvoxamine in heterozygote serotonin transporter knockout mice. *J Neurochem* **86**: 210–19.

Murphy D L, Lesch K P (2008). Targeting the murine serotonin transporter: insights into human neurobiology. *Nat Rev Neurosci* **9**: 85–96.

Murphy D L, Li Q, Engel S, *et al.* (2001). Genetic perspectives on the serotonin transporter. *Brain Res Bull* **56**: 487–94.

Murray C, Lopez A D, editors (1996). *The global burden of disease – Summary*. Boston: The World Health Organization and Harvard University Press.

Nemeroff C B, Owens M J (2002). Treatment of mood disorders. *Nat Neurosci* **5** (Suppl): 1068–70.

Nestler E J, Barrot M, DiLeone R J, Eisch A J, Gold S J, Monteggia L M (2002). Neurobiology of depression. *Neuron* **34**: 13–25.

North C S, Hong B A, Alpers D H (2007). Relationship of functional gastrointestinal disorders and psychiatric disorders: implications for treatment. *World J Gastroenterol* **13**: 2020–7.

O'Brien J (2005). Dementia associated with psychiatric disorders. *Int Psychogeriatr* **17** (Suppl 1): S207–21.

Olivier J D A, van der Hart M G C, van Swelm R P L, *et al.* (2008). A study in male and female serotonin transporter knockout rats: an animal model for anxiety and depression disorders. *Neuroscience* **152**: 573–84.

Parsey R V, Hastings R S, Oquendo M A, *et al.* (2006). Effect of a triallelic functional polymorphism of the serotonin-transporter-linked promoter region on expression of serotonin transporter in the human brain. *Am J Psychiatry* **163**: 48–51.

Pezawas L, Meyer-Lindenberg A, Drabant E M, *et al.* (2005). 5-HTTLPR polymorphism impacts human cingulate–amygdala interactions: a genetic susceptibility mechanism for depression. *Nat Neurosci* **8**: 828–34.

Ren-Patterson R F, Cochran L W, Holmes A, Lesch K P, Lu B, Murphy D L (2006). Gender-dependent modulation of brain monoamines and anxiety-like behaviors in mice with genetic serotonin transporter and BDNF deficiencies. *Cell Mol Neurobiol* **26**: 755–80.

Santarelli L, Saxe M, Gross C, *et al.* (2003). Requirement of hippocampal neurogenesis for the behavioral effects of antidepressants. *Science* **301**: 805–09.

Schmitt A, Mossner R, Gossmann A, *et al.* (2003). Organic cation transporter capable of transporting serotonin is up-regulated in serotonin transporter-deficient mice. *J Neurosci Res* **71**: 701–09.

Serretti A, Calati R, Mandelli L, De Ronchi D (2006). Serotonin transporter gene variants and behavior: a comprehensive review. *Curr Drug Targets* **7**: 1659–69.

Shioe K, Ichimiya T, Suhara T, *et al.* (2003). No association between genotype of the promoter region of serotonin transporter gene and serotonin transporter binding in human brain measured by PET. *Synapse* **48**: 184–8.

Sibille E, Lewis D A (2006). SERT-ainly involved in depression, but when? *Am J Psychiatry* **163**: 8–11.

Spiller R (2007). Serotonin, inflammation, and IBS: fitting the jigsaw together? *J Pediatr Gastroenterol Nutr* **45** (Suppl 2): S115–9.

Thakker D R, Natt F, Husken D, *et al.* (2005). siRNA-mediated knockdown of the serotonin transporter in the adult mouse brain. *Mol Psychiatry* **10**: 714, 782–9.

Tjurmina O A, Armando I, Saavedra J M, Goldstein D S, Murphy D L (2002). Exaggerated adrenomedullary response to immobilization in mice with targeted disruption of the serotonin transporter gene. *Endocrinology* **143**: 4520–6.

Vogel C, Mossner R, Gerlach M, *et al.* (2003). Absence of thermal hyperalgesia in serotonin transporter-deficient mice. *J Neurosci* **23**: 708–15.

Weissman M M, Klerman G L, Markowitz J S, Ouellette R (1989). Suicidal ideation and suicide attempts in panic disorder and attacks. *N Engl J Med* **321**: 1209–14.

Wellman C L, Izquierdo A, Garrett J E, *et al.* (2007). Impaired stress-coping and fear extinction and abnormal corticolimbic morphology in serotonin transporter knock-out mice. *J Neurosci* **27**: 684–91.

Willner P, Muscat R, Papp M (1992). Chronic mild stress-induced anhedonia: a realistic animal model of depression. *Neurosci Biobehav Rev* **16**: 525–34.

Zhao S, Edwards J, Carroll J, *et al.* (2006). Insertion mutation at the C-terminus of the serotonin transporter disrupts brain serotonin function and emotion-related behaviors in mice. *Neuroscience* **140**: 321–34.

Zorn B H, Montgomery H, Pieper K, Gray M, Steers W D (1999). Urinary incontinence and depression. *J Urol* **162**: 82–4.

DANIELA POPA, CHLOÉ ALEXANDRE, JOËLLE ADRIEN AND CLÉMENT LÉNA

5

The serotonin transporter and animal models of depression

ABSTRACT

The serotonin transporter (SERT), a membrane protein responsible for the reuptake of extracellular serotonin, is a prominent target of antidepressants. Moreover, a polymorphism of this gene that decreases serotonin uptake has been linked to depression. However, the role of SERT in depression is poorly understood. Several functional impairments, notably in behavior, sleep, and response to stress, are consistently found in animal models of depression, but consistent correlation with serotonergic dysfunction has not been demonstrated. Nevertheless, in certain genetic backgrounds, the same impairments are also found in mutant rodents in which serotonin transport has been abolished. These impairments are also observed in adult rodents after a transient disruption of serotonin transport during the first postnatal month. Conversely, they may be prevented in mutant rodents by normalizing serotonergic transmission postnatally. Therefore, the function of the serotonin transporter during postnatal development is critical for the proper maturation of brain circuits, while susceptibility to depression caused by reduced serotonin transporter function may be determined, in part, during development.

INTRODUCTION

Depression is one of the most common psychiatric disorders in developed countries. This disease affects mood, psychomotor activity, neurovegetative functions, and cognition (Fava and Kendler, 2000).

Experimental Models in Serotonin Transporter Research, eds. A. V. Kalueff and J. L. LaPorte. Published by Cambridge University Press.

Estimates indicate a lifetime prevalence up to 20% for major depression (Blazer, 2000; Fava and Kendler, 2000; Kornstein *et al.*, 2000), and the likelihood of experiencing this disorder is twice as high in women as in men (Kornstein *et al.*, 2000). Depression can be a lifelong episodic disorder with multiple recurrences. The first episode can occur during childhood, in adolescence, or as an adult. The chronic and recurrent course of depression is a critical clinical concern, often requiring long-term treatment (Fava and Kendler, 2000). Antidepressants acting on serotonergic and noradrenergic systems were introduced for the treatment of depression about 50 years ago (Kline, 1958) and are still used today. While there is a long history of involvement of the serotonergic system in this disease, the link between serotonin and depression is still far from resolved and is the subject of active investigations. The purpose of this chapter is to show how animal models may help to understand the connections between serotonin, serotonin transporter, and depression.

The serotonergic system is a complex neuromodulatory system composed of several brain nuclei and involving multiple receptor subtypes. The serotonin transporter (SERT) is a key component in this system and is in charge of removal of the serotonin from the extracellular space. The early proposal (Coppen, 1967) that depression results directly from reduced brain extracellular serotonin levels has been clearly shown to be simplistic (Lacasse and Leo, 2005). However, as shown below, several lines of evidence directly relate SERT to depression: SERT is the target of antidepressant drugs; there are reports of changes in SERT activity in depressed patients (although the literature is often contradictory); and a polymorphism of the SERT gene, leading to reduced SERT activity, has been proposed to be associated with vulnerability to depression.

The vast majority of the antidepressants currently prescribed affect serotonin and norepinephrine transporters or degradation enzymes (Berman and Charney, 1999; Nestler *et al.*, 2002b; Papakostas *et al.*, 2007). However, one of the most puzzling aspects of these medications is the onset of their effect, which develops slowly over weeks. This slow time course has been proposed to result from the fact that SERT inhibitors tend to increase the levels of serotonin, but this effect is counteracted by the negative feedback that serotonin exerts in the serotonergic neurons in the raphe nuclei via the serotonergic 5-HT1A receptors' subtypes. The gradual desensitization of these 5-HT1A autoreceptors over weeks could remove this inhibitory control over the firing rate of serotonergic neurons (Blier, 2003; Hensler, 2002). However, this interpretation has only received limited support since pharmacological studies investigating the role of 5-HT1A on selective SERT inhibitors efficacy yielded inconsistent results in humans (Artigas *et al.*, 2006; Geretsegger *et al.*, 2008) and in rodents (Guilloux *et al.*, 2006; Holick *et al.*, 2008; Moser and Sanger *et al.*, 1999; Redrobe *et al.*, 1996).

Studies on animals have suggested an alternative explanation for the late effects of selective SERT inhibitors by showing increased neurogenesis in the rodent hippocampus after chronic treatments (Malberg *et al.*, 2000; review in Paizanis *et al.*, 2007). Evidence from knock-out mice suggests that this serotonergic control of neurogenesis requires functional 5-HT1A receptors (Holick *et al.*, 2008; Santarelli *et al.*, 2003). Neurotrophins have also been proposed to play a central role in the effects of selective SERT inhibitors, notably via brain-derived neurotrophic factor (BDNF) and TrkB receptor (reviews in: Castren *et al.*, 2007; Kozisek *et al.*, 2008; Nestler *et al.*, 2002a). Therefore, SERT inhibitors would trigger corrective mechanisms in depressed patients rather than directly correct a deficit in brain extracellular serotonin. The link between serotonin, depression, and neurogenesis/growth factors is reviewed in a separate chapter of this book.

Finally, it should be noted that selective SERT inhibitors may be less beneficial than their frequent prescription to depressed patients suggests. While the efficacy of the antidepressants depends on the severity of initial depression scores (Matthews *et al.*, 2005), this effect might result from decreased responsiveness to placebo for severely depressed patients, rather than an increased responsiveness to medication (Kirsch *et al.*, 2008).

A number of studies have provided evidence for alterations of the serotonergic system in depressed patients (Owens and Nemeroff *et al.*, 1994), with changes in SERT binding (e.g. Perry *et al.*, 1983), altered sensitivity or binding to central 5-HT1A receptors (Drevets *et al.*, 2007) and worsening of symptoms following serotonin depletion caused by omission of its precursor, the amino acid tryptophan, from the diet (Delgado, 2006; Moreno *et al.*, 1999). However, the literature is often contradictory and the relevance of these observations to the pathology is still unclear. Therefore, the study of animal models of depression could be useful to clarify the impact of these alterations and discover the mechanisms by which they arise.

Another evidence for the involvement of the altered serotonin function in depression arises from genetic studies. A polymorphism in the promoter region of the SERT gene, possibly in association with a polymorphism in the middle region of this gene (Lazary *et al.*, 2008), has been linked to susceptibility to depression (Fava and Kendler, 2000;

Levinson, 2006 for a meta-analysis; Sham *et al.*, 2000; Sullivan *et al.*, 2000). It could predispose individuals to depression by reducing their ability to cope with stressful situations (Caspi *et al.*, 2003). This polymorphism would result in a reduction of serotonin uptake activity (Holmes *et al.*, 2003a; Lesch *et al.*, 1996; review in Mansour *et al.*, 2005). The recent advent of knock-out mice (Bengel *et al.*, 1998; Lira *et al.*, 2003; Zhao *et al.*, 2006) and rats (Homberg *et al.*, 2007) that do not express the SERT gene now allows detailed examination of the impact of permanently reduced serotonin uptake on brain function.

In the following sections, we will first discuss the multiple genetic and epigenetic manipulations used to induce depressive-like syndromes in rodents. This will help us to understand the behavioral and biological alterations (including in the serotonergic system) encountered in rodent models of depression. Then, we will review the link between SERT genetic alterations and depression-related disturbances in rodents and attempt to establish the extent (and the conditions) to which SERT mutants compare with other animal models of depression. Finally, we will examine the role of early life serotonin in depression and review evidence that developmental alterations are likely to be responsible for a significant proportion of the syndrome observed in mutant animals.

ANIMAL MODELS OF DEPRESSION

According to the DSM-IV-R (*Diagnostic and Statistical Manual of Mental Disorders*, American Psychiatric Association, 2000), the criteria for Major Depressive Disorder include the co-existence of the symptoms of depressed mood, loss of interest or pleasure, loss or gain in weight, sleep disturbances, psychomotor abnormalities, fatigue, feelings of worthlessness, impaired concentration, and recurrent thoughts of death or suicide. Thus, some of the symptoms used to diagnose depression cannot be identified or reproduced in animals (e.g. feelings of guilt, suicidal thoughts). However, animal models of depression, or of some aspects of depression, have been developed, and there is arguably much to learn from such models. Animal models are developed in order to study the neurobiological basis of human disorders and to develop novel treatments (Nestler *et al.*, 2002a). They should meet the following validity criteria (e.g. Willner and Mitchell, 2002): face validity (they resemble the human disorder), construct validity (they are consistent with a theoretical rationale), and predictive validity (e.g. they respond to the same treatment as patients).

Establishing the face validity of an animal model of depression is a complex challenge since the symptoms of this disease, as defined in the DSM-IV, cannot be easily reproduced in experimental models. Furthermore, not all depressed patients show all the symptoms, and individual symptoms may also be found in other disorders. Depression is rather characterized by the co-existence of specific symptoms for a certain amount of time. All these factors make depression even more difficult to reproduce in animals. In rodents, the face validity is most frequently assessed by tests which probe the behavioral responses of animals to stressful situations (tail-suspension test: Cryan *et al.*, 2005; Steru *et al.*, 1987; Porsolt forced swim test: Porsolt, 2000; Porsolt *et al.*, 1977), novelty-induced behavioral inhibition, sensitivity to reinforcers (preferential sucrose consumption, conditioned place preference, or intracranial self-stimulation (e.g. Bevins and Besheer, 2005; Nestler *et al.*, 2002b)). Longer immobility time in the tail suspension and forced swim tests is interpreted as a reduced drive to escape from a stressful situation; high latency to approach food and to begin feeding in the center of an open field is a sign of increased behavioral inhibition by a mildly stressful context. Absence of preference for sweetened water over unsweetened water and a higher threshold of intra-cranial self-stimulation are signs of increased insensitivity to reinforcers (hence anhedonia). All these tests may thus indicate increased stress-sensitivity, anhedonia, and reduced motivation in animal models. The corrective effects of chronic antidepressant treatment in these tests assess the relevance of the behavioral alterations in animal models to depression.

Depressive states are not simply associated with behavioral or cognitive modifications, but also with alterations of biological functions, which may be more accessible to objective analysis. The face value of animal models may also be enhanced by the presence of biological markers of depression (Hasler *et al.*, 2004; Nestler *et al.*, 2002b). These include changes in the hypothalamic–pituitary–adrenocortical (HPA) axis that regulates the hormonal response to stress; dysfunction in the regulation of cortisol or corticotropine-releasing hormone (CRH); alterations of sleep (Benca, 2000) and circadian rhythms (McClung, 2007); alterations in the serotonergic system (e.g. sensitivity to tryptophan depletion, reduced binding to 5-HT1A receptors, see above).

The theoretical rationale is important for building construct validity. Environmental, genetic, and pharmacological manipulations have been used to induce depression in animals, although incidental findings have also provided several models of depression. Over the years, a large number of rodent models of depression have been proposed and validated. Arguably, the use of multiple convergent models and tests increase the relevance of the conclusions that may be drawn from these models of human pathology (Cryan and Mombereau, 2004). A complete review of all existing models is beyond the scope of this chapter. For the sake of simplicity, we distinguish three classes of rodent models of depression.

Environmentally induced depression-like behavior in adults

A first class of models is obtained from treatment of adult "normal" animals. Depressive states are obtained by repeated exposure to stress, such as the models of "learned helplessness" (animals repetitively exposed to inescapable shock subsequently fail to escape when escape is possible: Adrien *et al.*, 1991; Chourbaji *et al.*, 2005; Maudhuit *et al.*, 1997; Seligman and Maier, 1967; review in Willner, 1984), "chronic mild stress" (animals are intermittently and repetitively exposed to uncontrollable stressors: isolation housing, disruption of light–dark cycles, food or water deprivation, wet bedding of home cages: Mineur *et al.*, 2006; Strekalova *et al.*, 2004; for mice, review in Willner, 1997; Willner, 2005 for rats), and "social defeat" (animals are repeatedly exposed to an aggressive/dominant animal, which is a naturalistic stress: Blanchard *et al.*, 2001). Sensory deprivation may also induce depression-like states, as observed in the olfactory bulbectomized rat (review in Song and Leonard, 2005). These models offer the greatest similarity with the conditions that induce depression in humans.

Selective breeding

A second class of models has been obtained from strains that are constitutively "depressive" (i.e. with high scores in rodent behavioral tests of depression) or depression-prone. These models are designed in reference to the genetic component of susceptibility to depression (Levinson, 2006) and are often obtained by selectively breeding animals using their score in a behavioral test of depression. Thus, "congenitally learned helpless" rats (Lachman *et al.*, 1992; Willner and Mitchell, 2002) were selectively bred from Sprague–Dawley rats for their high predisposition to develop learned helplessness; "swim low-active" rats (Weiss *et al.*, 1998) were selectively bred Sprague–Dawley rats with low activity in the forced swim test after exposure to uncontrollable electric tail-shock; "helpless mice" were selectively bred from CD1 mice for their high immobility in the tail suspension test (El Yacoubi *et al.*, 2003; Popa *et al.*, 2006).

The single gene mutation approach has achieved limited success in establishing animal models of depression (see below for the SERT mutants), but it provides opportunities to study specific dysfunctions (or endophenotypes: Hasler *et al.*, 2004) related to depression (review in Urani *et al.*, 2005). Interestingly, some strains generated using a criterion of pharmacological sensitivity turned out to be models of depression: "Flinders Sensitive Line" – selectively bred from Sprague–Dawley rats with hypersensitivity to cholinergic agonists (Overstreet, 1993, 2002; Overstreet *et al.*, 2005), and "High DPAT Sensitive" rats – selectively bred from Sprague–Dawley lines with hypersensitivity to 8-OH-DPAT (Overstreet, 2002). In the latter case, the criterion used for breeding was the hypothermia consecutive to 5-HT1A receptor activation. This mirrors the increased 5-HT1A agonist induced hypothermia found in "helpless mice" (El Yacoubi *et al.*, 2003; Popa *et al.*, 2006), and provides a strong indication of a contribution of the serotonergic system in constitutive models of depression.

Environmental manipulation during development

A third class of models has been obtained by manipulation during the perinatal period. These manipulations mainly fall in two categories: stress and block of the monoamine/serotonin transporter(s). In rodents, excess stress during the perinatal period has strong detrimental effects in adults: protocols of prenatal stress, early postnatal handling, or maternal separation produce a depression-like phenotype in adults (Caldji *et al.*, 2000; Francis *et al.*, 1996; Ladd *et al.*, 2000; Meaney, 2001; Pryce *et al.*, 2005; Stamatakis *et al.*, 2006; Vazquez *et al.*, 2005). Neonatal pharmacological treatments with clomipramine, which transiently increase brain monoamines, were initially motivated by the desire to probe the role of rapid-eye-movement (REM) sleep in brain development (Mirmiran *et al.*, 1981) and turned out to yield adult animals with behavioral and biological markers of depression (Frank and Heller, 1997; Hilakivi and Hilakivi, 1987; Velazquez-Moctezuma and Diaz Ruiz, 1992; Vogel *et al.*, 1990a). Later studies using drugs with better specificity than clomipramine demonstrated that the same effects were reproduced by selective SERT inhibitors: fluoxetine (Ansorge *et al.*, 2004, 2008), citalopram (Maciag *et al.*, 2006a), Lu 10–134-C (Hansen *et al.*, 1997), escitalopram (Popa *et al.*, 2008), but not noradrenergic transporter blockers (Ansorge *et al.*, 2008; Frank and Heller, 1997). These studies have established that postnatal serotonin has a strong influence on the development of the brain systems involved in depression. This aspect will be discussed in more detail in the last section of this chapter.

BIOLOGICAL MARKERS IN ANIMAL MODELS OF DEPRESSION

The analytic approach to depression may take advantage of other markers associated with depression, such as reactivity of the stress system, sleep regulation, or biochemical changes in the nervous system.

Stress-related markers

Stress is a pathogenic factor in the development of depressive episodes. The endocrinological response to stress is largely controlled by the hypothalamic–pituitary–adrenal (HPA) axis. Along this axis, stress triggers a sequential release of corticotropin-releasing factor (CRF), adrenocorticotropic hormone (ACTH), and glucocorticoids (cortisol in humans, corticosterone in rodents). The glucocorticoids then trigger a repressive (negative) feedback on the HPA axis, notably by the activation of receptors in the hippocampus. Depression is often associated with hypercortisolemia (Gillespie and Nemeroff, 2005), abnormally high levels of CRF (Arborelius *et al.*, 1999), and has been linked to a decreased negative feedback in the HPA axis (Heuser *et al.*, 1994; Holsboer, 2000) and to a decreased glucocorticoid receptor function in the hippocampus (Barden, 2004). Biological markers of stress have been mostly investigated in stress-related models of depression: hypercortisolemia has been found in models of chronic mild stress (Li *et al.*, 2008; Raone *et al.*, 2007; Stout *et al.*, 2000; Ushijima *et al.*, 2006) and helpless mice (El Yacoubi *et al.*, 2003). Increased levels of CRF and ACTH have also been reported in animals exposed to chronic mild stress (Li *et al.*, 2008; Stout *et al.*, 2000). Increases in the resting state of the HPA axis were not found in all stress-related models of depression such as social defeat (Berton *et al.*, 1999; Buwalda *et al.*, 1999) or prenatal stress (Dugovic *et al.*, 1999), but enhanced hormonal responses to stress or CRF injections in these models indicated an exaggerated responsiveness of the HPA axis, possibly due to a deficient regulatory negative feedback. Indeed, decreased glucocorticoid receptor density in the hippocampus has been reported in models of social defeat (Buwalda *et al.*, 1999), chronic stress (Raone *et al.*, 2007), maternal separation (Aisa *et al.*, 2007, 2008; Ladd *et al.*, 2004), and prenatal stress (Morley-Fletcher *et al.*, 2004). Similar alterations have been found in animal models of depression that were not based on stress, such as the neonatal treatments with clomipramine or a selective SERT inhibitor (Popa *et al.*, 2008; Prathiba *et al.*, 1998), therefore suggesting a direct link between the serotonin transporter (at least during development) and the dysfunction of the HPA axis observed in depression (Lanfumey *et al.*, 2008).

Sleep-related markers

Patients with depression frequently complain of insomnia, difficulty in falling asleep, and vivid, frequently unpleasant dreams (Benca *et al.*, 1997). These complaints are substantiated by polygraphic recordings demonstrating sleep fragmentation, less or lighter slow-wave sleep, reduced latency, and increased amounts of rapid-eye-movement sleep (REMS) during the first part of the night. These changes in REMS are characteristic in mood disorders, and, interestingly, there is only a partial normalization during periods of remission, suggesting that they could be a trait related to vulnerability to depression (Hasler *et al.*, 2004). Sleep disturbances are one of the criteria used for the diagnosis of depression, and indeed these anomalies have also been found in animal models. Shorter latency to REMS and/or increased amounts of REMS and sleep fragmentation have been found transiently in learned helplessness (Adrien *et al.*, 1991) and chronic mild stress (Cheeta *et al.*, 1997; Gronli *et al.*, 2004; Moreau *et al.*, 1995) paradigms. Permanent alterations in REMS are also found in Flinders rats (Overstreet, 1993; Shiromani *et al.*, 1988), helpless mice (Popa *et al.*, 2006), and prenatally stressed rats (Dugovic *et al.*, 1999), as well as after neonatal treatment with clomipramine or zimelidine (Frank and Heller, 1997; Vogel *et al.*, 1990b) and selective SERT inhibitors (Popa *et al.*, 2008). Interestingly, there is a clear correlation between individual values of REMS duration, sleep fragmentation, and plasma corticosterone after an acute stress in the model of prenatal stress (Dugovic *et al.*, 1999), suggesting the existence of a link between the factors that control REMS and sleep quality, and the factors that control the responsiveness of the HPA axis, as suggested previously by clinical studies (e.g. Hubain *et al.*, 1998; Rush *et al.*, 1982; Staner *et al.*, 2003). Finally, a global flattening of physiological circadian rhythms has been reported in several animal models of depression (Overstreet, 1993; Popa *et al.*, 2006; Solberg *et al.*, 2001), mimicking that observed in depressed patients (Avery *et al.*, 1999; Bunney and Bunney, 2000; Souetre *et al.*, 1989).

Biochemical markers in the central nervous system

Being the targets of most antidepressant compounds, the monoaminergic systems are suspected to play an important role in depression. Among them, the serotonergic system has been most amply studied.

Quantitative analyses of SERT levels in depressed subjects have provided inconsistent results. Postmortem binding studies of SERT ligands in subjects with recent symptoms of depression have failed to find changes in the raphe nuclei (Bligh-Glover *et al.*, 2000; Klimek *et al.*, 2003). On the other hand, binding in prefrontal areas and hippocampus has been found to be either reduced or unchanged in depressed subjects (review in Stockmeier, 2003). An alternate method to assess SERT availability is by binding of radiolabeled ligands in vivo (review in Meyer, 2007). Only a few studies have been performed so far, but evidence for regional increased availability of the transporter (suggestive of reduced extracellular serotonin levels) was found only for severe forms of depression (Meyer *et al.*, 2004).

In animal models of depression the results are also contradictory: increased cortical SERT binding has been found in helpless mice (El Yacoubi *et al.*, 2003; Naudon *et al.*, 2002) and in bulbectomized rats (Zhou *et al.*, 1998), while a decrease was observed in rats that received neonatal treatment with a selective SERT inhibitor (Maciag *et al.*, 2006a). Decreased levels of SERT mRNA in the raphe (Lee *et al.*, 2007), but no change in cortical binding (Vicentic *et al.*, 2006), have also been reported after maternal separation. Therefore, changes in SERT seem very heterogeneous and may depend strongly on the model.

5-HT1A autoreceptors in the raphe nuclei have also received much attention, since they are strong determinants of serotonergic neurotransmission and potentially important relays for the action of antidepressants. The status of these receptors has therefore been investigated in depressed patients and in several animal models of depression.

In humans, changes of 5-HT1A autoreceptor expression and binding have been observed in depressed patients, although the sign of these changes is not consistent across studies (Drevets *et al.*, 2007). Enhanced 5-HT1A autoreceptor-driven inhibition of serotonergic neurons has been observed, together with an increase in 5-HT1A receptor mRNA in the raphe of helpless mice (El Yacoubi *et al.*, 2003), and without such an increase after neonatal separation (Arborelius *et al.*, 2004). In contrast, the autoinhibition of raphe neurons in rats was decreased after neonatal clomipramine treatments (Maudhuit *et al.*, 1995).

Some authors have also proposed assessing the functionality of 5-HT1A autoreceptors by measuring the hypothermia induced by systemic injections of 5-HT1A agonists (Goodwin *et al.*, 1985). Although the general validity of this method to assess 5-HT1A autoreceptors is still disputed (e.g. Rausch *et al.*, 2006 for a recent discussion), evidence indicates that it depends on species (Bill *et al.*, 1991). In mice, the hypothermic response disappears after lesioning the presynaptic serotonergic compartments with 5,7-dihydroxytryptamine (Goodwin *et al.*, 1985), and the magnitude of the hypothermic response correlates with the sensitivity of raphe serotonergic neurons to 5-HT1A agonists (Alexandre *et al.*, 2006; Bouali *et al.*, 2003; El Yacoubi *et al.*, 2003). An enhanced hypothermic response to 5-HT1A agonists has been found in helpless mice (El Yacoubi *et al.*, 2003) and following neonatal treatment with a selective SERT inhibitor (Popa *et al.*, 2008).

Therefore, while evidence for changes in SERT and 5-HT1A receptors in various regions of the brain has been found in patients and in animal models, there is so far no evidence for consistent changes, indicating that these determinants of brain serotonin levels are not critical to the pathology, at least in the adult.

ANTIDEPRESSANT TREATMENTS IN ANIMAL MODELS OF DEPRESSION

To assess the predictive validity of animal models of depression, a number of studies examined whether the behavioral and/or biological abnormalities observed in these models can be reversed or prevented by adult chronic antidepressant treatment.

Behavior

A reversal of behavioral abnormalities has been found after chronic antidepressant therapy with one or more of the following types of compounds: selective SERT and monoamine oxidase inhibitors, tricyclics, and atypical drugs (or the less conventional lithium). For example, the beneficial effects of such treatments have been found in models of stress-induced depression (anhedonia in chronic mild stress [review in Willner, 2005]; increased immobility in forced swim test in prenatal stress model [Alonso *et al.*, 1999; Morley-Fletcher *et al.*, 2004]; decreased swimming in forced swim test in low-active rats (West and Weiss, 2005); development of learned helplessness [review in Henn and Vollmayr, 2005]), in Flinders rats (increase in immobility in forced swim test [review in Overstreet *et al.*, 2005]) or in olfactory bulbectomized rats (hyperactivity in open field [Breuer *et al.*, 2007]). The increased locomotor activity and the impaired sexual behavior were also reversed following chronic adult antidepressant (imipramine) treatment in a neonatal citalopram model (Maciag *et al.*, 2006b). Behavioral impairments in the tail suspension and/or forced swim tests were also improved by chronic treatment with the selective SERT inhibitor fluoxetine in helpless mice (El Yacoubi *et al.*, 2003; Naudon *et al.*, 2002) or in the escitalopram neonatal model (Popa *et al.*, 2008).

Furthermore, just as in depressed patients, for whom total sleep or selective REMS deprivation has a short-term antidepressant effect (review in Wirz-Justice and Van den Hoofdakker, 1999), depression-like behavior was reduced by a 6-h sleep deprivation in helpless mice (Popa, unpublished data) and by a 16-h REMS deprivation in helpless rats (Adrien, unpublished data).

Biological markers

Normalization of the hyperactive HPA axis has been observed after antidepressant therapy in a rat chronic stress model (Raone *et al.*, 2007) and after prenatal stress (Morley-Fletcher *et al.*, 2004), as described in humans (review in Barden, 2004; Barden *et al.*, 1995).

It is well known that most antidepressants reduce REMS in naïve animals either after acute or chronic administration (Gervasoni *et al.*, 2002; Maudhuit *et al.*, 1994; Monaca *et al.*, 2003; Neckelmann *et al.*, 1996), as in depressed patients (review in Mayers and Baldwin, 2005). The rapid time course of chronic antidepressant action on REMS indicates that the amount of REMS is reduced by a different pathway than behavior and mood. The correction by antidepressant treatments of REMS anomalies has not yet been studied in an animal model of depression.

Serotonergic dysfunctions (5-HT1A hypersensitivity) can be improved after chronic treatment with fluoxetine in helpless mice (El Yacoubi *et al.*, 2003; Naudon *et al.*, 2002) and in the neonatal escitalopram mouse model (Popa *et al.*, 2008), as well as with zimeldine in helpless rats (Maudhuit *et al.*, 1997), or with imipramine in prenatally stressed rats (Morley-Fletcher *et al.*, 2004). In contrast, neither chronic antidepressant treatment nor sleep deprivation was found to induce any change in the 5-HT1A-driven neuronal response of the nucleus raphe dorsalis in the neonatal clomipramine model, even though these treatments decreased the response in "normal" rats (Maudhuit *et al.*, 1996a, 1996b; Prevot *et al.*, 1996) and mice (Evrard *et al.*, 2006).

This brief overview of the biological signs of depression found in animal models of depression demonstrates that these models reproduce at least some of the biological alterations found in depressed patients. The general corrective effects of antidepressants, notably the SERT inhibitors, on behavioral and biological alterations contrast the limited evidence for a consistent serotonergic dysfunction in adult animal models of depression.

SERT MUTANT RODENTS

Since a polymorphism of the SERT gene predisposes to the development of depression, it is of interest to study mutant mice with genetic impairments of the SERT gene to examine the impact of permanently altered serotonin uptake on behavior and biological signs of depression. A number of genetically modified mice with altered expression of the SERT gene have been generated. Two lines of constitutive SERT knock-out mice were generated by homologous recombination with similar targeting constructs directed towards the second exon (N-terminus) of the SERT gene (*slc6a4*), by replacing it with a neomycin cassette (Bengel *et al.*, 1998; Lira *et al.*, 2003). Another line of knock-out mice has been generated by trapping of the sequence encoding the C-terminus of SERT (Zhao *et al.*, 2006). A knock-down (reduction of expression) of SERT has also been performed in adult animals using short interfering RNA (siRNA) (Thakker *et al.*, 2005). A line of mice has been produced to over-express the human SERT gene from a yeast artificial chromosome construct (Jennings *et al.*, 2006). Finally, SERT knock-out Wistar rats have been obtained by chemical mutagenesis (Homberg *et al.*, 2007). A large number of studies have been performed in these mutants. Here we will focus on the results relevant to depression.

Behavioral alterations in SERT mutants

Genetic differences across mouse strains have been demonstrated for numerous behavioral tests (review in Crawley and Paylor, 1997; Voikar *et al.*, 2001). The penetrance of a genetic mutation may also depend on the strain (Gerlai, 1996). The influence of the genetic background on immobility time in tail suspension tests and forced swim tests has been amply documented (Crowley *et al.*, 2005; Cryan *et al.*, 2005; Liu and Gershenfeld, 2001; Lucki *et al.*, 2001; Montkowski *et al.*, 1997; Trullas *et al.*, 1989; van der Heyden *et al.*, 1987; Vaugeois *et al.*, 1997), and indeed, the scores of SERT mutants in these tests (and discrepancies across studies) strongly depend on the breeding strategies used. The results in these tests may also be related to measures of locomotor activity, which may be viewed as a measure of the propensity for immobility.

Tail suspension, forced swim tests, and anhedonia

SERT knock-out mice on a C57BL/6J background show normal baseline performance in the acute tail suspension test and the forced swim test (Holmes *et al.*, 2002b), despite reduced locomotor activity in both the home cage (Holmes *et al.*, 2002a) and a novel environment (Holmes *et al.*, 2003b). In contrast, SERT knock-out mice on a 129 background show decreased immobility in the tail suspension test, but increased immobility in the forced swim test (Holmes *et al.*, 2002a; Lira *et al.*, 2003), and no change of locomotor activity in a novel environment (Lira *et al.*, 2003). Thus, the 129 SERT mutant exhibits opposite responses in two putatively similar behavioral tests: tail suspension test and forced swim test. The SERT knock-out mice, kept on a mixed 129 × C57BL/6J background, exhibit increased immobility in the acute tail suspension test (Zhao *et al.*, 2006). Mutant rats also exhibit increased immobility in the forced swim test (Olivier *et al.*, 2008). Finally, SERT knock-out rodents on CD1 background exhibit increased immobility both in tail suspension test and forced swim test, as well as a reduced locomotor activity in the home cage and in a novel environment (Alexandre *et al.*, 2006; after neonatal saline injections: Popa *et al.*, 2008). Tests of anhedonia provided results consistent with a depressive phenotype in SERT knock-out mice with a CD1 (Popa *et al.*, 2008), but not a C57BL/6J (Kalueff *et al.*, 2006) genetic background. Therefore, the CD1 and 129 genetic backgrounds favored the expression of a depressive phenotype in SERT knock-out mice, while the C57BL/6J background did not.

Interestingly, C57BL/6J SERT knock-out mice exhibit increased immobility in tail suspension and forced swim tests following repeated exposure to these tests (Wellman *et al.*, 2007; Zhao *et al.*, 2006). These results are in line with the recent data suggesting that low-expressing isoforms of Rhesus macaque SERT genes are associated with increased emotionality and reactivity to stress, especially following prolonged or repeated exposure to stressors (Barr *et al.*, 2004; Champoux *et al.*, 2002) and studies in humans (Caspi *et al.*, 2003). Thus, C57BL/6J mice may be less relevant for the study of the behavioral expression of depression following SERT mutations, but more appropriate for the study of the increased sensitivity to stress consecutive to such alterations, as observed in species other than rodents. Taken together, these results indicate that the genetic background interacts strikingly with the SERT mutation in behavioral paradigms of response to an inescapable stress, as well as in anhedonia. The behavioral consequences of SERT gene deletion in classical tests of depression thus seem to depend critically on interactions with other genes (e.g. Kaufman *et al.*, 2006; Wichers *et al.*, 2008).

Shock avoidance, novelty suppressed feeding, and fear conditioning

SERT mutant mice have also been subjected to other behavioral tests of response to stress. In the shock avoidance test, a paradigm that examines the response to an escapable stress (foot shocks), high rates of escape failures are not observed in normal animals, but may be induced by repeated exposure to inescapable foot shocks. However, 129 SERT knock-out mice exhibited longer latencies to escape foot shocks and a higher rate of escape failures than wildtype mice (Ansorge *et al.*, 2004; Lira *et al.*, 2003). These mice therefore exhibit a constitutive learned helplessness.

The novelty suppressed feeding paradigm resembles the exploration-conflict tests used to assess anxiety (see below), although hunger is the primary drive rather than exploration. The latencies to approach the food and begin feeding in the center of an open field are sensitive to anxiolytic drugs, such as benzodiazepines, but also to antidepressant treatments (Lira *et al.*, 2003). In this test, SERT knock-out mice on a 129 background exhibit longer latencies to begin feeding than wildtype mice (Ansorge *et al.*, 2004; Lira *et al.*, 2003). A similar result has been found in knock-out SERT rats (Olivier *et al.*, 2008).

SERT knock-out mice have also been subjected to a Pavlovian fear conditioning, extinction, and extinction recall paradigm and they showed significant and selective impairment in extinction recall (Wellman *et al.*, 2007). These findings suggest that loss of SERT function compromises the capacity to cope adaptively with environmental stress. A deficit in the extinction is a cardinal feature of anxiety disorders such as post-traumatic stress disorder (PTSD), and humans carrying the polymorphic variant of the promoter region of the SERT gene leading to reduced SERT function show elevated rates of PTSD (Lee *et al.*, 2005).

In summary, SERT gene invalidation affects the behavior of mice in tests of depression and sensitivity to stress, but the choice of the genetic background will be of crucial importance in future studies aimed at understanding the contribution of SERT in these different aspects.

Biological signs of depression in SERT mutant mice

Biological alterations of SERT in response to stress

We describe above how SERT knock-out mice display increased behavioral sensitivity to stressors as well as increased depression-related behaviors. At the biological level, these mutants also have altered responses to various stressors. Indeed, SERT knock-out mice exhibit augmented neuroendocrine and catecholamine responses to strong stressors like immobilization stress. Immobilization (15 min) increases the plasma levels of catecholamines, ACTH, and corticosterone similarly in normal and mutant mice, but C57BL/6J SERT mutants exhibit increased responses of plasma epinephrine to immobilization and significant depletion of adrenal epinephrine, norepinephrine, and serotonin compared to wildtype mice (Tjurmina *et al.*, 2002). Additionally, an enhanced depletion of pituitary ACTH has been observed after immobilization in the SERT knock-out mice. Increased plasma ACTH levels, compared to wildtype controls, have also been observed after saline injection in 129 × CD1 SERT knock-out, indicating an increased sensitivity to stress in these mice (Li *et al.*, 1999).

A delayed REMS rebound is classically observed after an immobilization stress (Boutrel *et al.*, 2002; Bouyer *et al.*, 1998; Lena *et al.*, 2004; Rampin *et al.*, 1991) and is related to the serum corticosterone level (Lena *et al.*, 2004; Marinesco *et al.*, 1999; Popa *et al.*, 2006, 2008). A prolonged increase of corticosterone after immobilization stress prevents the occurrence of the REMS rebound which would occur at the return of corticosterone to baseline levels. The CD1 SERT knock-out mice expressed no increase of REMS associated with a long-lasting elevation of plasma corticosterone levels in the 24 h following 90 min of immobilization stress. A similar response was found in an animal model of depression, the helpless mice (Popa *et al.*, 2006). In summary, there is an increased responsiveness of the HPA axis in SERT mutants, as has been also observed in other models of depression (see above).

REMS and circadian rhythms

Increases in amounts and decreases in latencies of REMS (other biological markers found in animal models of depression – see above) have been observed in SERT knock-out mice on both C57BL/6J and CD1 genetic backgrounds (Alexandre *et al.*, 2006; Popa *et al.*, 2008; Wisor *et al.*, 2003). Indeed, SERT mutants exhibited an increase of about 40% in REMS amounts and episode frequency, and a shortened spontaneous

REMS latency compared to wildtype mice (Alexandre *et al.*, 2006; Popa *et al.*, 2008; Wisor *et al.*, 2003). Additional slow-wave sleep alterations (indicative of sleep fragmentation) have also been observed in the CD1 genetic background (Popa *et al.*, 2008). Interestingly, the mechanisms underlying this REMS over-expression following SERT invalidation may depend on the genetic background. The increase in REMS is mainly due to prolonged REMS episodes (compared to wildtype controls) in knock-out mice with a C57BL/6J background (Wisor *et al.*, 2003), and more frequent episodes (but of similar duration compared to wildtype controls) in knock-out mice with a CD1 background (Alexandre *et al.*, 2006; Popa *et al.*, 2008).

Circadian rhythms of activity and temperature in SERT knock-out mice have also been examined on a CD1 background. Both SERT knock-out and control wildtype mice exhibit a diurnal rhythm of locomotor activity and body temperature characterized by higher levels during the dark than during the light period. However, SERT knock-out mice exhibit a decrease in locomotor activity and in body temperature during the dark period compared to wildtype mice. The absence of a peak in temperature and activity at the beginning of the dark period has also been observed in the mutants (Figure 5.1; Popa, unpublished data). These results are similar to those reported for animal models of depression (Overstreet, 1993; Popa *et al.*, 2006; Solberg *et al.*, 2001).

Altered serotonergic system

SERT knock-out mice exhibit marked disturbances in the serotonergic system itself, notably low levels of brain-tissue serotonin content, enhanced serotonin synthesis and turnover (Bengel *et al.*, 1998; Kim *et al.*, 2005), and marked increases in the extracellular serotonin concentration (Fabre *et al.*, 2000). The mutants exhibit reduced mRNA expression and protein binding of the 5-HT1A receptor in raphe nuclei and some forebrain areas (amygdala, hypothalamus) (Alexandre *et al.*, 2006; Bouali *et al.*, 2003; Fabre *et al.*, 2000; Li *et al.*, 2000; Lira *et al.*, 2003). In contrast, 5-HT1A receptor mRNA expression and protein binding is increased in the hippocampus (Alexandre *et al.*, 2006; Fabre *et al.*, 2000). 5-HT1A autoreceptors have been consistently found to be desensitized in SERT knock-out mice, as shown by the attenuated response of dorsal raphe neurons to 5-HT1A agonists (Bouali *et al.*, 2003; Gobbi *et al.*, 2001; Mannoury la Cour *et al.*, 2001). In agreement with these data, SERT knock-out mice exhibited abnormal neuroendocrine responses to 5-HT1A receptor agonists (review in Fox *et al.*, 2007). The 5-HT1A agonist

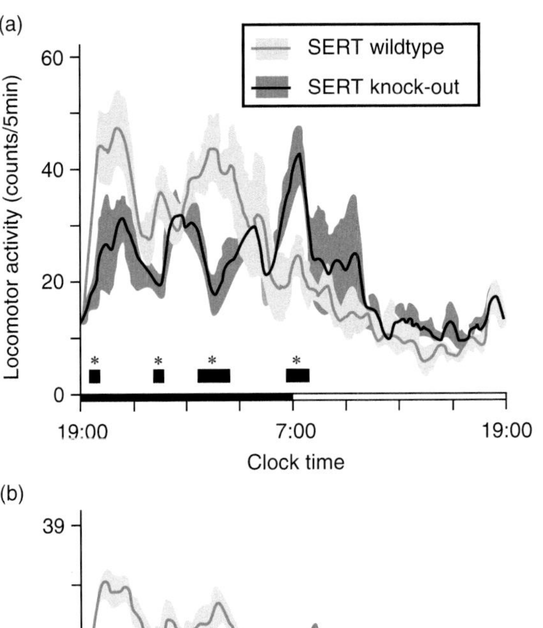

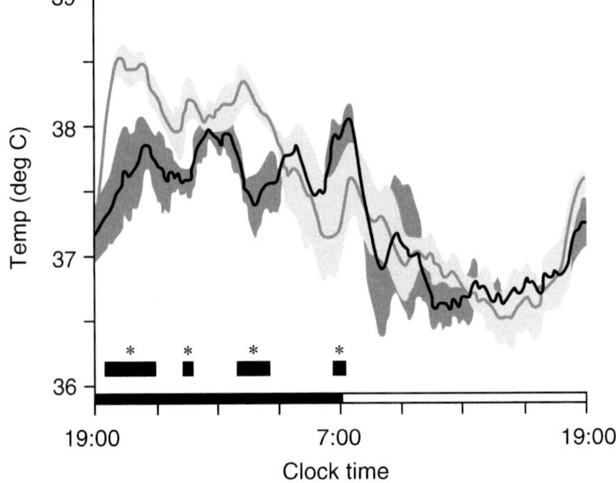

Figure 5.1 Flattening of circadian rhythms of activity and temperature in CD1 SERT knock-out mice. (a) Locomotor activity, and (b) body temperature in CD1 SERT wildtype female mice (gray line) and SERT knock-out mice (black line), recorded during 8 days using a telemetry mini-emitter. Data (mean ± SEM of 4 animals in each group) are expressed every 5 min for 24 h as counts for the activity and as degrees Celsius for the temperature. Note the rapid rise of temperature and activity at the beginning of the dark period (19:00–7:00) in wildtype mice but not in mutant mice. *$p<0.05$, significantly different between groups, unpaired Student's t test. (For methods, see Popa *et al.*, 2006.)

8-OH-DPAT failed to raise plasma oxytocin and corticosterone levels (Li *et al.*, 1999), an effect that could indicate desensitization of 5-HT1A receptors in the paraventricular nucleus of the hypothalamus (Bagdy, 1996). This only elicited an attenuated decrease in the body temperature of knock-out mice compared to wildtype mice (Bouali *et al.*, 2003; Li *et al.*, 1999), in agreement with the desensitization of 5-HT1A autoreceptors. These results contrast the enhanced hypothermic response observed in some models of depression (El Yacoubi *et al.*, 2003; Popa *et al.*, 2008), but rather seem reminiscent of the 5-HT1A autoreceptor desensitization observed after chronic treatment with a selective SERT antagonist in adult rodents (Blier, 2003; Le Poul *et al.*, 1995). Since behavioral signs of depression may be observed in knock-out mice in the presence of desensitized 5-HT1A autoreceptors, this suggests that these mice could be used to investigate the effects of antidepressants that operate by another mechanism than SERT inhibition and the desensitization of these autoreceptors.

Morphological changes

There is growing evidence for altered connectivity between the prefrontal cortex and amygdala in the pathophysiology of depression and anxiety disorders (Phelps *et al.*, 2004; Siegle *et al.*, 2002). The search for morphological anomalies has been quite limited in animal models of depression, but has been performed recently in SERT knock-out mice. Changes have been found in both basolateral amygdala and ventromedial prefrontal cortex (infralimbic) of SERT knock-out mice (Wellman *et al.*, 2007). Higher spine density has been observed on the high-order dendritic branches in the amygdala, and, while the density of spines is normal in pyramidal neurons in the prefrontal cortex, the dendrites of pyramidal cells in this area are significantly elongated compared to wildtype mice. The investigation of such abnormalities in animal models of depression will offer the opportunity to compare them with the SERT knock-out animals.

SERT heterozygous mutant mice

Mice that lack only one copy of the SERT gene might provide a closer equivalent to the human SERT promoter variant associated with anxio-depressive traits (Kalueff *et al.*, 2007). However, only a few studies reported data obtained in these heterozygous mutants, and they generally showed a pattern intermediate between wildtype and homozygous

SERT knock-out mice (review in Fox *et al.*, 2007; Kalueff *et al.*, 2007). This is notably the case for the reduced density of SERT and 5-HT1A receptors (Bengel *et al.*, 1998; Fabre *et al.*, 2000), as well as 8-OH-DPAT-induced inhibition of raphe neuron activity (Gobbi *et al.*, 2001). Small or mild differences from wildtype mice have been found in emotional behaviors (Ansorge *et al.*, 2004; Holmes *et al.*, 2002b), sleep patterns (Adrien, unpublished results), or 5-HT1A receptor agonist-induced hypothermia (Li *et al.*, 1999). However, SERT heterozygous mutant mice exhibit gender differences consistent with those found in humans, and they could thus be particularly suitable for the analysis of such differences (Kalueff *et al.*, 2007).

In light of the results exposed above, it appears that SERT knock-out mice may express a combination of behavioral and biological signs of depression, and thus share a number of characteristics with animal models of depression and, more generally, to stress vulnerability. These studies also underpin the importance of genetic background, and thus highlight the need for further studies to identify other genes involved in the expression of the detrimental effects of SERT reduction.

PERSPECTIVE: THE DEVELOPMENTAL HYPOTHESIS OF SERT DYSFUNCTION

Neonatal treatments with antidepressant drugs (like clomipramine) have long been known to produce adult animals with a depressive phenotype. However, only the recent advent of highly selective pharmacological tools has allowed the demonstration that these effects are reproduced, at least to some extent, by a specific inhibition of SERT during development (Ansorge *et al.*, 2004, 2008; Maciag *et al.*, 2006a, 2006b; Popa *et al.*, 2008). As in SERT knock-out mice, the effects of neonatal treatments depend in part on the genetic background (e.g. Popa *et al.*, 2008, for discussion). These studies then raise the possibility that some of the detrimental effects of SERT gene deletion result from developmental alterations, and, indeed, combined studies (Ansorge *et al.*, 2004; Popa *et al.*, 2008) demonstrated a substantial similarity between the phenotype of adult SERT knock-out mice and mice (with the same genetic background) that had received a neonatal treatment with a selective SERT inhibitor (Figure 5.2A).

The developmental origin of the dysfunctions observed in the adult after neonatal treatment has been demonstrated with treatments of similar duration in adult animals, and by the failure of such adult treatments to induce delayed effects on behavior (Ansorge *et al.*,

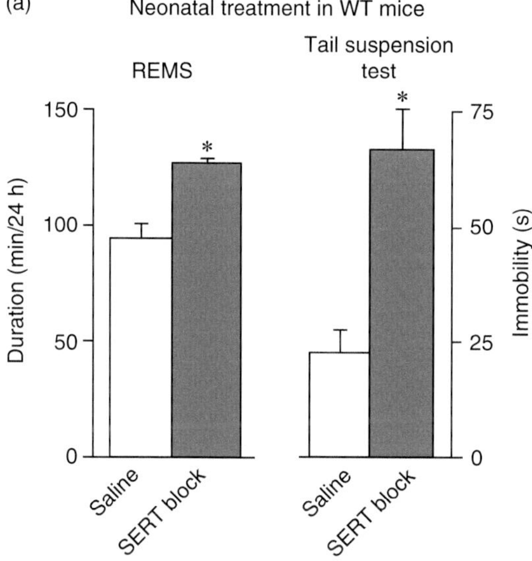

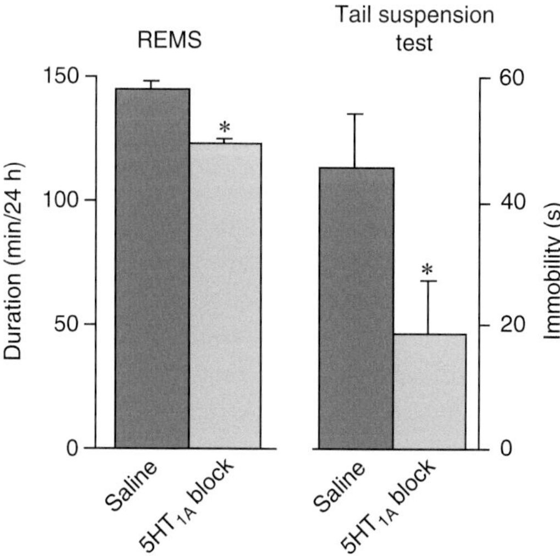

Figure 5.2 Bidirectional effects of neonatal treatments in SERT wildtype and knock-out adult mice. REMS amounts and time of immobilization in tail suspension test in (a) WT female mice after neonatal saline (white bars) or selective SERT inhibition by escitalopram (gray bars) treatments; (b) SERT knock-out female mice after neonatal saline (dark gray bars), or after the 5-HT1A antagonist WAY 100635 (light gray bars) treatments (data from (Alexandre *et al.*, 2006; Popa *et al.*, 2008)). An increase in REMS

2008; Popa *et al.*, 2008) or biological markers (Popa *et al.*, 2008). Similarly, knock-down of SERT in the adult fails to produce the major alterations found in life-long knock-out mice (Thakker *et al.*, 2005). More strikingly, the neonatal treatment of SERT knock-out mice (with a CD1 genetic background) with an inhibitor of 5-HT synthesis or a 5-HT1A receptor antagonist reversed, at least partially, the abnormal sleep patterns, depression-related behavior, and 5-HT$_{1A}$ autoreceptor binding in adult animals (Alexandre *et al.*, 2006) (Figure 5.2B). These results indicate that several of the main depression-related phenotypes caused by SERT gene invalidation are established during the first postnatal month in the rodent, and may involve 5-HT1A receptors. Interestingly, the anxious phenotype of 5-HT1A receptor knock-out mice (Heisler *et al.*, 1998; Parks *et al.*, 1998; Ramboz *et al.*, 1998) can be corrected by the re-expression of 5-HT1A receptors in the tele-encephalon of these mutants during the first 3 postnatal weeks, while the re-expression of these same receptors later during development does not restore a normal phenotype (Gross *et al.*, 2002; Kusserow *et al.*, 2004). Conversely, beneficial effects of reduced serotonin transporter function during development have been demonstrated in an animal model of depression. Treatment with a selective SERT inhibitor during the first postnatal month, but not later, normalized several abnormalities in adult mice that received a prenatal stress, notably the plasma corticosterone levels in response to restraint stress (Ishiwata *et al.*, 2005).

The specific neuronal alterations produced by anomalous brain serotonin levels during the first postnatal month in the rodent, and the mechanisms by which they arise, still need to be identified. A large body of evidence indicates that serotonin regulates many developmental processes in the brain, including differentiation, cell migration, and synaptogenesis (review in Azmitia, 2001; Lauder, 1990; Rubenstein, 1998; Whitaker-Azmitia, 2001), as well as neuronal differentiation and

Caption for Figure 5.2 (cont.)
amounts and in immobilization time in tail suspension test are observed in mice after neonatal block of SERT function (a) and after the deletion of the SERT-encoding gene (b). These increases in SERT knock-out mice are reduced by a neonatal treatment with the 5-HT1A receptor antagonist WAY 100635. Therefore, increases of the serotoninergic transmission during early development leads to depression-like abnormalities (increased REMS and immobility time in tail suspension test, (a), and reciprocally, the reduction of serotoninergic transmission can prevent these depression-like dysfunctions in adult SERT knock-out mice (b).

maturation of postsynaptic neurons (Emerit *et al.*, 1992; Lavdas *et al.*, 1997). Thus, the serotonin may play a prominent role in regulating neuronal architecture and connectivity in addition to its classical role in neurotransmission. Targeted genetic and neurochemical approaches will probably help to define the developmental effects of serotonin relevant to depression.

Moreover, brain serotonin levels control the vigilance state, which may indirectly but strongly affect brain wiring. High brain serotonin levels, such as those encountered after neonatal treatments with selective SERT inhibitors, substantially reduce REMS during the treatment (Mirmiran *et al.*, 1981, 1983; Vogel *et al.*, 1990a), and an instrumental REMS deprivation preserving the SERT function during the first postnatal month has been shown to produce a depressive phenotype (Feng and Ma, 2003). Further studies will hopefully help to understand the role of REMS in the maturation of brain circuits involved in depression, anxiety, and reactivity to stress.

In conclusion, there is now ample evidence for a link between the SERT and the intricate systems involved in depression, anxiety, and vulnerability to stress. The observation of consistent changes in the serotonergic system in depressed patients and in animal models of depression has eluded researchers' efforts. In contrast, clear alterations of the emotional systems have been found in mice with altered SERT expression, and the strong contribution of the genetic background in the phenotypes of mutant mice now calls for further studies aimed at discovering the other genes interacting with the SERT. The first postnatal month in rodents is a critical period for the impact of SERT functional alterations, suggesting that the phenotype of SERT knockout mice is largely established during this period of time. Further studies focusing on the neurobiological events during this period should help to resolve the mechanisms at work.

Animal studies have clearly established that anomalous brain serotonin levels during development produce deleterious long-term effects in the adult. Whether the vulnerability to depression found in humans with a genetic variant(s) of the SERT gene yielding a low uptake of serotonin is caused by developmental alterations remains to be established. Long-term studies of children exposed to antidepressants during their early life are lacking, and could provide a first hint. However, the greatest caution should be exerted for the prescription of selective SERT inhibitors before adulthood, until the presence, or absence, in humans of the alterations found by animal studies is established. Finally, the reversal of anomalies in animal models of depression or in SERT mutant mice by neonatal treatments normalizing the serotonergic transmission also indicate that studies of the neonatal period might open perspectives for novel preventive therapeutic strategies.

ACKNOWLEDGMENTS

The authors would like to thank Boris Barbour for the critical reading of the manuscript and gratefully acknowledge funding from la Fondation pour la Recherche Médicale, and support from the INSERM and CNRS.

REFERENCES

Adrien J, Dugovic C, Martin P (1991). Sleep-wakefulness patterns in the helpless rat. *Physiol Behav* **49**: 257–62.

Aisa B, Tordera R, Lasheras B, Del Rio J, Ramirez M J (2007). Cognitive impairment associated to HPA axis hyperactivity after maternal separation in rats. *Psychoneuroendocrinology* **32**: 256–66.

Aisa B, Tordera R, Lasheras B, Del Rio J, Ramirez M J (2008). Effects of maternal separation on hypothalamic–pituitary–adrenal responses, cognition and vulnerability to stress in adult female rats. *Neuroscience* **154**: 1218–26.

Alexandre C, Popa D, Fabre V, *et al.* (2006). Early life blockade of 5-hydroxytryptamine 1A receptors normalizes sleep and depression-like behavior in adult knock-out mice lacking the serotonin transporter. *J Neurosci* **26**: 5554–64.

Alonso S J, Castellano M A, Quintero M, Navarro E (1999). Action of antidepressant drugs on maternal stress-induced hypoactivity in female rats. *Methods Find Exp Clin Pharmacol* **21**: 291–5.

Ansorge M S, Morelli E, Gingrich J A (2008). Inhibition of serotonin but not norepinephrine transport during development produces delayed, persistent perturbations of emotional behaviors in mice. *J Neurosci* **28**: 199–207.

Ansorge M S, Zhou M, Lira A, Hen R, Gingrich J A (2004). Early-life blockade of the 5-HT transporter alters emotional behavior in adult mice. *Science* **306**: 879–81.

Arborelius L, Hawks B W, Owens M J, Plotsky P M, Nemeroff C B (2004). Increased responsiveness of presumed 5-HT cells to citalopram in adult rats subjected to prolonged maternal separation relative to brief separation. *Psychopharmacology (Berl)* **176**: 248–55.

Arborelius L, Owens M J, Plotsky P M, Nemeroff C B (1999). The role of corticotropin-releasing factor in depression and anxiety disorders. *J Endocrinol* **160**: 1–12.

Artigas F, Adell A, Celada P (2006). Pindolol augmentation of antidepressant response. *Curr Drug Targets* **7**: 139–47.

Avery D H, Shah S H, Eder D N, Wildschiodtz G (1999). Nocturnal sweating and temperature in depression. *Acta Psychiatr Scand* **100**: 295–301.

Azmitia E C (2001). Modern views on an ancient chemical: serotonin effects on cell proliferation, maturation, and apoptosis. *Brain Res Bull* **56**: 413–24.

Bagdy G (1996). Role of the hypothalamic paraventricular nucleus in 5-HT1A, 5-HT2A and 5-HT2C receptor-mediated oxytocin, prolactin and ACTH/corticosterone responses. *Behav Brain Res* **73**: 277–80.

Barden N (2004). Implication of the hypothalamic–pituitary–adrenal axis in the physiopathology of depression. *J Psychiatry Neurosci* **29**: 185–93.

Barden N, Reul J M, Holsboer F (1995). Do antidepressants stabilize mood through actions on the hypothalamic–pituitary–adrenocortical system? *Trends Neurosci* **18**: 6–11.

Barr C S, Newman T K, Shannon C, *et al.* (2004). Rearing condition and rh5-HTTLPR interact to influence limbic–hypothalamic–pituitary–adrenal axis response to stress in infant macaques. *Biol Psychiatry* **55**: 733–8.

Benca R (2000). Mood disorders. In Kryger M, Roth T, Dement W, editors. *Principles and practice of sleep medecine*. Philadelphia: Saunders, pp. 1140–58.

Benca R M, Okawa M, Uchiyama M, (1997). Sleep and mood disorders. *Sleep Med Rev* **1**: 45–56.

Bengel D, Murphy D L, Andrews A M, *et al.* (1998). Altered brain serotonin homeostasis and locomotor insensitivity to 3,4-methylenedioxymethamphetamine ("Ecstasy") in serotonin transporter-deficient mice. *Mol Pharmacol* **53**: 649–55.

Berman R M, Charney D S (1999). Models of antidepressant action. *J Clin Psychiatry* **60** (Suppl 14): 16–20; discussion 31–15.

Berton O, Durand M, Aguerre S, Mormede P, Chaouloff F (1999). Behavioral, neuroendocrine and serotonergic consequences of single social defeat and repeated fluoxetine pretreatment in the Lewis rat strain. *Neuroscience* **92**: 327–41.

Bevins R A, Besheer J (2005). Novelty reward as a measure of anhedonia. *Neurosci Biobehav Revi* **29**: 707–14.

Bill D J, Knight M, Forster E A, Fletcher A (1991). Direct evidence for an important species difference in the mechanism of 8-OH-DPAT-induced hypothermia. *Br J Pharmacol* **103**: 1857–64.

Blanchard R J, McKittrick C R, Blanchard D C (2001). Animal models of social stress: effects on behavior and brain neurochemical systems. *Physiol Behav* **73**: 261–71.

Blazer D G (2000). Mood disorders: epidemiology. In Sadock B J, Sadock V A, editors. *Comprehensive textbook of psychiatry*. New York: Lippincott, Williams & Wilkins, pp. 1298–308.

Blier P (2003). The pharmacology of putative early-onset antidepressant strategies. *Eur Neuropsychopharmacol* **13**: 57–66.

Bligh-Glover W, Kolli T N, Shapiro-Kulnane L, *et al.* (2000). The serotonin transporter in the midbrain of suicide victims with major depression. *Biol Psychiatry* **47**: 1015–24.

Bouali S, Evrard A, Chastanet M, Lesch K P, Hamon M, Adrien J (2003). Sex hormone-dependent desensitization of 5-HT1A autoreceptors in knockout mice deficient in the 5-HT transporter. *Eur J Neurosci* **18**: 2203–12.

Boutrel B, Monaca C, Hen R, Hamon M, Adrien J (2002). Involvement of 5-HT1A receptors in homeostatic and stress-induced adaptive regulations of paradoxical sleep: studies in 5-HT1A knock-out mice. *J Neurosci* **22**: 4686–92.

Bouyer J J, Vallee M, Deminiere J M, Le Moal M, Mayo W (1998). Reaction of sleep–wakefulness cycle to stress is related to differences in hypothalamo–pituitary–adrenal axis reactivity in rat. *Brain Res* **804**: 114–24.

Breuer M E, Groenink L, Oosting R S, Westenberg H G, Olivier B (2007). Long-term behavioral changes after cessation of chronic antidepressant treatment in olfactory bulbectomized rats. *Biol Psychiatry* **61**: 990–5.

Bunney W E, Bunney B G (2000). Molecular clock genes in man and lower animals: possible implications for circadian abnormalities in depression. *Neuropsychopharmacology* **22**: 335–45.

Buwalda B, de Boer S F, Schmidt E D, *et al.* (1999). Long-lasting deficient dexamethasone suppression of hypothalamic–pituitary–adrenocortical activation following peripheral CRF challenge in socially defeated rats. *J Neuroendocrinol* **11**: 513–20.

Caldji C, Francis D, Sharma S, Plotsky P M, Meaney M J (2000). The effects of early rearing environment on the development of GABAA and central benzodiazepine receptor levels and novelty-induced fearfulness in the rat. *Neuropsychopharmacology* **22**: 219–29.

Caspi A, Sugden K, Moffitt T E, *et al.* (2003). Influence of life stress on depression: moderation by a polymorphism in the 5-HTT gene. *Science* **301**: 386–9.

Castren E, Voikar V, Rantamaki T (2007). Role of neurotrophic factors in depression. *Curr Opin Pharmacol* **7**: 18–21.

Champoux M, Bennett A, Shannon C, Higley J D, Lesch K P, Suomi S J (2002). Serotonin transporter gene polymorphism, differential early rearing, and behavior in rhesus monkey neonates. *Mol Psychiatry* **7**: 1058–63.

Cheeta S, Ruigt G, van Proosdij J, Willner P (1997). Changes in sleep architecture following chronic mild stress. *Biol Psychiatry* **41**: 419–27.

Chourbaji S, Zacher C, Sanchis-Segura C, Dormann C, Vollmayr B, Gass P (2005). Learned helplessness: validity and reliability of depressive-like states in mice. *Brain Res Brain Res Protoc* **16**: 70–8.

Coppen A (1967). The biochemistry of affective disorders. *Br J Psychiatry* **113**: 1237–64.

Crawley J N, Paylor R (1997). A proposed test battery and constellations of specific behavioral paradigms to investigate the behavioral phenotypes of transgenic and knockout mice. *Horm Behav* **31**: 197–211.

Crowley J J, Blendy J A, Lucki I (2005). Strain-dependent antidepressant-like effects of citalopram in the mouse tail suspension test. *Psychopharmacology (Berl)* **183**: 257–64.

Cryan J F, Mombereau C (2004). In search of a depressed mouse: utility of models for studying depression-related behavior in genetically modified mice. *Mol Psychiatry* **9**: 326–57.

Cryan J F, Mombereau C, Vassout A (2005). The tail suspension test as a model for assessing antidepressant activity: review of pharmacological and genetic studies in mice. *Neurosci Biobehav Rev* **29**: 571–625.

Delgado P L (2006). Monoamine depletion studies: implications for antidepressant discontinuation syndrome. *J Clin Psychiatry* **67** (Suppl 4): 22–6.

Drevets W C, Thase M E, Moses-Kolko E L, *et al.* (2007). Serotonin-1A receptor imaging in recurrent depression: replication and literature review. *Nucl Med Biol* **34**: 865–77.

Dugovic C, Maccari S, Weibel L, Turek F W, Van Reeth O (1999). High corticosterone levels in prenatally stressed rats predict persistent paradoxical sleep alterations. *J Neurosci* **19**: 8656–64.

El Yacoubi M, Bouali S, Popa D, *et al.* (2003). Behavioral, neurochemical, and electrophysiological characterization of a genetic mouse model of depression. *Proc Natl Acad Sci USA* **100**: 6227–32.

Emerit M B, Riad M, Hamon M (1992). Trophic effects of neurotransmitters during brain maturation. *Biol Neonate* **62**: 193–201.

Evrard A, Barden N, Hamon M, Adrien J (2006). Glucocorticoid receptor-dependent desensitization of 5-HT1A autoreceptors by sleep deprivation: studies in GR-i transgenic mice. *Sleep* **29**: 31–6.

Fabre V, Beaufour C, Evrard A, *et al.* (2000). Altered expression and functions of serotonin 5-HT1A and 5-HT1B receptors in knock-out mice lacking the 5-HT transporter. *Eur J Neurosci* **12**: 2299–310.

Fava M, Kendler K S (2000). Major depressive disorder. *Neuron* **28**: 335–41.

Feng P, Ma Y (2003). Instrumental REM sleep deprivation in neonates leads to adult depression-like behaviors in rats. *Sleep* **26**: 990–6.

Fox M A, Andrews A M, Wendland J R, Lesch K P, Holmes A, Murphy D L (2007). A pharmacological analysis of mice with a targeted disruption of the serotonin transporter. *Psychopharmacology (Berl)* **195**: 147–66.

Francis D, Diorio J, LaPlante P, Weaver S, Seckl J R, Meaney M J (1996). The role of early environmental events in regulating neuroendocrine development. Moms, pups, stress, and glucocorticoid receptors. *Ann NY Acad Sci* **794**: 136–52.

Frank M G, Heller H C (1997). Neonatal treatments with the serotonin uptake inhibitors clomipramine and zimelidine, but not the noradrenaline uptake inhibitor desipramine, disrupt sleep patterns in adult rats. *Brain Res* **768**: 287–93.

Geretsegger C, Bitterlich W, Stelzig R, Stuppaeck C, Bondy B, Aichhorn W (2008). Paroxetine with pindolol augmentation: a double-blind, randomized, placebo-controlled study in depressed in-patients. *Eur Neuropsychopharmacol* **18**: 141–6.

Gerlai R (1996). Gene-targeting studies of mammalian behavior: is it the mutation or the background genotype? *Trends Neurosci* **19**: 177–81.

Gervasoni D, Panconi E, Henninot V, *et al.* (2002). Effect of chronic treatment with milnacipran on sleep architecture in rats compared with paroxetine and imipramine. *Pharmacol Biochem Behav* **73**: 557–63.

Gillespie C F, Nemeroff C B (2005). Hypercortisolemia and depression. *Psychosom Med* **67** (Suppl 1): S26–8.

Gobbi G, Murphy D L, Lesch K, Blier P (2001). Modifications of the serotonergic system in mice lacking serotonin transporters: an in vivo electrophysiological study. *J Pharmacol Exp Ther* **296**: 987–95.

Goodwin G M, De Souza R J, Green A R (1985). The pharmacology of the hypothermic response in mice to 8-hydroxy-2-(di-*n*-propylamino)tetralin (8-OH-DPAT). A model of presynaptic 5-HT1 function. *Neuropharmacology* **24**: 1187–94.

Gronli J, Murison R, Bjorvatn B, Sorensen E, Portas C M, Ursin R (2004). Chronic mild stress affects sucrose intake and sleep in rats. *Behav Brain Res* **150**: 139–47.

Gross C, Zhuang X, Stark K, *et al.* (2002). Serotonin1A receptor acts during development to establish normal anxiety-like behavior in the adult. *Nature* **416**: 396–400.

Guilloux J P, David D J, Guiard B P, *et al.* (2006). Blockade of 5-HT1A receptors by (+/−)-pindolol potentiates cortical 5-HT outflow, but not antidepressant-like activity of paroxetine: microdialysis and behavioral approaches in 5-HT1A receptor knockout mice. *Neuropsychopharmacology* **31**: 2162–72.

Hansen H H, Sanchez C, Meier E (1997). Neonatal administration of the selective serotonin reuptake inhibitor Lu 10-134-C increases forced swimming-induced immobility in adult rats: a putative animal model of depression? *J Pharmacol Exp Ther* **283**: 1333–41.

Hasler G, Drevets WC, Manji H K, Charney D S (2004). Discovering endophenotypes for major depression. *Neuropsychopharmacology* **29**: 1765–81.

Heisler L K, Chu H M, Brennan T J, *et al.* (1998). Elevated anxiety and antidepressant-like responses in serotonin 5-HT1A receptor mutant mice. *Proc Natl Acad Sci USA* **95**: 15 049–54.

Henn F A, Vollmayr B (2005). Stress models of depression: forming genetically vulnerable strains. *Neurosci Biobehav Rev* **29**: 799–804.

Hensler J G (2002). Differential regulation of 5-HT1A receptor-G protein interactions in brain following chronic antidepressant administration. *Neuropsychopharmacology* **26**: 565–73.

Heuser I, Yassouridis A, Holsboer F (1994). The combined dexamethasone/CRH test: a refined laboratory test for psychiatric disorders. *J Psychiatr Res* **28**: 341–56.

Hilakivi L A, Hilakivi I (1987). Increased adult behavioral 'despair' in rats neonatally exposed to desipramine or zimeldine: an animal model of depression? *Pharmacol Biochem Behav* **28**: 367–9.

Holick K A, Lee D C, Hen R, Dulawa S C (2008). Behavioral effects of chronic fluoxetine in BALB/cJ mice do not require adult hippocampal neurogenesis or the serotonin 1A receptor. *Neuropsychopharmacology* **33**: 406–17.

Holmes A, Lit Q, Murphy D L, Gold E, Crawley J N (2003a). Abnormal anxiety-related behavior in serotonin transporter null mutant mice: the influence of genetic background. *Genes Brain Behav* **2**: 365–80.

Holmes A, Murphy D L, Crawley J N (2002a). Reduced aggression in mice lacking the serotonin transporter. *Psychopharmacology (Berl)* **161**: 160–7.

Holmes A, Yang R J, Lesch K P, Crawley J N, Murphy D L (2003b). Mice lacking the serotonin transporter exhibit 5-HT(1A) receptor-mediated abnormalities in tests for anxiety-like behavior. *Neuropsychopharmacology* **28**: 2077–88.

Holmes A, Yang R J, Murphy D L, Crawley J N (2002b). Evaluation of antidepressant-related behavioral responses in mice lacking the serotonin transporter. *Neuropsychopharmacology* **27**: 914–23.

Holsboer F (2000). The corticosteroid receptor hypothesis of depression. *Neuropsychopharmacology* **23**: 477–501.

Homberg J R, Olivier J D, Smits B M, *et al.* (2007). Characterization of the serotonin transporter knockout rat: a selective change in the functioning of the serotonergic system. *Neuroscience* **146**: 1662–76.

Hubain P P, Staner L, Dramaix M, *et al.* (1998). The dexamethasone suppression test and sleep electroencephalogram in nonbipolar major depressed inpatients: a multivariate analysis. *Biol Psychiatry* **43**: 220–9.

Ishiwata H, Shiga T, Okado N (2005). Selective serotonin reuptake inhibitor treatment of early postnatal mice reverses their prenatal stress-induced brain dysfunction. *Neuroscience* **133**: 893–901.

Jennings K A, Loder M K, Sheward W J, *et al.* (2006). Increased expression of the 5-HT transporter confers a low-anxiety phenotype linked to decreased 5-HT transmission. *J Neurosci* **26**: 8955–64.

Kalueff A V, Gallagher P S, Murphy D L (2006). Are serotonin transporter knockout mice 'depressed'? Hypoactivity but no anhedonia. *Neuroreport* **17**: 1347–51.

Kalueff A V, Ren-Patterson R F, Murphy D L (2007). The developing use of heterozygous mutant mouse models in brain monoamine transporter research. *Trends Pharmacol Sci* **28**: 122–7.

Kaufman J, Yang B Z, Douglas-Palumberi H, *et al.* (2006). Brain-derived neurotrophic factor-5-HTTLPR gene interactions and environmental modifiers of depression in children. *Biol Psychiatry* **59**: 673–80.

Kim D K, Tolliver T J, Huang S J, *et al.* (2005). Altered serotonin synthesis, turnover and dynamic regulation in multiple brain regions of mice lacking the serotonin transporter. *Neuropharmacology* **49**: 798–810.

Kirsch I, Deacon B J, Huedo-Medina T B, Scoboria A, Moore T J, Johnson B (2008). Initial severity and antidepressant benefits: a meta-analysis of data submitted to the Food and Drug Administration. *PLoS Med* **5**: e45.

Klimek V, Roberson G, Stockmeier C A, Ordway G A (2003). Serotonin transporter and MAO-B levels in monoamine nuclei of the human brainstem are normal in major depression. *J Psychiatr Res* **37**: 387–97.

Kline N S (1958). Clinical experience with iproniazid (marsilid). *J Clin Exp Psychopathol* **19**: 72–8; discussion 78–9.

Kornstein S G, Schatzberg A F, Thase M E, *et al.* (2000). Gender differences in chronic major and double depression. *J Affect Disord* **60**: 1–11.

Kozisek M E, Middlemas D, Bylund D B (2008). Brain-derived neurotrophic factor and its receptor tropomyosin-related kinase B in the mechanism of action of antidepressant therapies. *Pharmacol Ther* **117**: 30–51.

Kusserow H, Davies B, Hortnagl H, *et al.* (2004). Reduced anxiety-related behavior in transgenic mice overexpressing serotonin 1A receptors. *Brain Res Mol Brain Res* **129**: 104–16.

Lacasse J R, Leo J (2005). Serotonin and depression: a disconnect between the advertisements and the scientific literature. *PLoS Med* **2**: e392.

Lachman H M, Papolos D F, Weiner E D, *et al.* (1992). Hippocampal neuropeptide Y mRNA is reduced in a strain of learned helpless resistant rats. *Brain Res Mol Brain Res* **14**: 94–100.

Ladd C O, Huot R L, Thrivikraman K V, Nemeroff C B, Meaney M J, Plotsky P M (2000). Long-term behavioral and neuroendocrine adaptations to adverse early experience. *Prog Brain Res* **122**: 81–103.

Ladd C O, Huot R L, Thrivikraman K V, Nemeroff C B, Plotsky P M (2004). Long-term adaptations in glucocorticoid receptor and mineralocorticoid receptor mRNA and negative feedback on the hypothalamo–pituitary–adrenal axis following neonatal maternal separation. *Biol Psychiatry* **55**: 367–75.

Lanfumey L, Mongeau R, Cohen-Salmon C, Hamon M (2008). Corticosteroid–serotonin interactions in the neurobiological mechanisms of stress-related disorders. *Neurosci Biobehav Rev* **32**: 1174–84.

Lauder J M (1990). Ontogeny of the serotonergic system in the rat: serotonin as a developmental signal. *Ann NY Acad Sci* **600**: 297–313; discussion 314.

Lavdas A A, Blue M E, Lincoln J, Parnavelas J G (1997). Serotonin promotes the differentiation of glutamate neurons in organotypic slice cultures of the developing cerebral cortex. *J Neurosci* **17**: 7872–80.

Lazary J, Lazary A, Gonda X, *et al.* (2008). New evidence for the association of the serotonin transporter gene (SLC6A4) haplotypes, threatening life events, and depressive phenotype. *Biol Psychiatry* **64**: 498–504.

Le Poul E, Laaris N, Doucet E, Laporte A M, Hamon M, Lanfumey L (1995). Early desensitization of somato-dendritic 5-HT$_{1A}$ autoreceptors in rats treated with fluoxetine or paroxetine. *Naunyn Schmiedebergs Arch Pharmacol* **352**: 141–8.

Lee H J, Lee M S, Kang R H, *et al.* (2005). Influence of the serotonin transporter promoter gene polymorphism on susceptibility to posttraumatic stress disorder. *Depress Anxiety* **21**: 135–9.

Lee J H, Kim H J, Kim J G, *et al.* (2007). Depressive behaviors and decreased expression of serotonin reuptake transporter in rats that experienced neonatal maternal separation. *Neurosci Res* **58**: 32–9.

Lena C, Popa D, Grailhe R, Escourrou P, Changeux J P, Adrien J (2004). Beta2-containing nicotinic receptors contribute to the organization of sleep and regulate putative micro-arousals in mice. *J Neurosci* **24**: 5711–8.

Lesch K P, Bengel D, Heils A, *et al.* (1996). Association of anxiety-related traits with a polymorphism in the serotonin transporter gene regulatory region. *Science* **274**: 1527–31.

Levinson D F (2006). The genetics of depression: a review. *Biol Psychiatry* **60**: 84–92.

Li Q, Wichems C, Heils A, Lesch K P, Murphy D L (2000). Reduction in the density and expression, but not G-protein coupling, of serotonin receptors (5-HT1A) in 5-HT transporter knock-out mice: gender and brain region differences. *J Neurosci* **20**: 7888–95.

Li Q, Wichems C, Heils A, Van De Kar L D, Lesch K P, Murphy D L (1999). Reduction of 5-hydroxytryptamine (5-HT)(1A)-mediated temperature and neuroendocrine responses and 5-HT(1A) binding sites in 5-HT transporter knockout mice. *J Pharmacol Exp Ther* **291**: 999–1007.

Li S, Wang C, Wang W, Dong H, Hou P, Tang Y (2008). Chronic mild stress impairs cognition in mice: from brain homeostasis to behavior. *Life Sci* **82**: 934–42.

Lira A, Zhou M, Castanon N, *et al.* (2003). Altered depression-related behaviors and functional changes in the dorsal raphe nucleus of serotonin transporter-deficient mice. *Biol Psychiatry* **54**: 960–71.

Liu X, Gershenfeld H K (2001). Genetic differences in the tail-suspension test and its relationship to imipramine response among 11 inbred strains of mice. *Biol Psychiatry* **49**: 575–81.

Lucki I, Dalvi A, Mayorga A J (2001). Sensitivity to the effects of pharmacologically selective antidepressants in different strains of mice. *Psychopharmacology (Berl)* **155**: 315–22.

Maciag D, Simpson K L, Coppinger D, *et al.* (2006a). Neonatal antidepressant exposure has lasting effects on behavior and serotonin circuitry. *Neuropsychopharmacology* **31**: 47–57.

Maciag D, Williams L, Coppinger D, Paul I A (2006b). Neonatal citalopram exposure produces lasting changes in behavior which are reversed by adult imipramine treatment. *Eur J Pharmacol* **532**: 265–9.

Malberg J E, Eisch A J, Nestler E J, Duman R S (2000). Chronic antidepressant treatment increases neurogenesis in adult rat hippocampus. *J Neurosci* **20**: 9104–10.

Mannoury la Cour C, Boni C, Hanoun N, Lesch K P, Hamon M, Lanfumey L (2001). Functional consequences of 5-HT transporter gene disruption on 5-$HT_{(1A)}$ receptor-mediated regulation of dorsal raphe and hippocampal cell activity. *J Neurosci* **21**: 2178–85.

Mansour H A, Talkowski M E, Wood J, *et al.* (2005). Serotonin gene polymorphisms and bipolar I disorder: focus on the serotonin transporter. *Ann Med* **37**: 590–602.

Marinesco S, Bonnet C, Cespuglio R (1999). Influence of stress duration on the sleep rebound induced by immobilization in the rat: a possible role for corticosterone. *Neuroscience* **92**: 921–33.

Matthews K, Christmas D, Swan J, Sorrell E (2005). Animal models of depression: navigating through the clinical fog. *Neurosci Biobehav Rev* **29**: 503–13.

Maudhuit C, Hamon M, Adrien J (1995). Electrophysiological activity of raphe dorsalis serotoninergic neurones in a possible model of endogenous depression. *Neuroreport* **6**: 681–4.

Maudhuit C, Hamon M, Adrien J (1996a). Effects of chronic treatment with zimelidine and REM sleep deprivation on the regulation of raphe neuronal activity in a rat model of depression. *Psychopharmacology (Berl)* **124**: 267–74.

Maudhuit C, Jolas T, Chastanet M, Hamon M, Adrien J (1996b). Reduced inhibitory potency of serotonin reuptake blockers on central serotoninergic neurons in rats selectively deprived of rapid eye movement sleep. *Biol Psychiatry* **40**: 1000–07.

Maudhuit C, Jolas T, Lainey E, Hamon M, Adrien J (1994). Effects of acute and chronic treatment with amoxapine and cericlamine on the sleep-wakefulness cycle in the rat. *Neuropharmacology* **33**: 1017–25.

Maudhuit C, Prevot E, Dangoumau L, Martin P, Hamon M, Adrien J (1997). Antidepressant treatment in helpless rats: effect on the electrophysiological activity of raphe dorsalis serotonergic neurons. *Psychopharmacology (Berl)* **130**: 269–75.

Mayers A G, Baldwin D S (2005). Antidepressants and their effect on sleep. *Hum Psychopharmacol* **20**: 533–59.

McClung C A (2007). Circadian genes, rhythms and the biology of mood disorders. *Pharmacol Ther* **114**: 222–32.

Meaney M J (2001). Maternal care, gene expression, and the transmission of individual differences in stress reactivity across generations. *Annu Rev Neurosci* **24**: 1161–92.

Meyer J H (2007). Imaging the serotonin transporter during major depressive disorder and antidepressant treatment. *J Psychiatry Neurosci* **32**: 86–102.

Meyer J H, Houle S, Sagrati S, *et al.* (2004). Brain serotonin transporter binding potential measured with carbon 11-labeled DASB positron emission tomography: effects of major depressive episodes and severity of dysfunctional attitudes. *Arch Gen Psychiatry* **61**: 1271–9.

Mineur Y S, Belzung C, Crusio W E (2006). Effects of unpredictable chronic mild stress on anxiety and depression-like behavior in mice. *Behav Brain Res* **175**: 43–50.

Mirmiran M, Scholtens J, van de Poll N E, Uylings H B, van der Gugten J, Boer G J (1983). Effects of experimental suppression of active (REM) sleep during early development upon adult brain and behavior in the rat. *Brain Res* **283**: 277–86.

Mirmiran M, van de Poll N E, Corner M A, van Oyen H G, Bour H L (1981). Suppression of active sleep by chronic treatment with chlorimipramine during early postnatal development: effects upon adult sleep and behavior in the rat. *Brain Res* **204**: 129–46.

Monaca C, Boutrel B, Hen R, Hamon M, Adrien J (2003). 5-HT 1A/1B receptor-mediated effects of the selective serotonin reuptake inhibitor, citalopram, on sleep: studies in 5-HT 1A and 5-HT 1B knockout mice. *Neuropsychopharmacology* **28**: 850–6.

Montkowski A, Poettig M, Mederer A, Holsboer F (1997). Behavioural performance in three substrains of mouse strain 129. *Brain Res* **762**: 12–18.

Moreau J L, Scherschlicht R, Jenck F, Martin J R (1995). Chronic mild stress-induced anhedonia model of depression; sleep abnormalities and curative effects of electroshock treatment. *Behav Pharmacol* **6**: 682–7.

Moreno F A, Gelenberg A J, Heninger G R, *et al.* (1999). Tryptophan depletion and depressive vulnerability. *Biol Psychiatry* **46**: 498–505.

Morley-Fletcher S, Darnaudery M, Mocaer E, *et al.* (2004). Chronic treatment with imipramine reverses immobility behavior, hippocampal corticosteroid receptors and cortical 5-HT(1A) receptor mRNA in prenatally stressed rats. *Neuropharmacology* **47**: 841–7.

Moser P C, Sanger D J (1999). 5-HT1A receptor antagonists neither potentiate nor inhibit the effects of fluoxetine and befloxatone in the forced swim test in rats. *Eur J Pharmacol* **372**: 127–34.

Naudon L, El Yacoubi M, Vaugeois J M, Leroux-Nicollet I, Costentin J (2002). A chronic treatment with fluoxetine decreases 5-HT(1A) receptors labeling in mice selected as a genetic model of helplessness. *Brain Res* **936**: 68–75.

Neckelmann D, Bjorvatn B, Bjorkum A A, Ursin R (1996). Citalopram: differential sleep/wake and EEG power spectrum effects after single dose and chronic administration. *Behav Brain Res* **79**: 183–92.

Nestler E J, Barrot M, DiLeone R J, Eisch A J, Gold S J, Monteggia L M (2002a). Neurobiology of depression. *Neuron* **34**: 13–25.

Nestler E J, Gould E, Manji H, *et al.* (2002b). Preclinical models: status of basic research in depression. *Biol Psychiatry* **52**: 503–28.

Olivier J D, Van Der Hart M G, Van Swelm R P, *et al.* (2008). A study in male and female 5-HT transporter knockout rats: an animal model for anxiety and depression disorders. *Neuroscience* **152**: 573–84.

Overstreet D H (1993). The Flinders sensitive line rats: a genetic animal model of depression. *Neurosci Biobehav Rev* **17**: 51–68.

Overstreet D H (2002). Behavioral characteristics of rat lines selected for differential hypothermic responses to cholinergic or serotonergic agonists. *Behav Genet* **32**: 335–48.

Overstreet D H, Friedman E, Mathe A A, Yadid G (2005). The Flinders Sensitive Line rat: a selectively bred putative animal model of depression. *Neurosci Biobehav Rev* **29**: 739–59.

Owens M J, Nemeroff C B (1994). Role of serotonin in the pathophysiology of depression: focus on the serotonin transporter. *Clin Chem* **40**: 288–95.

Paizanis E, Hamon M, Lanfumey L (2007). Hippocampal neurogenesis, depressive disorders, and antidepressant therapy. *Neural Plasticity* **2007**: 73 754.

Papakostas G I, Thase M E, Fava M, Nelson J C, Shelton R C (2007). Are antidepressant drugs that combine serotonergic and noradrenergic mechanisms of action more effective than the selective serotonin reuptake inhibitors in treating major depressive disorder? A meta-analysis of studies of newer agents. *Biol Psychiatry* **62**: 1217–27.

Parks C L, Robinson P S, Sibille E, Shenk T, Toth M (1998). Increased anxiety of mice lacking the serotonin1A receptor. *Proc Natl Acad Sci USA* **95**: 10 734–9.

Perry E K, Marshall E F, Blessed G, Tomlinson B E, Perry R H (1983). Decreased imipramine binding in the brains of patients with depressive illness. *Br J Psychiatry* **142**: 188–92.

Phelps E A, Delgado M R, Nearing K I, LeDoux J E (2004). Extinction learning in humans: role of the amygdala and vmPFC. *Neuron* **43**: 897–905.

Popa D, El Yacoubi M, Vaugeois J M, Hamon M, Adrien J (2006). Homeostatic regulation of sleep in a genetic model of depression in the mouse: effects of muscarinic and 5-HT1A receptor activation. *Neuropsychopharmacology* **31**: 1637–46.

Popa D, Lena C, Alexandre C, Adrien J (2008). Lasting syndrome of depression produced by reduction in serotonin uptake during postnatal development: evidence from sleep, stress, and behavior. *J Neurosci* **28**: 3546–54.

Porsolt R D (2000). Animal models of depression: utility for transgenic research. *Rev Neurosci* **11**: 53–8.

Porsolt R D, Le Pichon M, Jalfre M (1977). Depression: a new animal model sensitive to antidepressant treatments. *Nature* **266**: 730–2.

Prathiba J, Kumar K B, Karanth K S (1998). Hyperactivity of hypothalamic pituitary axis in neonatal clomipramine model of depression. *J Neural Transm* **105**: 1335–9.

Prevot E, Maudhuit C, Le Poul E, Hamon M, Adrien J (1996). Sleep deprivation reduces the citalopram-induced inhibition of serotoninergic neuronal firing in the nucleus raphe dorsalis of the rat. *J Sleep Res* **5**: 238–45.

Pryce C R, Ruedi-Bettschen D, Dettling A C, *et al.* (2005). Long-term effects of early-life environmental manipulations in rodents and primates: potential animal models in depression research. *Neurosci Biobehav Rev* **29**: 649–74.

Ramboz S, Oosting R, Amara D A, *et al.* (1998). Serotonin receptor 1A knockout: an animal model of anxiety-related disorder. *Proc Natl Acad Sci USA* **95**: 14 476–81.

Rampin C, Cespuglio R, Chastrette N, Jouvet M (1991). Immobilisation stress induces a paradoxical sleep rebound in rat. *Neurosci Lett* **126**: 113–8.

Raone A, Cassanelli A, Scheggi S, Rauggi R, Danielli B, De Montis M G (2007). Hypothalamus–pituitary–adrenal modifications consequent to chronic stress exposure in an experimental model of depression in rats. *Neuroscience* **146**: 1734–42.

Rausch J L, Johnson M E, Kasik K E, Stahl S M (2006). Temperature regulation in depression: functional 5HT1A receptor adaptation differentiates antidepressant response. *Neuropsychopharmacology* **31**: 2274–80.

Redrobe J P, MacSweeney C P, Bourin M (1996). The role of 5-HT1A and 5-HT1B receptors in antidepressant drug actions in the mouse forced swimming test. *Eur J Pharmacol* **318**: 213–20.

Rubenstein J L (1998). Development of serotonergic neurons and their projections. *Biol Psychiatry* **44**: 145–50.

Rush A J, Giles D E, Roffwarg H P, Parker C R (1982). Sleep EEG and dexamethasone suppression test findings in outpatients with unipolar major depressive disorders. *Biol Psychiatry* **17**: 327–41.

Santarelli L, Saxe M, Gross C, *et al.* (2003). Requirement of hippocampal neurogenesis for the behavioral effects of antidepressants. *Science* **301**: 805–09.

Seligman M E, Maier S F (1967). Failure to escape traumatic shock. *J Exp Psychol* **74**: 1–9.

Sham P C, Sterne A, Purcell S, *et al.* (2000). GENESiS: creating a composite index of the vulnerability to anxiety and depression in a community-based sample of siblings. *Twin Res* **3**: 316–22.

Shiromani P J, Overstreet D, Levy D, Goodrich C A, Campbell S S, Gillin J C (1988). Increased REM sleep in rats selectively bred for cholinergic hyperactivity. *Neuropsychopharmacology* **1**: 127–33.

Siegle G J, Steinhauer S R, Thase M E, Stenger V A, Carter C S (2002). Can't shake that feeling: event-related fMRI assessment of sustained amygdala activity in response to emotional information in depressed individuals. *Biol Psychiatry* **51**: 693–707.

Solberg L C, Olson S L, Turek F W, Redei E (2001). Altered hormone levels and circadian rhythm of activity in the WKY rat, a putative animal model of depression. *Am J Physiol Regul Integr Comp Physiol* **281**: R786–94.

Song C, Leonard B E (2005). The olfactory bulbectomised rat as a model of depression. *Neurosci Biobehav Rev* **29**: 627–47.

Souetre E, Salvati E, Belugou J L, *et al.* (1989). Circadian rhythms in depression and recovery: evidence for blunted amplitude as the main chronobiological abnormality. *Psychiatry Res* **28**: 263–78.

Stamatakis A, Mantelas A, Papaioannou A, Pondiki S, Fameli M, Stylianopoulou F (2006). Effect of neonatal handling on serotonin 1A sub-type receptors in the rat hippocampus. *Neuroscience* **140**: 1–11.

Staner L, Duval F, Haba J, Mokrani M C, Macher J P (2003). Disturbances in hypothalamo pituitary adrenal and thyroid axis identify different sleep EEG patterns in major depressed patients. *J Psychiatr Res* **37**: 1–8.

Steru L, Chermat R, Thierry B, *et al.* (1987). The automated Tail Suspension Test: a computerized device which differentiates psychotropic drugs. *Prog Neuropsychopharmacol Biol Psychiatry* **11**: 659–71.

Stockmeier C A (2003). Involvement of serotonin in depression: evidence from postmortem and imaging studies of serotonin receptors and the serotonin transporter. *J Psychiatr Res* **37**: 357–73.

Stout S C, Mortas P, Owens M J, Nemeroff C B, Moreau J (2000). Increased corticotropin-releasing factor concentrations in the bed nucleus of the stria terminalis of anhedonic rats. *Eur J Pharmacol* **401**: 39–46.

Strekalova T, Spanagel R, Bartsch D, Henn F A, Gass P (2004). Stress-induced anhedonia in mice is associated with deficits in forced swimming and exploration. *Neuropsychopharmacology* **29**: 2007–17.

Sullivan P F, Neale M C, Kendler K S (2000). Genetic epidemiology of major depression: review and meta-analysis. *Am J Psychiatry* **157**: 1552–62.

Thakker D R, Natt F, Husken D, *et al.* (2005). siRNA-mediated knockdown of the serotonin transporter in the adult mouse brain. *Mol Psychiatry* **10**: 714, 782–9.

Tjurmina O A, Armando I, Saavedra J M, Goldstein D S, Murphy D L (2002). Exaggerated adrenomedullary response to immobilization in mice with targeted disruption of the serotonin transporter gene. *Endocrinology* **143**: 4520–6.

Trullas R, Jackson B, Skolnick P (1989). Genetic differences in a tail suspension test for evaluating antidepressant activity. *Psychopharmacology (Berl)* **99**: 287–8.

Urani A, Chourbaji S, Gass P (2005). Mutant mouse models of depression: candidate genes and current mouse lines. *Neurosci Biobehav Rev* **29**: 805–28.

Ushijima K, Morikawa T, To H, Higuchi S, Ohdo S (2006). Chronobiological disturbances with hyperthermia and hypercortisolism induced by chronic mild stress in rats. *Behav Brain Res* **173**: 326–30.

van der Heyden J A, Molewijk E, Olivier B (1987). Strain differences in response to drugs in the tail suspension test for antidepressant activity. *Psychopharmacology (Berl)* **92**: 127–30.

Vaugeois J M, Passera G, Zuccaro F, Costentin J (1997). Individual differences in response to imipramine in the mouse tail suspension test. *Psychopharmacology (Berl)* **134**: 387–91.

Vazquez V, Farley S, Giros B, Dauge V (2005). Maternal deprivation increases behavioural reactivity to stressful situations in adulthood: suppression by the CCK2 antagonist L365,260. *Psychopharmacology (Berl)* **181**: 706–13.

Velazquez-Moctezuma J, Diaz Ruiz O (1992). Neonatal treatment with clomipramine increased immobility in the forced swim test: an attribute of animal models of depression. *Pharmacol Biochem Behav* **42**: 737–9.

Vicentic A, Francis D, Moffett M, *et al.* (2006). Maternal separation alters serotonergic transporter densities and serotonergic 1A receptors in rat brain. *Neuroscience* **140**: 355–65.

Vogel G, Neill D, Hagler M, Kors D (1990a). A new animal model of endogenous depression: a summary of present findings. *Neurosci Biobehav Rev* **14**: 85–91.

Vogel G, Neill D, Kors D, Hagler M (1990b). REM sleep abnormalities in a new animal model of endogenous depression. *Neurosci Biobehav Rev* **14**: 77–83.

Voikar V, Koks S, Vasar E, Rauvala H (2001). Strain and gender differences in the behavior of mouse lines commonly used in transgenic studies. *Physiol Behav* **72**: 271–81.

Weiss J M, Cierpial M A, West C H (1998). Selective breeding of rats for high and low motor activity in a swim test: toward a new animal model of depression. *Pharmacol Biochem Behav* **61**: 49–66.

Wellman C L, Izquierdo A, Garrett J E, *et al.* (2007). Impaired stress-coping and fear extinction and abnormal corticolimbic morphology in serotonin transporter knock-out mice. *J Neurosci* **27**: 684–91.

West C H, Weiss J M (2005). A selective test for antidepressant treatments using rats bred for stress-induced reduction of motor activity in the swim test. *Psychopharmacology (Berl)* **182**: 9–23.

Whitaker-Azmitia P M (2001). Serotonin and brain development: role in human developmental diseases. *Brain Res Bull* **56**: 479–85.

Wichers M, Kenis G, Jacobs N, *et al.* (2008). The BDNF Val(66)Met × 5-HTTLPR × child adversity interaction and depressive symptoms: an attempt at replication. *Am J Med Genet B Neuropsychiatr Genet* **147B**: 120–3.

Willner P (1984). The validity of animal models of depression. *Psychopharmacology (Berl)* **83**: 1–16.

Willner P (1997). Validity, reliability and utility of the chronic mild stress model of depression: a 10-year review and evaluation. *Psychopharmacology (Berl)* **134**: 319–29.

Willner P (2005). Chronic mild stress (CMS) revisited: consistency and behavioural–neurobiological concordance in the effects of CMS. *Neuropsychobiology* **52**: 90–110.

Willner P, Mitchell P J (2002). The validity of animal models of predisposition to depression. *Behav Pharmacol* **13**: 169–88.

Wirz-Justice A, Van den Hoofdakker R H (1999). Sleep deprivation in depression: what do we know, where do we go? *Biol Psychiatry* **46**: 445–53.

Wisor J P, Wurts S W, Hall F S, *et al.* (2003). Altered rapid eye movement sleep timing in serotonin transporter knockout mice. *Neuroreport* **14**: 233–8.

Zhao S, Edwards J, Carroll J, *et al.* (2006). Insertion mutation at the C-terminus of the serotonin transporter disrupts brain serotonin function and emotion-related behaviors in mice. *Neuroscience* **140**: 321–34.

Zhou D, Grecksch G, Becker A, Frank C, Pilz J, Huether G (1998). Serotonergic hyperinnervation of the frontal cortex in an animal model of depression, the bulbectomized rat. *J Neurosci Res* **54**: 109–16.

JOCELIEN OLIVIER, ALEXANDER COOLS, BART ELLENBROEK, EDWIN CUPPEN AND JUDITH HOMBERG

6

The serotonin transporter knock-out rat: a review

ABSTRACT

This chapter dicusses the most recent data on the serotonin transporter knock-out rat, a unique rat model that has been generated by target-selected *N*-ethyl-*N*-nitrosourea (ENU) driven mutagenesis. The knock-out rat is the result of a premature stopcodon in the serotonin transporter gene, and the absence of the serotonin transporter has been confirmed at mRNA, protein, and functional levels. The serotonin transporter (SERT) plays a crucial role in serotonin reuptake and its absence has a huge effect on serotonin neurotransmission – exemplified by increased extracellular serotonin levels, reduced serotonin tissue/platelet/blood levels, and reduced evoked serotonin release – yet the animals appear normal and do not differ from wildtype littermates in respect to breeding and health. Behavioral phenotypes are only apparent when the animals are exposed to certain stimuli. For instance, the serotonin transporter knock-out rat displays increased stress sensitivity in a variety of anxiety- and depression-like tests, such as the elevated plus maze test and the forced swim test. Also remarkable, while general activity is not changed, the knock-out rats show a "neurotic-like" exploratory pattern. In line with the serotonin hypothesis of impulsivity, which argues that there is an inverse relationship between the two, serotonin transporter knock-out rats show reduced motor impulsivity in the five-choice serial reaction time task, and a reduction in social interaction during play and aggressive encounters. Interestingly, abdominal fat seems to be increased in the knock-out rat, despite normal body weight. Pharmacological compounds also elicit genotype-dependent responses

Experimental Models in Serotonin Transporter Research, eds. A. V. Kalueff and J. L. LaPorte. Published by Cambridge University Press.

in the knock-out rats. For instance, the animals are supersensitive to cocaine, regarding cocaine's psychomotor effects, cocaine-induced place preference, and intravenous cocaine self-administration. Further, the responsivity to 5-HT1A receptor ligands is changed, as is the effect of these ligands on the psychomotor effects of cocaine, suggesting that compensatory adaptations in the serotoninergic system contribute to the behavioral profile of the knock-out rats. Are all central serotonin-mediated processes affected in the knock-out rat? Clearly not, since some serotonin-mediated behaviors, such as cognitive flexibility, prepulse inhibition, spontaneous alternation, and food intake are surprisingly unaffected by the constitutive absence of the serotonin transporter. Together, these data will help in the understanding of the relationship between serotonin-mediated processes and, importantly, will complement serotonin transporter mouse studies, based on each species' research advantages.

THE MAKING OF KNOCK-OUT RATS

The laboratory rat is one of the most extensively studied model organisms for various aspects of human health and disease. The wealth of literature on the rat makes it easier to interpret novel findings. Further, many behavioral tests have been developed and validated for rats, and rat behavioral repertoires and related neural correlates have been well-described. Among behavioral models that are well developed for rats are tasks assessing executive functioning (Dalley *et al.*, 2004), social behavior (Pellis and Pasztor, 1999; Poole and Fish, 1975) and intravenous drug self-administration (Griffith *et al.*, 1980). Rats are also preferred because of their relatively large size, which allows for the effective use of a wide variety of tools to study the brain, such as imaging, micromanipulation, and in vivo sampling. In 2004, the rat joined the mouse and human as the third vertebrate species for which the complete genome sequence (more than 90% coverage) has been determined (Gibbs *et al.*, 2004). For these reasons, knock-out rats would be valuable models in, among others, neuroscience research, and could complement knock-out mice studies to dissect gene–behavior associations.

In October 2007, the Nobel Prize in Physiology or Medicine was awarded to Mario R. Capecchi, Martin J. Evans, and Oliver Smithies for their discoveries of "principles for introducing specific gene modifications in mice by the use of embryonic stem cells". Their discoveries led to the immensely powerful gene targeting technology in mice. It is now being applied to virtually all areas of biomedicine – from basic research to the development of new therapies. Nowadays, thousands of mouse genes have been knocked out. The first report in which homologous recombination in embryonic stem (ES) cells were used to generate gene-targeted mice were published in 1989. Since then, the number of reported knock-out mouse lines has risen exponentially. However, as a genetic model, the rat is clearly lagging behind the mouse, primarily because gene knock-out technology using pluripotent embryonic stem cells is still lacking due to the lack of suitable ES cell lines. An alternative approach to the ES cell technique to make genetic knock-outs is target-selected mutagenesis or TILLING (targeting induced local lesions in genomes). This universal approach has been developed for various model organisms, such as *Caenorhabditis elegans* (Jansen *et al.*, 1997), *Drosophila* (Bentley *et al.*, 2000), zebrafish *Danio rerio* (Wienhols *et al.*, 2002), *Arabidopsis* (McCallum *et al.*, 2000), maize (Till *et al.*, 2004), and *Lotus* (Perry *et al.*, 2003). Recently, *N*-ethyl-*N*-nitrosourea (ENU)-driven target selected mutagenesis was successfully established for the rat (Smits *et al.*, 2004, 2006; Zan *et al.*, 2003). The approach starts with inducing mutagenesis of the male germline by intraperitoneal injection of ENU. ENU induces random point mutations, primarily in spermatogonial stem cells. These mutations become fixed in the sperm cells during spermatogenesis, which lasts approximately 12 weeks in rats. Mutagenized males are mated with untreated females to generate a large population of F1 animals that harbor many random heterozygous point mutations in their genome. Next, DNA samples are extracted from each F1 individual, which are subsequently screened for induced mutations in exons of interest (Figure 6.1). The most deleterious type of mutation is the non-sense mutation or premature stopcodon, which interrupts the translation process. Mutations can also involve missense mutations, amino acid changes that could lead to structural and/or functional changes of the protein, e.g. when the amino acid change is located in a conserved region of the protein. Splice-site mutations affect alternative splicing processes and are of interest as well. Silent mutations are not expected to have any phenotypic effects (Smits and Cuppen, 2005).

The efficacy of the procedure is largely dependent on the frequency of induced mutations, as well as the efficiency and throughput of the mutation method. Outbred strains such as Sprague–Dawley and Wistar tend to give the highest mutation frequency and have superior reproductive performances as compared to inbred strains, making outbred strains particularly suited for ENU-driven mutagenesis (Smits *et al.*, 2006; Zan *et al.*, 2003). In relation to the human genetic heterogeneity,

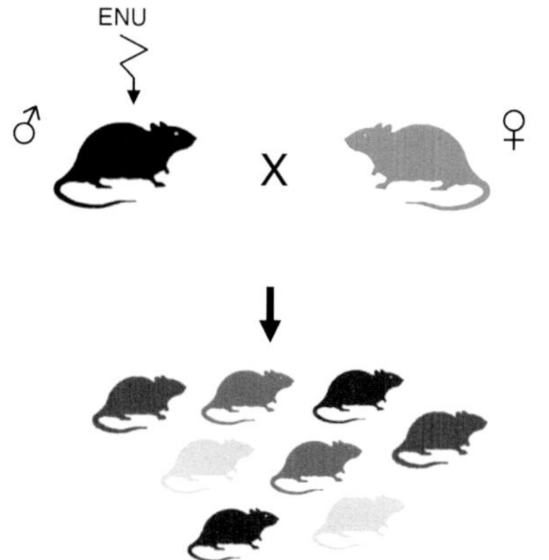

Figure 6.1 Schematic representation of ENU-driven target-selected mutagenesis. Male rats are injected with ENU and crossed with untreated females. A cohort of animals (F1) with random point mutations is generated, and their DNA is isolated for high-throughput screening resequencing of genes of interest.

outbred strains are also more relevant to humans than inbred strains. The first line of Sprague–Dawley knock-out rats was produced using a yeast-based screening assay that only identifies truncated mRNAs, which focuses on non-sense mutations (Zan *et al.*, 2003). In comparison, dideoxy resequencing allows for the detection of all types of mutations. This method is more costly, but by several adaptations in the standard protocol the costs can be reduced (Smits *et al.*, 2004, 2006). The dideoxy resequencing method, applied to approximately 400 amplicons (~200 genes) in 1500 rats (mainly Wistars), resulted in the identification of more than 120 ENU-induced mutations, including 56 missense and 6 non-sense mutations, among which is a premature stopcodon in the serotonin transporter (SERT) gene (Figure 6.2). To be precise, the ENU-induced mutagenesis caused a C to A transversion at position 3924 in the third exon encoding the second extracellular loop of the SERT (ENSRNOG0000003476) in a female F1 rat with a Wistar/Crl background, which resulted in a premature stopcodon (TGC > TGA) (Figure 6.2; Smits *et al.*, 2006).

To generate a homozygous SERT knock-out rat line and to simultaneously get rid of other potential induced mutations, rats carrying

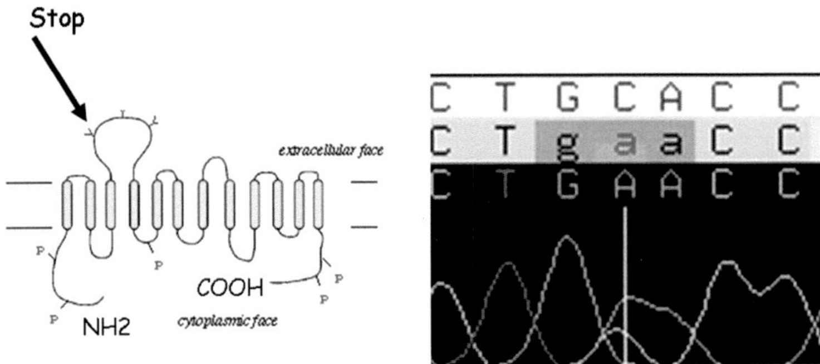

Figure 6.2 Schematic representation of the SERT gene and the induced knock-out mutation (Slc6a4^{1Hubr}) achieved by target-selected mutagenesis. The arrow indicates the location of the ENU-induced C to A mutation that results in the change of amino acid 209 from a cysteine to a stopcodon. Reused from Homberg *et al.* (2007a), with kind permission of Elsevier Limited.

the SERT gene premature stopcodon were first outcrossed on commercially available wildtype rats (Harlan, The Netherlands) for five generations before the first experiments began. Of note is that outcrossing may not eliminate all additional induced mutations. Mutations closely linked to the SERT gene (that is, within a region of less than 10–20 cm) may co-segregate with the stopcodon in the SERT gene. However, based on the mutation rate of non-sense mutations within a 20 cm region, the chance of having a second premature stopcodon is less than 2% (E. Cuppen, unpublished data). Nevertheless, this chance should not be ignored. Therefore, experiments have been designed such that knock-out rats were compared to control littermates rather than unrelated commercial wildtype Wistar rats. The possibility for additional mutations may seem to be a disadvantage of this rat knock-out approach, but thus far target-selected mutagenesis is the only method available to generate knock-out rats. Because several phenotypes of the SERT knock-out rat are stable across generations and laboratories, and several phenotypes are concurrent with literature findings and SERT knock-out mouse phenotypes, it is assumed that any phenotype in the knock-out rat is most likely attributable to the absence of the SERT and not other induced mutations.

CONFIRMATION OF THE SERT KNOCK-OUT RAT AT THE MOLECULAR LEVEL

The nature of non-transgenic ENU-induced gene knock-outs is fundamentally different from the homologous recombination method commonly used to generate mouse knock-outs. In the latter models, genomic fragments encoding important protein domains or the complete protein are replaced by a selection cassette, whereas the model presented here is induced by a single point mutation that introduces a premature stopcodon. It is theoretically possible for an almost intact protein to be made, presumably from an alternative spliced transcript. However, Northern blot analysis (Homberg *et al.*, 2007a) and sequencing of RT-PCR products (J. Homberg, unpublished observations) reveals that the SERT transcript is almost completely absent in homozygous SERT knock-out (SERT−/−) rats. This is most likely due to a process called "non-sense mediated decay" (Baker and Parker, 2004), a mechanism by which non-sense transcripts are degraded. The expression level of the SERT transcript in heterozygous SERT knock-out (SERT+/−) rats is intermediate to that of SERT−/− and wildtype (SERT+/+) rats. Autoradiography, using the tritium labeled form of the highly selective serotonin reuptake inhibitor (SSRI) citalopram, reveals that SERT binding is completely absent in SERT−/− rats (Figure 6.3). In SERT+/− rats, SERT binding is reduced by approximately 40% as compared to SERT+/+ littermates (Homberg *et al.*, 2007a). At the functional level, *d*-fenfluramine-induced hypothermia, which can be blocked by citalopram (J. Olivier, unpublished observations), is completely absent in SERT−/− rats, and reduced in SERT+/− rats relative to SERT+/+ littermates. Finally, the in vitro maximum rate (V_{max}) of [^{3}H]5-HT uptake in synaptosomes prepared from the hippocampus is reduced by 13.4% in SERT+/− rats, and by 72.2% in SERT−/− rats. From these data it can be concluded that the premature stopcodon in the SERT gene results in a full knock-out of the SERT. Furthermore, the SERT+/− rat studies show that there is a gene–dose effect for these molecular and neurochemical findings.

GENERAL APPEARANCE OF SERT KNOCK-OUT RATS

Despite the important role of 5-HT in the development of the nervous system (Lauder, 1990), SERT−/− and SERT+/− knock-out rats appear normal, and score similarly to SERT+/+ littermates on measures of health and neurological functions. This has been shown by use of an adapted SHIRPA protocol. The SHIRPA protocol has been developed to characterize the phenotype of transgenic and knock-out mice (Rogers *et al.*, 1997; mammalian genome). Several components of this protocol have been adapted, and an experimenter blind to genotype evaluated the rats. Behaviors in the viewing jar (body position,

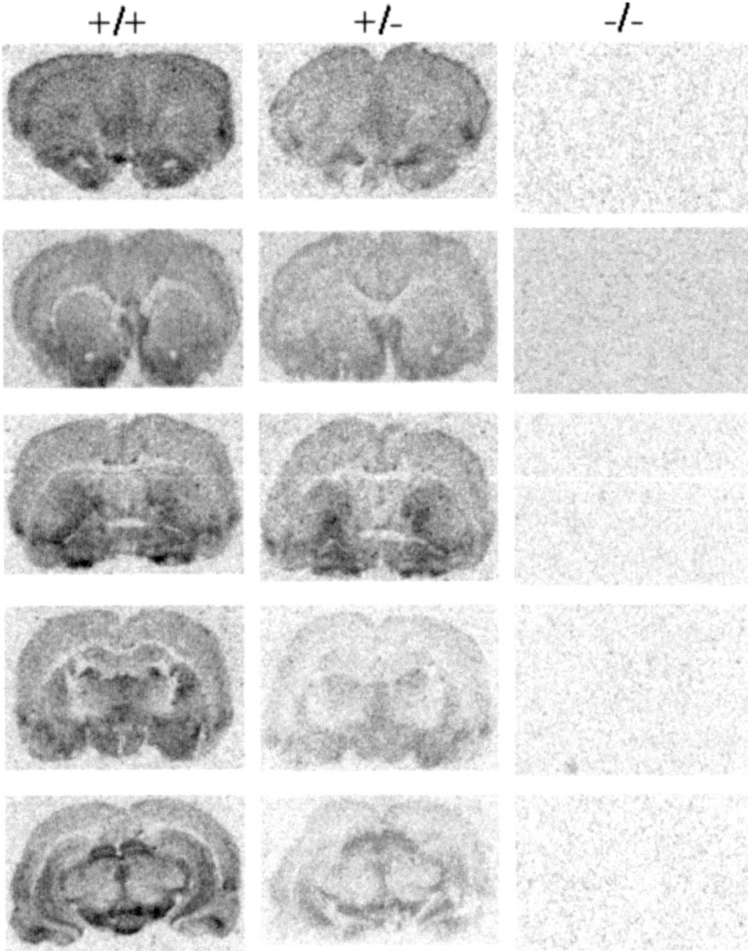

Figure 6.3 Representative [^{3}H]citalopram autoradiograms of coronal brain sections from male SERT+/+, SERT+/−, and SERT−/− rats show that SERT protein is completely absent in homozygous knock-out animals and is reduced in heterozygous animals. Areas include amygdala, bed nucleus stria terminals, caudate putamen, dorsal raphe nuclei, hippocampus, hypothalamus, median raphe nuclei, nucleus accumbens, prefrontal cortex, substantia nigra, somatosensory cortex, thalamus. Reused from Homberg *et al.* (2007a), with kind permission of Elsevier Limited.

spontaneous activity, respiration rate, and tremor), behavior in an open arena (transfer arousal, locomotor activity, palpebral closure, piloerection, startle response, gait, pelvic elevation, tail elevation, touch escape, and positional passivity), behaviors recorded on or above the arena (trunk curl, limb grasping, visual placing, grip strength, body tone, pinna reflex, corneal reflex, toe pinch, and wire movement) were not different between genotypes. In addition, during supine restraint several physiological and behavioral measurements were made (skin color, heart rate, limb tone, abdominal tone, lacrimation, salivation, provoked biting, righting reflex, contact righting reflex, negative geotaxis, fear, irritability, aggression, vocalization, and body temperature). No differences were found in the general appearance of male SERT+/+ and SERT−/− rats (J. Olivier, unpublished observations). However, the body weight of female SERT−/− rats compared to female SERT+/+ rats is reduced by 10% from the age of 3 weeks, while the weight of male SERT−/− rats is not different from SERT+/+ rats (Homberg *et al.*, 2007a).

To generate experimental animals, SERT+/− × SERT+/− crossings are maintained, with litter sizes of 10 on average and a Mendelian distribution of +/+, −/− and +/− alleles. After 8–10 generations of outcrossings it is possible to perform SERT−/− × SERT−/− and SERT+/+ × SERT+/+ crossings to maintain the line and produce proper control animals, although the reproductivity may be slightly reduced in SERT−/− × SERT−/− crossings (J. Homberg and J. Olivier, unpublished observations). However, one should realize that the genetic background of SERT−/− rats and control SERT+/+ rats may differ in a more systematic way than when using littermates as controls, which may confound measurements.

SEROTONIN HOMEOSTASIS

Presynaptic adaptations

Throughout development, neuroplastic events are likely to have taken place which compensate for the lifelong reduced 5-HT uptake in SERT+/− and SERT−/− rats. An overview of the possible adaptations that have been studied in the SERT−/− rats are listed in Table 6.1. The most obvious consequence of the absence of the SERT is that extraneuronal 5-HT levels are strongly increased in both male and female SERT−/− rats, as measured by microdialysis with the dialysis probe located in the hippocampus (Figure 6.4; Homberg *et al.*, 2007a; J. Olivier, manuscript submitted), a strongly serotonergic innervated region of interest for many types of behavior.

Table 6.1. *An overview of serotonin homeostasis and adaptive presynaptic processes tested in SERT−/− rats. All results are indicated as SERT−/− rats versus SERT+/+ rats*

Measurement	Tissue	Method	Results: SERT−/− rats versus SERT+/+ rats
Extraneuronal 5-HT levels	Hippocampus	Microdialyses	Ninefold higher
Tryptophan hydroxylase	Several brain regions	Enzymatic reactivity	No difference
Tryptophan hydroxyase	DRN	Immunoreactivity	No difference
MAO-A activity	Various brain regions	Enzymatic reactivity	No difference
5-HT tissue levels	Various brain areas	HPLC	55–75% reduced
5-HIAA tissue levels	Various brain areas	HPLC	45–50% reduced
Ca^{2+}-dependent 5-HT release	Superfused brain slices	Superfused electrically evoked [^{3}H]5-HT release	Reduced
5-HT levels	CSF	HPLC	Reduced
5-HIAA/5-HT ratio	CSF	HPLC	Increased
5-HT uptake with DAT blocker	Hippocampal synaptosomes	[^{3}H]5-HT uptake	Residual 5-HT uptake in SERT−/− rats
5-HT uptake with DAT and NET blocker	Hippocampal synaptosomes	[^{3}H]5-HT uptake	Residual uptake abolished in SERT−/− rats
Ca^{2+}-dependent DA release	Various brain areas	Superfused electrically evoked [^{3}H]DA release	No difference
Ca^{2+}-dependent NE release	Various brain areas	Superfused electrically evoked [^{3}H]NE release	No difference
SERT binding	Various brain areas	Autoradiography	Completely absent

DAT binding	Various brain areas	Autoradiography	No difference
NET binding	Various brain areas	Autoradiography	No difference
DA tissue level	Various brain areas	HPLC	No difference
NE tissue levels	Various brain areas	HPLC	Decreased in amygdala only
HVA tissue levels	Various brain areas	HPLC	Decreased in amygdala only
DOPAC tissue levels	Various brain areas	HPLC	No difference
Ca^{2+}-dependent ACH, GABA, glutamate release	Various brain areas	Superfused electrically/4-AP evoked [^{3}H] neurotransmitter release	No difference

Notes: 5-HT, serotonin (5-hydroxytryptamine); 5-HIAA, 5-hydroxyindoleacetic acid; CSF, cerebro-spinal fluid; DA, dopamine; DAT, dopamine transporter; DOPAC, 3,4-dihydroxyphenylacetic acid; DRN, dorsal raphe nuclei; HAC, high-performance liquid chromatography; HVA, homovanillic acid; MAO, monoamine oxidase; NE, norepinephrine; SERT, serotonin transporter.

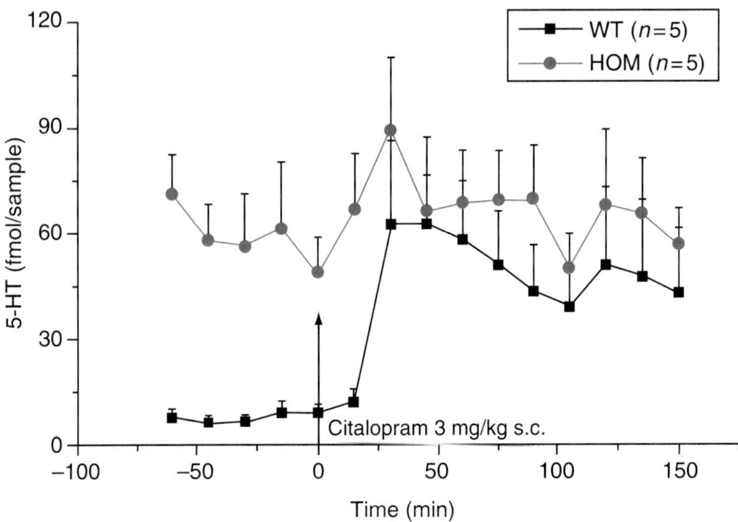

Figure 6.4 Extracellular 5-HT levels in the ventral hippocampus of male SERT+/+ and SERT−/− rats as measured by in vivo microdialysis. Basal dialysate 5-HT levels are ninefold increased in SERT−/− rats. Citalopram (3 mg/kg) increased 5-HT levels in SERT+/+ rats to that of SERT−/− rats, while citalopram had no effect in SERT−/− rats. Data represent mean (± SEM) extracellular 5-HT (fmol/sample). Reused from Homberg *et al.* (2007a), with kind permission of Elsevier Limited.

Compensatory adaptations are likely to have taken place to enable the organism to "cope" with this extreme condition. Presynaptically, the serotonergic system would be expected to be "silenced", as the serotonergic tone is already high. Tryptophan hydroxylase (5-HT synthesis) and monoamine oxidase (MAO-A; 5-HT degradation) enzymatic activity are not different between genotypes across several brain regions, including the raphe nuclei. These findings are supported by the absence of genotype differences in tryptophan hydroxylase immunoreactivity in the dorsal raphe nuclei (Homberg *et al.*, 2007a). While the 5-HT synthesis and degradation machinery seem to function normally, 5-HT tissue levels are reduced by approximately 55–75% and 5-hydroxyindoleacetic acid (5-HIAA) levels by approximately 45–50% in various brain regions (Homberg *et al.*, 2007a, 2007c). We assume that 5-HT tissue levels predominantly reflect intracellular 5-HT content. Thus, intracellular 5-HT levels are decreased in neurons of SERT−/− rats, while extracellular 5-HT levels are increased. If less 5-HT is available for release and 5-HT release will have little effect on neurotransmission processes because of the high endogenous 5-HT tone, it is expected that 5-HT release would be attenuated. That is exactly what has been found for electrically evoked Ca^{2+}-dependent 5-HT release in superfused brain slices (Homberg *et al.*, 2007a). Together, the findings of substantially reduced 5-HT uptake and release, and reduced 5-HT tissue levels indicate that 5-HT recylcing might be attenuated in SERT−/− rats, which further implies that the serotonergic system has lost its dynamics and flexibility. Thus, it is tempting to suggest that 5-HT homeostasis may be changed in such a way that the animal is able to function normally under basal conditions, but when exposed to challenges or stimuli, this system may not be able to adapt appropriately, resulting in aberrant behavioral responses.

Interestingly, 5-HT levels in CSF are significantly reduced and the 5-HIAA/5-HT ratio in CSF is increased in SERT−/− knock-out rats (Homberg *et al.*, 2007c). Because selected subsets of serotonergic dorsal raphe neurons project to the ependymal wall of the ventricular system in the rat (Simpson *et al.*, 1998), CSF 5-HIAA and 5-HT levels may particularly reflect 5-HT homeostasis processes in the raphe nuclei. Otherwise, the CSF may collect the freely diffusible 5-HIAA from diverse brain regions. Overall, the CSF measurements suggest that 5-HT turnover is increased in SERT−/− rats, which is in line with the increased serotonergic tone in this mutant rat model (Homberg *et al.*, 2007a). This notion is very valuable in the interpretation of CSF 5-HIAA measurements in humans and non-human primates in relation to central serotonergic activity (Fairbanks *et al.*, 2001; Linnoila *et al.*, 1983).

Despite a 40% reduction in SERT binding (Homberg *et al.*, 2007a), there are no differences in 5-HT tissue levels and 5-HT release in SERT+/− rats, probably because 5-HT uptake (Homberg *et al.*, 2007a) and extraneuronal 5-HT levels (J. Homberg and J. Olivier, unpublished observations) are only slightly reduced and increased, respectively, in these animals compared to SERT+/+ rats. Hence, there may be at least a redundancy of 40–50% in SERT availability. 5-HT uptake in hippocampal synaptosomes is strongly decreased in SERT−/− rats, but not completely absent, which suggests that there are alternative routes by which 5-HT can be taken up from the synaptic cleft. The monoamine transporters are neuron-specific, but not neurotransmitter-specific, and have low affinity and reuptake capacity for monoamines that do not match the monoamine transporter. Under extreme conditions; e.g. high levels of monoamines, the high affinity "monoamine-own" uptake process will be over-ruled by the abundancy of other monoamines, resulting in the uptake of "false" neurotransmitters (Vizi *et al.*, 2004). The hippocampus is noradrenaline-enriched. In this region, combined dopamine (DAT) and noradrenaline (NET) transporter blockade, but not DAT blockade alone, prevents the reuptake of residual 5-HT in SERT−/− rats (Homberg *et al.*, 2007a), suggesting that the NET is responsible for residual 5-HT uptake in the hippocampus of SERT−/− rats. In dopamine-rich regions, e.g. the striatum, it is expected that residual 5-HT uptake will take place via the DAT, as has been reported in SERT−/− mice (Zhou *et al.*, 2002). Due to false 5-HT uptake, DAT or NET blockade in SERT−/− models will not only result in increases in extracellular DA or NE levels, but also 5-HT levels (Shen *et al.*, 2004).

The 5-HT system interacts with several other (neurotransmitter) systems, and secondary to the changes in 5-HT homeostasis in the knock-out rat, these systems may adapt as well. The presynaptic function of dopaminergic and noradrenergic neurons has been studied by measuring the electrically evoked Ca^{2+}-dependent dopamine (DA) and noradrenaline (NE) release. Despite the high endogenous 5-HT tonus, no change is observed in DA and NE release. The absence of presynaptic adaptations in dopaminergic and noradrenergic neuron function is further supported by the lack of genotype differences in DAT and NET binding and tissue levels of DA, NE, and their metabolites homovanillic acid (HVA) and 3,4-dihydroxyphenylacetic acid (DOPAC). The exception is NE levels in the amygdala, which are decreased in SERT−/− rats, along with HVA levels. Also, the reactivity of cholinergic, glutamatergic, and GABAergic neurons are not changed in SERT−/− rats (Homberg *et al.*, 2007a). Together, these data suggest that compensatory adaptations in response to the constitutive absence of the SERT are found predominantly in the serotonergic system. This observation makes the SERT−/− rat very valuable for studying the role of the serotonergic system in any system of interest, although it should be kept in mind that, due to the lifelong increased 5-HT tonus, the SERT−/− condition is not directly comparable to the consequences of acute rises in 5-HT.

LOCOMOTOR ACTIVITY

Analysis of locomotor activity and related parameters, under novel and habituated conditions, is highly informative in obtaining a general behavioral profile of animals, and is relevant to the interpretation of more specified behavioral tests in which locomotor activity is unequivocally involved. The Phenotyper® (Noldus Technology, Wageningen, The Netherlands), an automated behavioral observation system that monitors behavior of individually housed animals for 24 h/7 d (de Visser *et al.*, 2006), is ideal to measure both responses towards novelty and habituated behavior. SERT−/− rats do not show abnormalities in novelty-induced

Table 6.2. *The effects of 5-HT_{1A} agonists and antagonist on hypothermia and stress-induced hyperthermia (SIH). Results are indicated as SERT−/− rats versus SERT+/+ rats*

Drug	Dose	Hypothermia SERT−/− rats vs. SERT+/+ rats	SIH SERT−/− rats vs. SERT+/+ rats
8-OHDPAT	0.25 mg/kg	↓	SIH ↓
Flesinoxan	3 and 10 mg/kg	Completely absent	SIH ↓
S-15535	2.5 and 5 mg/kg	–	SIH ↑
WAY100635	0.1 and 1 mg/kg	–	SIH ↑

locomotor activity (Homberg *et al.*, manuscript submitted). However, while SERT+/+ rats explore the entire cage, SERT−/− rats avoid the center of the cage and show thigmotaxis. This phenotype is maintained over 6 days (J. Homberg, unpublished observations), and also observed on a large open field (J. Olivier, manuscript submitted), suggesting that SERT−/− rats consistently show anxiety-like exploratory behavior. Finally, in the Phenotyper® SERT−/− rats spend more time in the shelter – which the animals use as sleep localization – than SERT+/+ rats (J. Homberg, unpublished observations), which may be related to increased anxiety or changes in sleeping behavior.

PHARMACOLOGICAL RESPONSES

5-HT_{1A} receptor ligands

SERT−/− rats exhibit ninefold increases in extraneuronal 5-HT levels (Homberg *et al.*, 2007a) that could affect the functioning or responsivity of 5-HT receptors, as has been reported after chronic SSRI treatment (Blier *et al.*, 1990; Briley and Moret, 1993). To address this issue, the effect of flesinoxan (5-HT_{1A} receptor agonist), 8-OHDPAT (5-$HT_{1A/7}$ receptor agonist) and S-15535 (selective somatodendritic 5-HT_{1A} receptor agonist and weak partial postsynaptic 5-HT_{1A} receptor agonist (de Boer *et al.*, 2000; Millan *et al.*, 1993a; Newman-Tancredi *et al.*, 1999)) on body temperature and stress-induced hyperthermia (SIH) have been measured, processes that are well known to be modulated by 5-HT_{1A} receptor ligands (Bouwknecht *et al.*, 2000; Cryan *et al.*, 1999; Olivier *et al.*, 1998). Results of the 5-HT_{1A} receptor (ant)agonists on hypothermia and SIH are summarized in Table 6.2. In the SERT−/− rat, 0.25 mg/kg 8-OHDPAT-induced hypothermia is significantly decreased, but not completely abolished (Homberg *et al.*, manuscript submitted). In contrast, flesinoxan-induced (10 mg/kg) hypothermia is completely absent in SERT−/− rats (Olivier *et al.*, manuscript submitted). The 8-OHDPAT dose may have been too low to completely block the hypothermic response in SERT−/− rats. Otherwise, 8-OHDPAT and flesinoxan may exert their effects via distinct populations of 5-HT receptors. As the effect of flesinoxan in SERT+/+ rats is antagonized by the selective 5-HT_{1A} receptor antagonist WAY100635 (Olivier *et al.*, manuscript submitted), the different responses to 8-OHDPAT as opposed to flesinoxan may be related to activation of 5-HT_7 receptors by 8-OHDPAT. While flesinoxan dose-dependently (0.3–10 mg/kg) inhibits SIH and additionally induces hypothermia in SERT+/+ rats, a threefold higher dose is needed to inhibit SIH in SERT−/− rats, and no additional hypothermia is observed (Olivier *et al.*, manuscript submitted). This higher dose needed to reduce SIH may be due to the absence of an additional effect of hypothermia as found in SERT+/+. S-15535 (2.5 and 5.0 mg/kg) attenuates SIH in SERT+/+ and SERT+/− rats, but in SERT−/− rats the same doses facilitates SIH (Homberg *et al.*, manuscript submitted). Finally, WAY100635 alone strongly enhances SIH in SERT−/− rats, but not in SERT+/+ rats (Olivier *et al.*, manuscript submitted). These findings clearly indicate that the responsivity to 5-HT_{1A} receptor ligands is changed in SERT−/− rats. The lower responsivity to 5-HT_{1A} receptor agonists may be explained either by constitutive occupation of 5-HT_{1A} receptors due to the high endogenous 5-HT tonus, or by desensitization of the receptors as a compensatory adaptive response to the high endogenous 5-HT tonus, or both.

The remarkable response to WAY100635 in SERT−/− rats is most likely explained by the high endogenous 5-HT tonus, such that WAY100635 is competing with endogenous 5-HT occupation of 5-HT_{1A} receptors. Likewise, the S-15535-mediated facilitation of SIH in SERT−/− rats may be the result of 5-HT_{1A} receptor antagonistic effects of the compound, as partial agonists function as antagonists when neurotransmitter levels are high. In rats (e.g. Bill *et al.*, 1991; Goodwin *et al.*, 1987; Millan *et al.*, 1993b) and humans (Blier *et al.*, 2002), 5-HT_{1A} receptor-mediated hypothermia is thought to be mediated by postsynaptic 5-HT_{1A} receptors, while in mice the somatodendritic 5-HT_{1A} receptors seem to be involved (Goodwin *et al.*, 1985; Martin *et al.*, 1992). However, some studies also suggest that 5-HT_{1A} receptor-mediated hypothermia in rats is mediated by somatodendritic 5-HT_{1A} receptors (Higgins *et al.*, 1988; Hillegaart, 1991).

As S-15535, which has predominantly somatodendritic 5-HT_{1A} receptor effects, lacks hypothermic effects (de Boer *et al.*, 2000; Millan *et al.*, 1993a), the 8-OHDPAT- and flesinoxan-mediated hypothermic responses may be exerted via postsynaptic 5-HT_{1A} receptors. Hence, the response profile of SERT−/− rats may suggest that postsynaptic 5-HT_{1A} receptors are fully occupied in SERT−/− rats and/or (slightly) desensitized. This is further supported by the finding that 8-OHDPAT induces locomotor activity and 5-HT syndrome symptoms less strongly in SERT−/− rats compared to SERT+/+ rats when habituated, responses that have been attributed to postsynaptic 5-HT_{1A} receptors consistently (Yamada *et al.*, 1988). Regarding the SIH, it is not clear whether this short-lasting thermogenic effect is mediated by somatodendritic or postsynaptic 5-HT_{1A} receptors, or both. The fact that S-15535 dose-dependently attenuates SIH in SERT+/+ and SERT+/− rats (Homberg *et al.*, manuscript submitted) indicates that somatodendritic sites are involved. Whether the failure of S-15535 to reduce SIH in SERT−/− rats reflects somatodendritic 5-HT_{1A} receptors desensitization or whether the postsynaptic antagonistic effects of S-15535 – due to the high endogenous 5-HT tonus – completely over-rule the somatodendritic effects of this compound cannot be deduced from these data. However, the finding that flesinoxan reduces the SIH in SERT−/− rats suggests that 5-HT_{1A} receptors involved in SIH may be more or less sensitive to 5-HT_{1A} agonists and represent a different population of 5-HT_{1A} receptors than those involved in hypothermia.

While the 5-HT_{1A} receptor-mediated autonomic responses have not provided sufficient data from which a firm conclusion can be drawn regarding enhanced 5-HT_{1A} receptor occupation or receptor desensitization, autoradiography studies reveal slight, but significant, decreases in 5-HT_{1A} receptor density in the raphe nuclei and several terminal regions (Homberg *et al.*, manuscript submitted). Hence, reduced expression of the 5-HT_{1A} receptor may partially explain the reduced responsivity to 5-HT_{1A} receptor agonists in SERT−/− rats.

Cocaine

Cocaine exerts its behavioral effects primarily via inhibition of the DAT, NET, and SERT (Heikkila *et al.*, 1975), with approximately equal affinity for each transporter (Reith *et al.*, 1980). While DA has been the primary focus in research on the rewarding effects of cocaine (Koob, 1992; Pierce and Kumaresan, 2006), accumulating evidence suggests that 5-HT plays an important modulatory role in cocaine reward, although this process is not understood fully. For example, chronic treatment with the SSRI fluoxetine in preclinical and clinical trials results in both positive and negative effects on cocaine self-administration and cocaine's subjective effects (Walsh and Cunningham, 1997). To extend our insight into the serotonergic mechanisms that mediate the rewarding effects of cocaine, the SERT−/− rat has been tested in three distinct paradigms, which measure different aspects of cocaine's behavioral effects. In the open field test, the motor-stimulating effect of 20 mg/kg cocaine occurs more rapidly and lasts longer in SERT−/− rats compared to SERT+/+ rats. Further, cocaine-induced conditioned place preference is increased in SERT−/− rats, such that the dose–response curve (5, 7.5, 10 mg/kg cocaine) is shifted to the left. SERT−/− rats have also been tested for intravenous cocaine self-administration, a paradigm that is especially well-established in the rat (Griffith *et al.*, 1980). During acquisition (fixed ratio 1; FR1) SERT−/− rats self-administer higher amounts of cocaine when a low dose is available (0.3 mg/kg/infusion), but not when a high dose is available (0.6 mg/kg/infusion). During a progressive ratio (PR) schedule, in which the number of responses required to obtain a drug infusion is exponentially increased (Hodos, 1961; Richardson and Roberts, 1996), SERT−/− are highly motivated to self-administer cocaine, particularly when a high dose is available (0.9 mg/kg/infusion) (Homberg *et al.*, manuscript submitted). These data indicate that the SERT−/− rat is hypersensitive to the rewarding and motivational properties of cocaine. The number of inactive (non-rewarded) responses during the PR, but not FR1, schedule is also significantly increased in SERT−/− rats. As SERT−/− rats fail to stop responding towards the previously rewarded nose poke hole, increased rewarded and non-rewarded responding during the PR schedule may reflect persistence, driven by the initial cocaine hypersensitivity.

The neurochemical responses to cocaine have been studied using microdialysis, with dialysis probes positioned in the rostral part of the nucleus accumbens shell and the ventral part of the hippocampus. Upon receiving a 10 mg/kg cocaine challenge, the percentage of DA and NE release is similar in SERT+/+ and SERT−/− rats, whereas the 5-HT response is significantly lower in SERT−/− rats compared to SERT+/+ rats (unpublished observations). This finding may be attributed to the absence of the SERT in SERT−/− rats, such that cocaine-induced 5-HT release via inhibition of the SERT cannot take place. False 5-HT release by dopaminergic and/or noradrenergic neurons may contribute to the small serotonergic response to cocaine in SERT−/− rats. These data suggest that 5-HT dampens the rewarding effects of cocaine, which is consistent with findings that acute SSRIs, which result in an increase in extraneural 5-HT levels, reduce cocaine self-administration

Table 6.3. *An overview of the responsiveness of SERT+/+ and SERT−/− rats to cocaine in distinct behavioral paradigms, with or without 5-HT$_{1A/1B}$ receptor (ant)agonist pretreatment*

Test	Drug doses	Responsivity of SERT−/− and SERT+/+ rats
Open field	20 mg/kg cocaine	Latency hyperactivity decreased in SERT−/− rats. Duration hyperactivity increased in SERT−/− rats
Conditioned place preference	5, 7.5, and 10 mg/kg cocaine	Increased conditioned place preference in SERT−/− rats
Self-administration (FR1)	0.3 mg/kg cocaine	Higher rate of self-administration in SERT−/− rats
Self-administration (FR1)	0.6 mg/kg cocaine	No difference between SERT+/+, SERT+/−, and SERT−/−
Self-administration (PR schedule)	0.9 mg/kg cocaine	Increased motivation to self-administer cocaine in SERT−/− rats
Microdialysis	10 mg/kg cocaine	Decreased 5-HT response in SERT−/− rats. No differences in NE and DA responses between SERT+/+, SERT+/− and SERT−/−

(Carroll *et al.*, 1990; Homberg *et al.*, 2004; Peltier and Schenk, 1993; Richardson and Roberts, 1991).

The mechanism underlying this 5-HT dampening is not understood. As the responsivity to 5-HT receptor ligands, and possibly 5-HT receptor function, is altered in SERT−/− rats, downstream neurotransmission processes may contribute to this 5-HT dampening. To study whether changes in 5-HT$_{1A}$ receptor function/responsivity contribute to the cocaine hypersensitivity, the effect of the 5-HT$_{1A}$ receptor agonists 8-OHDPAT, S-15535 and the selective 5-HT$_{1A}$ receptor antagonist WAY100635 on the locomotor effects of cocaine have been tested. The results are summarized in Table 6.3. When rats are challenged with 10 mg/kg cocaine, a dose which fails to induce a significant locomotor response in SERT+/+ and SERT−/− rats, both 8-OHDPAT (0.25 mg/kg) and S-15535 (2.5 mg/kg) pretreatment potentiate locomotor activity in SERT−/− rats only. When rats are challenged with 20 mg/kg cocaine, 8-OHDPAT strongly enhances cocaine-induced hyperactivity in SERT+/+ rats, such that SERT+/+ rats are more active than 8-OHDPAT and saline pretreated SERT−/− rats. S-15535 pretreatment potentiates cocaine-induced locomotor activity in SERT+/+ rats, and their locomotor response reaches the response level of SERT−/− rats. Neither 8-OHDPAT nor S-15535 affects locomotor activity in SERT−/− rats at the 20 mg/kg cocaine dose. Because WAY100635, at 0.25 mg/kg (inhibiting postsynaptic 5-HT_{1A} receptors) and at 0.05 mg/kg (inhibiting somatodendritic 5-HT_{1A} receptors) reduces cocaine-induced locomotor activity (20 mg/kg cocaine dose) in SERT−/− rats only (Homberg *et al.*, manuscript submitted), the failure of 8-OHDPAT and S-15535 to further increase cocaine-induced activity in SERT−/− rats is likely to be explained by the maximum activation of 5-HT_{1A} receptors – due to receptor desensitization or full occupation of receptor under high 5-HT tonus. The message that can be drawn from these findings is that secondary reduced function/responsivity of 5-HT_{1A} receptors contributes to cocaine hypersensitivity, such that the effects of low cocaine doses are facilitated, and a ceiling effect is obtained at high cocaine doses. Holding the (underpinned) assumption that the effect of S-15535 is predominantly mediated via somatodendritic 5-HT_{1A} receptors and the effect of 8-OHDPAT predominantly via postsynaptic 5-HT_{1A} receptors (Homberg *et al.*, manuscript submitted), the data suggest that somatodendritic and postsynaptic 5-HT_{1A} receptor-mediated effects on cocaine-induced locomotor activity follow the same direction. This observation is rather remarkable, considering that S-15535 mediated reduction in raphe firing rate via inhibitory 5-HT_{1A} autoreceptors (Millan *et al.*, 1993b), and 8-OHDPAT mediated facilitation of 5-HT neurotransmission via postsynaptic 5-HT_{1A} receptors. Other 5-HT receptors may also contribute to the cocaine hypersensitivity of SERT−/− rats. For instance, the 5-HT_{1B} receptor, the agonist CP94,253 potentiates cocaine's locomotor activating effects at 20 mg/kg in SERT+/+ rats. As is seen for S-15535, a reduction in the response latency and an increase in the response duration is observed. The failure of SERT−/− rats to respond to CP94,253 suggests that 5-HT_{1B} receptors might be subresponsive/desensitized in these animals as well. Autoradiography does not indicate genotype differences in 5-HT_{1B} receptor binding (J. Homberg, unpublished observations), at least implying that the underlying mechanism does not involve receptor downregulation.

Although no differences are observed in DA and NE release upon a cocaine challenge between SERT+/+ and SERT−/− rats, in view of the complex interactions between central 5-HT, DA, and NA systems, a contribution of the dopaminergic and noradrenergic systems, secondary to the changes in the serotonergic system, cannot be ruled out. The generally held assumption is that 5-HT mediates the aversive effects of cocaine, while DA mediates its rewarding effects. If 5-HT mediated the anxiogenic effects of cocaine (Paine *et al.*, 2002), the reduced cocaine-induced 5-HT release in SERT−/− rats (unpublished observations) may explain the cocaine hypersensitivity. Otherwise, under homeostasis 5-HT and DA levels are in balance. A possibility is that when the change in 5-HT is small after a cocaine challenge in SERT−/− rats, cocaine hypersensitivity can be indirectly the result of a more dopaminergic type of response to cocaine (Carey *et al.*, 2004, 2005).

Alcohol

Studies in rodents have shown that ethanol significantly elevates extracellular levels of forebrain 5-HT (Daws *et al.*, 2006; Le Marquand *et al.*, 1994; McBride *et al.*, 1993). Further supporting a functional relationship between ethanol and the SERT, significant reductions in SERT binding have been found in the living and postmortem brains of alcoholics (Heinz *et al.*, 2000; Kranzler *et al.*, 2002), and SSRIs attenuate ethanol intake in animal models of alcoholism (LeMarquand *et al.*, 1994; Maurel *et al.*, 1999; Naranjo *et al.*, 1990). Hence, under conditions of elevated extraneuronal 5-HT levels, the rewarding effects of ethanol are expected to be diminished. When SERT−/− rats are allowed to drink increasing concentrations of alcohol (2–12%) presented on alternate days in free choice with water, alcohol consumption and preference is decreased at 4–6% alcohol concentration, but not at higher concentrations (J. Homberg, unpublished observations). As alcohol is still palatable at 4–6%, but the amount of alcohol consumption is less than 1.5 g/kg – which is insufficient to exert pharmacological relevant effects – reduced alcohol drinking in SERT−/− rats may not reflect changes in the rewarding property of the alcohol solution, but rather is due to differences in palability of the solution.

ANXIETY AND DEPRESSION-RELATED BEHAVIOR

It is widely accepted that disturbances in the 5-HT system are involved in the onset of depression (reviewed in Jans *et al.*, 2007). Several alterations in the 5-HT system have been reported in depression, including decreased plasma tryptophan levels (Coppen *et al.*, 1973; Cowen *et al.*, 1989) and decreased levels of 5-HIAA in CSF (Asberg *et al.*, 1976a, 1976b; Owens and Nemeroff, 1998), suggesting an association between decreased central 5-HT metabolism and depressive symptoms. Moreover, brain imaging studies have reported a reduction in 5-HT_{1A}

receptor binding in depression (Drevets *et al.*, 1999; Sargent *et al.*, 2000). In humans, women experience depression about twice as often as men (Gorman, 2006). Possible explanations for this phenomenon are linked directly or indirectly to 5-HT neurotransmission. For example, in vivo measurements of 5-HT synthesis in the brain by positron emission tomography (PET) showed that whole brain rates of 5-HT synthesis is lower in women than in men (Nishizawa *et al.*, 1997). Moreover, women have lower SERT binding in the prefrontal cortex than do men (Mann *et al.*, 2000). Finally, depressed women show a decrease of SERT availability, while almost no decrease has been reported in men. In the SERT−/− rat, anxiety- and depression-related behaviors have been analyzed in both male and female rats to find out if females are more sensitive to the loss of the SERT compared to males. All anxiety- and depression-related behaviors of the SERT−/− rats are summarized in Table 6.4.

Anxiety-related behavior

To determine whether SERT−/− rats have an increased level of anxiety, they have been subjected to the open field test and the elevated plus maze. Decreases in time spent in the central part of the open field and on the open arm of the elevated plus maze are considered as indicators of anxiety-like behavior (Hogg, 1996; Prut and Belzung, 2003). Both male and female SERT−/− rats spend significantly less time in the central part of the open field and less time on the open arms of the elevated plus maze compared to their SERT+/+ littermates. SERT−/− rats have also been subjected to the novelty suppressed feeding (NSF) assay. The latency to approach the brightly lit center and start eating is considered to be an indication of anxiety (Shephard and Broadhurst, 1982). In this test, only male SERT−/− rats show a longer latency to start eating compared to SERT+/+ controls. The home cage emergence test has been used as a last assay to assess anxiety-related behaviors in the SERT−/− rats. In this test, an increased latency to escape the home cage is thought to reflect a heightened level of anxiety (Prickaerts *et al.*, 1996). Both male and female SERT−/− rats show a higher escape latency than SERT+/+ littermates. Together, these results indicate increases in anxiety levels in SERT−/− rats.

Depression-related behavior

Loss of interest or pleasure in events that are usually enjoyed (anhedonia) is a core symptom of depression. In animal studies

Table 6.4. *An overview of mood disorder-related symptoms and cognitive processes in SERT−/− and SERT+/+ rats. ↑ indicates increased behavioral performance of SERT−/− rats compared to SERT+/+ rats; ↓ indicates decreased behavioral performance of SERT−/− compared to SERT+/+ rats; – indicates no difference between SERT−/− and SERT+/+ rats*

Test	Behavior response measured	Symptomatology	Results: SERT−/− rats vs. SERT+/+ rats
Open field	Time center open field	Anxiety	↑ Thigomaxis (locomotor activity unchanged)
Elevated plus maze	Time open arm	Anxiety	↑
Novelty suppressed feeding	Latency to start eating	Anxiety	↑
Home cage emergence	Latency to leave the home cage	Anxiety	↑
Sucrose preference	Sucrose intake	Depression	↓
Forced swim test	Immobility	Depression	↑
Social play in juveniles		Social behavior	↓
Aggression	Attack latency	Social behavior	↑
Sexual behavior	Mount and intromission latency	Social behavior	↑
5-CSRTT (serial) reversal learning task	Premature responding	Motor impulsivity Cognitive flexibility	↓
PPI	Prepulse inhibition (3, 5, 10 dB)	Sensory gating	–
Startle habituation	Basal startle	Attention	–
Morris water maze	Latency time to find platform	Memory	↓
Spontaneous alternation test	Frequency of alternation	Perseverative behavior	–

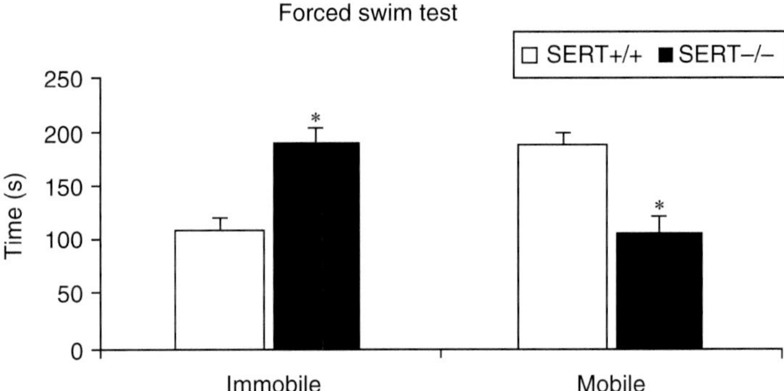

Figure 6.5 Immobility is increased and mobility is decreased in SERT–/– rats compared to SERT+/+ rats. The data represent mean ± SEM of the immobility time during a 5 min test. *$p<0.05$. Adapted from Olivier *et al.* (2008), with kind permission of Elsevier Limited.

a decreased consumption of palatable solutions is used to measure anhedonia. Antidepressants are effective against anhedonia (Muscat *et al.*, 1992; Willner *et al.*, 1987). In a two-bottle paradigm, SERT–/– rats consume less sucrose compared to SERT+/+ rats. Another measure of depression-like behavior is the immobility response in the forced swim test (FST). This response to the inescapable situation is considered as a state of behavioral despair, which is liable to antidepressant treatment (Connor *et al.*, 2000). Naïve SERT–/– rats show increased immobility compared to SERT+/+ rats (Olivier *et al.*, in press), suggesting an increased depression-like state in SERT–/– rats (Figure 6.5). Despite a higher general activity of females, no sex differences in anxiety- and depression-related behaviors have been found. Statistical analysis revealed no genotype × gender interactions (Olivier *et al.*, in press). If anything, male rats show a slightly increased expression of anxiety-related behaviors, since the latency to initiate food consumption in the NSF test is increased in male, but not female, SERT–/– rats compared to SERT+/+ rats. Thus, regardless of the basal 5-HT differences between males and females (Carlsson and Carlsson, 1988; Dominguez *et al.*, 2003; Haleem *et al.*, 1990; Watts and Stanley, 1984), these data show that lifelong absence of SERT in rats leads to a sex-independent increase of anxiety- or depression-like behavior. Apparently, the behavioral consequences of genetic inactivation of the SERT are so robust that any difference between male and female knock-out rats might be completely masked. This is in line with a human study, which reported that both male and female individuals with a short version of the SERT gene polymorphism are more prone to develop depression than those with the longer version (Mann *et al.*, 2000).

SOCIAL BEHAVIOR

There is a large body of literature associating 5-HT signaling with social behaviors in humans and animals. For instance, CSF 5-HIAA levels are inversely related to aggression in humans, primates, and rodents (Fairbanks *et al.*, 2001; Higley and Linnoila, 1997). SSRIs reduce impulsive aggression as well as sexual behavior in humans (New *et al.*, 2004; Olivier *et al.*, 2006).

Furthermore, depending on the social structure of the community, serotonergic drugs are able to interchange the dominant and subordinate status of primate community members (Edwards and Kravitz, 1997; Larson and Summers, 2001). It has been proposed that individual differences in 5-HT neurotransmission are an important neural underpinning of personality (Serretti *et al.*, 2006), based on the finding that central 5-HT levels are relatively stable over a lifetime (Higley and Linnoila, 1997). Studies showing that polymorphisms in 5-HT-related genes are linked to impulsive aggression in humans (Ferrari *et al.*, 2005; Haberstick *et al.*, 2006; Popova, 2006) provide support to the idea that the serotonergic modulation of social behavior is heritable (Higley and Linnoila, 1997). Social behavior and cognitive performance of SERT−/− rats are illustrated in Table 6.4.

Social play

Social play behavior is the earliest form of non-mother-directed social behavior in young mammals. Social play behavior consists of behavioral forms which are also found in adult sexual, affiliative, and aggressive encounters (Bolles and Woods, 1964; Poole and Fish, 1975). However, during social play, these behaviors are displayed in an out-of-context fashion (Poole and Fish, 1975). Social play is thought to promote social and cognitive development, because play deprivation (i.e. social isolation during periadolescence when social play peaks) has been found to result in behavioral disturbances, most prominently in the domain of social behaviors (e.g. Hol *et al.*, 1999; Van den Berg *et al.*, 1999). Because social play in rats is clearly manifested and has been well characterized, the rat is the preferred rodent species to study age-specific patterns of social behavior (Bolles and Woods, 1964; Poole and Fish, 1975; Vanderschuren *et al.*, 1997). Despite the well-recognized

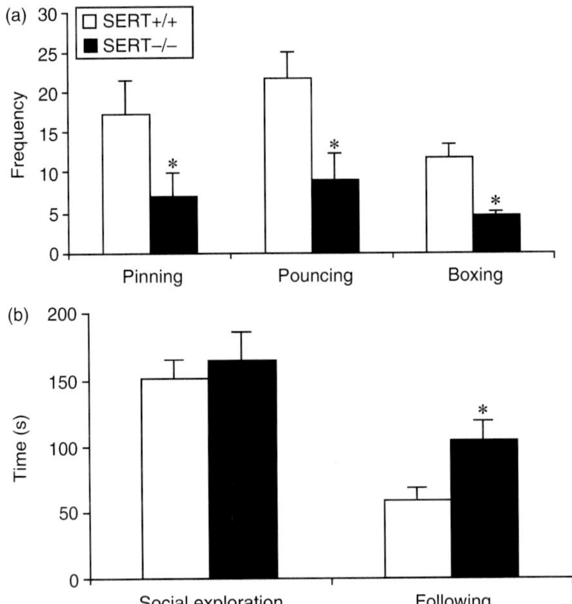

Figure 6.6 Social play behavior is reduced in juvenile male SERT−/− rats compared to SERT+/+ rats. The data represent mean ± SEM of the number of pins, pounces, and boxing/wrestling episodes (a) and mean ± SEM of the duration of social interactions, following/chasing and social grooming (b) during a 15 min test. *$p<0.05$ SERT−/− vs. SERT+/+. Reused from Homberg *et al.* (2007b), with kind permission of Springer Science and Business Media.

association between 5-HT and social behaviors, surprisingly little attention has been paid to the role of the serotonergic system in rat social play. Interestingly, periadolescent (aged between 28 and 35 days) SERT−/− rats play significantly less than SERT+/+ rats, while play-independent social behavior is unaffected in SERT−/− rats (Figure 6.6). However, following or chasing behavior – whose nature as a play behavior has not been agreed on among researchers – is increased in SERT−/− rats, suggesting that there is interest in the play partner, but that the animals for some reason are inhibited from engaging in full-blown social play. Acute treatment with fluoxetine and 3, 4-methylenedioxy-methamphetamine (MDMA or "ecstasy"), which are well known to induce an acute rise in extraneuronal 5-HT levels, similarly decrease social play in periadolescent wildtype rats, suggesting that reduced social play in SERT−/− rats is due to the high endogeous 5-HT tonus rather than to compensatory adaptations, e.g. in 5-HT receptor function (Homberg *et al.*, 2007b).

Aggression and sexual behavior

In line with the hypothesis that individual differences in 5-HT neurotransmission are an important neural underpinning of personality (Serretti *et al.*, 2006), the social inhibition in SERT−/− is extended into adulthood, as exemplified by reduced aggressive behavior (Homberg *et al.*, 2007c) and reduced sexual behavior (J. Homberg, unpublished observations). In particular, the attack latency, and the mount and intromission latencies, are increased in SERT−/− rats, possibly reflecting reduced social impulsivity (Fairbanks *et al.*, 2001). Together, the finding that 5-HT similarly modulates social behavior during periadolescence and adulthood indicates that 5-HT affects social behavior throughout development, consistent with the proposed trait-like relationship between 5-HT and social behavior (Higley and Linnoila, 1997).

COGNITION

"Motor" impulsivity

The five-choice serial reaction time task (5-CSRTT; Carli *et al.*, 1983) is a well-validated animal model to measure, among other parameters, "motor" impulsivity. In this task, animals have to respond to a cue light that is emitted from one of five holes within a limited period, and a correct response is rewarded by a food pellet. Responding before the presentation of the cue light is termed premature responding and is thought to reflect "motor" impulsivity. In line with the reduced social play, aggression, and sexual behaviors, SERT−/− rats display a decrease in premature responding. Concomitantly, the correct response latency is increased in SERT−/− rats. In contrast, attentional and motivational measurements are not affected in the SERT−/− rat. These data indicate that the increased behavioral inhibition displayed by SERT−/− rats in the 5-CSRTT is a selective phenotype (Figure 6.7). The improved inhibitory control of SERT−/− rats in the 5-CSRTT is in line with previous data indicating a modulatory role of 5-HT in inhibitory control processes. For instance, central 5-HT depletions have been found to increase premature responding (Harrison *et al.*, 1997; Winstanley *et al.*, 2004), whereas administration of the 5-HT releasing agent *d*-fenfluramine has been shown to decrease premature responding in the 5-CSRTT (Carli and Samanin, 1992). Taken together with data which show involvement of the serotonergic system in the medial prefrontal cortex (mPFC) in inhibitory control as measured in the 5-CSRTT (Chudasama *et al.*, 2003; Muir *et al.*, 1996; Passetti *et al.*, 2003; Winstanley *et al.*, 2003), these data

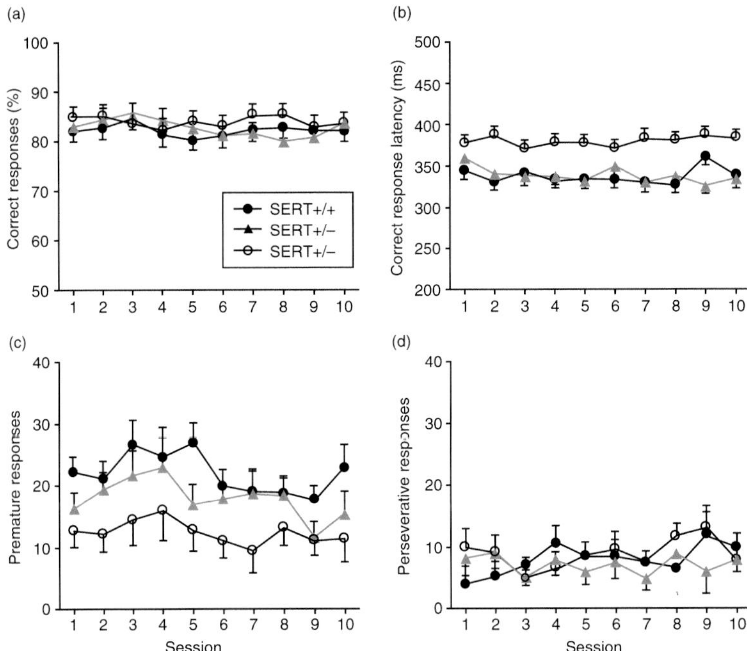

Figure 6.7 Premature responding in the 5-CSRTT is reduced in SERT−/− rats. Data depict mean (± SEM) percentage of accurate responding (a), latency to make a correct choice (b), number of premature responses (c) and number of perseverative responses after correct choice (d) during 10 consecutive baseline sessions. *$p<0.05$, SERT−/− different from SERT+/+ and SERT+/−. Reused from Homberg *et al.* (2007c), with kind permission of Blackwell Publishing.

suggest the possibility that 5-HT-mediated alteration in mPFC function underlies the improved behavioral control in SERT−/− rats. However, from the available data it cannot be deduced whether this modulatory role involves increased 5-HT tonus in the PFC, or compensatory 5-HT receptor adaptations, or both. Attentional processes, response selection, planning, and working memory, on the other hand, have been attributed to dorsal prefrontal cortical DA (Murphy *et al.*, 2002; Robbins, 2005; Winstanley *et al.*, 2006). Hence, the absence of genotype differences in attentional measurements in the 5-CSRTT is in line with the absence of genotype-related differences in DA tissue levels in, among others, the PFC (Homberg *et al.*, 2007c). These data are consistent with accumulating evidence that, at least within the PFC, inhibitory control and attentional function are neurochemically dissociable (for review, see Robbins, 2005).

Cognitive flexibility

Cognitive flexibility involves the adaptation of behavior according to changes in stimulus–reward contingencies. A test commonly used to measure cognitive flexibility is the (serial) reversal learning task, which requires the subject to reverse a visual discriminative operant (nose pose) response (de Bruin *et al.*, 2000; Rogers *et al.*, 1999) rewarded by three food pellets. As with motor impulsivity, negative correlations between 5-HT and reversal learning exist (Clarke *et al.*, 2004, 2005; Masaki *et al.*, 2006; Rogers *et al.*, 1999). Unexpectedly, behavioral flexibility is unaffected in SERT−/− rats (Homberg *et al.*, 2007c). A possibility is that there is a ceiling effect for the 5-HT to exert modulatory effects on behavioral flexibility, in which case further increases in serotonergic tone cannot further improve behavioral performance in the reversal learning paradigm. The integrity of the orbitofrontal cortex (OFC) is critical for flexible responding in reversal learning in rats (Boulougouris *et al.*, 2007). SERT−/− rats display reduced OFC tissue levels of 5-HT (Homberg *et al.*, 2007c), but whether this is related to altered OFC function in SERT−/− rats remains to be studied. Together with the 5-CSRRT findings, these data imply that there is a serotonergic dissociation between behavioral flexibility and inhibitory control, which is in line with earlier observations (Winstanley *et al.*, 2004).

Startle habituation, prepulse inhibition, spontaneous alteration, and Morris water maze

Cognitive deficits, which are notoriously resistant to treatment (Cannon *et al.*, 1994), are among the core symptoms of a large number of psychiatric disorders, especially schizophrenia (Saykin *et al.*, 1994). Although schizophrenic patients have a global deficit in all aspects of cognition, the deficit is particularly pronounced in a few specific areas, most notably sensory gating (automatic filtering of sensory information), attention, memory, and executive functioning (which is essential for planning and anticipation; Saykin *et al.*, 1994). Several different paradigms have been developed to assess these specific aspects of cognition. With respect to sensory gating, prepulse inhibition (PPI) is a well-validated model (Braff and Geyer, 1990). For attention, the habituation of the startle response is a suitable model, and with respect to memory, the Morris water maze is often used (Myers *et al.*, 2004). The spontaneous alternation test (Birrell and Brown, 2000) is accepted as a model to measure perseverative behavior.

Alterations in 5-HT neurotransmission have been reported to affect prepulse inhibition (Geyer *et al.*, 2001), startle habituation (Geyer and Tapson, 1988), and spontaneous alternation (Abel *et al.*, 1998; Seibell *et al.*, 2003). However, the exact role of 5-HT in these aspects of cognition still remains to be investigated. In the startle habituation test, both SERT−/− and SERT+/+ rats show a reduction in startle magnitude over time, without genotype differences (J. Olivier *et al.*, unpublished observations). In the prepulse inhibition test, the basal startle response, and PPI (3, 5, and 10 dB before 120 dB), are similar in SERT+/+ and SERT−/− rats. Also regarding spontaneous alteration, no differences have been found between SERT+/+ and SERT−/− rats (J. Olivier *et al.*, unpublished observations). Finally, in the Morris water maze, in which rats have four trials to find the platform, for four days in a row, SERT−/− rats show a longer latency to find the invisible platform compared to SERT+/+ rats. Especially in the first trial on the second day, SERT−/− rats need more time finding the platform. A visible platform test reveals that no motor coordination and vision differences between SERT+/+ and SERT-/- rats exist (J. Olivier *et al.*, unpublished observations). Moreover, no differences are found between SERT+/+ and SERT−/− in the probe trial. Overall, these results suggest that, in general, the SERT knock-out is not associated with changes in sensory gating, attention, memory, and perseverative behavior, with the exception of a modest effect in the Morris water maze.

PERIPHERAL MEASUREMENTS

Several lines of evidence suggest the involvement of 5-HT in the control of systemic blood pressure (Chon *et al.*, 2004; Ni *et al.*, 2006), but the role of 5-HT is far from clear (Watts, 2005). 5-HT in blood platelets plays a crucial role in vasoconstriction and has mitogenic activity in vascular smooth muscle (Watts, 2005). Along with SERT as the only mechanism available for 5-HT reuptake in platelets, SERT−/− rats almost completely lack 5-HT in blood platelets (Homberg *et al.*, 2006); nevertheless, no changes in basal systolic blood pressure have been found in SERT−/− rats. Further, the development of hypertension and renal damage upon nitric oxygen (NO) synthesis inhibition (LNNA) is comparable in SERT−/−, SERT+/−, and SERT+/+ rats. Left ventricular weight/body weight, proteinurea, plasma urea, plasma creatinine, and renal morphology under basal conditions and during LNNA treatment are also similar in SERT+/+, SERT+/−, and SERT−/− rats (Homberg *et al.*, 2006). From these findings it appears that the integrative role of the SERT in blood pressure control by systemic hemodynamics and by the kidney to protect against the hypertensive effects of NO shortage is limited.

5-HT has also been implicated in eating behavior and body weight regulation (Leibowitz and Alexander, 1998). A major concern of abdominal obesity is the association with metabolic syndrome and the increased risk for cardiovascular disease and diabetes mellitus in humans. While body weight of the SERT−/− rat is unaffected (males) or tends to be reduced (females), abdominal, but not subcutaneous, fat deposition is significantly enhanced. This is associated with increased plasma leptin and adiponectin levels, while glucose and insulin levels and total free lipids are unaltered in the knock-out rats (J. Homberg, unpublished observations). These data suggest that although SERT deficiency sex-specifically results in abdominal obesity, this occurs without the development of metabolic syndrome in the SERT−/− rat.

SYNTHESIS

Adaptive processes

The SERT−/− rat is one of the various genetic and pharmacological models available to study the role of 5-HT, and SERT, in any process in which 5-HT is potentially involved. A major concern of knock-out models is that the absence of a gene affects early development and that compensatory processes could have taken place. As such, phenotypes of a knock-out model may not be exclusively attributable to the gene that has been knocked-out, but also to secondary adaptations in interacting systems. Studying the function of the SERT itself may be best accomplished by using selective serotonin reuptake inhibitors (SSRIs), e.g. citalopram. Considering stable (genetic) individual differences in central serotonergic activity as an endophenotype underlying personality, such as harm avoidance (Gerra *et al.*, 2000) and social impulsivity (Fairbanks *et al.*, 2001), and those associated with the SERT promoter polymorphism (Dragan and Oniszczenko, 2006), SERT−/− models, including their adaptive mechanisms, are of major relevance. Insight into these processes is of importance because they may increase our understanding of interactions between systems, and adaptive capabilities of the central nervous system. Further, due to such adaptive processes, the impact of pharmacological compounds may change. Hence, individual differences in genetic, and consequently neurochemical, make-up may determine the efficacy of pharmacotherapies. When considering the SERT−/− rat as a potential model for inherited increased 5-HT levels, the pharmacological profile of these animals may have predictive value for pharmacological effects in humans exhibiting inherited increased central serotonergic activity.

Rat vs. mouse

Until now, rat genetic tools have clearly lagged behind those available for mice. Homologous recombination in embryonic stem (ES) cells, which is used to generate knock-out mice (for review see Capecchi, 1989), fails in rats. As an alternative, target-selected ENU-driven mutagenesis has been used to generate knock-out rats (Smits *et al.*, 2004, 2006; Zan *et al.*, 2003). ENU induces random point mutations, and the currently available mutation-detection techniques are insufficient to screen the entire genome for mutations, raising the possibility that additional mutations in the SERT−/− rats could have gone undetected. Using the homologous recombination technique in ES cells, the first SERT−/− mouse was generated 10 years ago (Bengel *et al.*, 1998), which has been characterized extensively afterwards (this book). To confirm that a premature stopcodon in the SERT gene results in a SERT−/− rat, and to establish whether rats and mice similarly adapt to the absence of the SERT, many measurements done in the SERT−/− mouse have been replicated in the SERT−/− rat. Interestingly, several phenotypes in SERT−/− mice and rats are comparable. For instance, both SERT−/− mice (Boyce-Rustay *et al.*, 2006; Carroll *et al.*, 2007; Fabre *et al.*, 2000; Fox *et al.*, 2007; Holmes *et al.*, 2002a, 2002b, 2003a, 2003b; Kalueff *et al.*, 2007a, 2007b; Kelaï *et al.*, 2003; Kim *et al.*, 2005; Lira *et al.*, 2003; Mathews *et al.*, 2004; Montañez *et al.*, 2003; Shen *et al.*, 2004; Sora *et al.*, 1998, 2001; Zhao *et al.*, 2006) and rats (Homberg *et al.*, 2007a–c; Homberg *et al.*, manuscript submitted; Olivier *et al.*, manuscript submitted) display strongly enhanced extraneuronal 5-HT levels; no change in in vitro MAO-A and TPH activity; reduced 5-HT and 5-HIAA tissue levels; unchanged NET density; no changes in DA, NE, DOPAC, and HVA tissue levels in the PFC, nucleus accumbens and caudate putamen; reduced responsivity to 5-HT$_{1A}$ ligands and reduced 5-HT$_{1A}$ receptor binding; thigmotaxis; increased anxiety and depression-related symptoms; increased cocaine-induced conditioned place preference; decreased cocaine-induced 5-HT release in the nucleus accumbens; reduced alcohol intake; and decreased aggression. These similarities in neurochemistry and behaviors indicate that phenotypes of SERT−/− rats are valid in the sense that the phenotypes in SERT−/− rats generally meet our expectations and are consistent with the literature. Moreover, they indicate that the influence of unknown additional mutations, if any are present, is minimal. Furthermore, these similarities between SERT−/− rat and mice models strengthen the assumption that gene function is conserved among species and thereby highlight the value of genetic animal models to understand gene function in humans. Differences between SERT−/− mice and rats also exist. For example, in contrast to SERT−/− rats (Homberg *et al.*, 2007a), there is no compensatory 5-HT uptake in hippocampal synaptosomes of SERT−/− mice (Bengel *et al.*, 1998); cocaine-induced locomotor activity is increased in SERT−/− rats (Homberg *et al.*, manuscript submitted) and decreased in SERT−/− mice (Wichems *et al.*, 1998); oral free-choice sucrose intake is decreased in SERT−/− rats (Olivier *et al.*, manuscript submitted), but not in SERT−/− mice (Kalueff *et al.*, 2006); and no changes in 5-HT_{1B} receptor binding are found in SERT−/− rats (Homberg *et al.*, unpublished findings), while regional changes in 5-HT_{1B} receptor binding have been found in SERT −/− mice (Fabre *et al.*, 2000). Finally, there are no differences in the number of immunopositive 5-HT neurons in the dorsal raphe nuclei between SERT−/− and SERT+/+ rats (J. Olivier *et al.*, manuscript submitted), while a 50% reduction of serotonergic cell number has been found in the SERT−/− mouse. It should be noted that techniques or experimental conditions used in mice and rat studies differ, which hamper direct rat–mouse comparisons. In addition, the SERT−/− has been generated in two different mouse inbred lines, which differ among themselves (Adamec *et al.*, 2006; Altamura *et al.*, 2007; Holmes *et al.*, 2003a), thereby further complicating comparisons with the SERT−/− rat that has been generated on an outbred Wistar background. Whether and how SERT−/− rat phenotypes are affected by genetic background is currently being investigated. Together, studying similarities and differences between SERT−/− rats and mice is highly informative for cross-species translation of results obtained in different rodent models and/or the extrapolation to the human situation.

Behavioral profile of SERT−/− rats

5-HT is involved in widespread central and peripheral processes and accordingly, the SERT−/− rat displays various phenotypes. Apparently, all these phenotypes can co-exist in one animal model, and combining these phenotypes may provide us with information regarding the inter-relationships between phenotypes. In summary, the SERT−/− rat displays anxiety- and depression-related symptoms, reduced social play, aggressive and sexual behavior, reduced impulsivity, improved long-term decision-making, cocaine hypersensitivity, and reduced alcohol intake. Overall, these phenotypes are not secondary effects of altered activity levels, motor, sensory, autonomic, or neurological deficits, as SERT−/− rats appear and behave normally, until exposure to stimuli that cannot be appropriately processed. Considering social behavior (Vanderschuren *et al.*, 1997) and sucrose as natural rewards, the SERT−/− rat may be generally hyposensitive to natural rewards. Social behavior, in particular the latency to initiate a social act, also reflects social impulsivity (Homberg *et al.*, 2007c). Improved behavioral control, as measured in the five-choice serial reaction time task (Homberg *et al.*, 2007c), therefore fits with the social reservation of SERT−/− rats.

Although the forced swim test is considered a depression model, immobility after experience of inescapable stress may be explained as impaired stress coping. Likewise, SERT−/− rats do not bury the shock prod in the shock prod burying test as do their SERT+/+ counterparts (S. de Boer, unpublished observations). Impaired stress coping may facilitate emotional responses to novel and stressful conditions and promote anxiety-like behaviors. While the anxiety models in which the SERT−/− rat has been tested involve acute models, in which the animals have been acutely exposed to novel and stressful conditions, the FST requires retesting of animals after an initial inescapable stress experience. Hence, the increased immobility response during the test, 24 h after the initial stress exposure, may actually reflect an enhanced conditioned response or improved recall of fear memory, as was found for SERT−/− mice in the fear conditioning test (Wellman *et al.*, 2007). As such, SERT−/− rats may well be capable of acquiring stimulus–response conditioned responses. This may not be true only for negative reinforcers such as inescapable stress, but may also apply to positive reinforcers. Thus, SERT−/− rats show enhanced cocaine-induced conditioned place preference, and are extremely motivated to self-administer cocaine under high effort/cost conditions. Nevertheless, this explanation does not resolve the finding that SERT−/− rats are less sensitive to natural rewards, including social behavior and sucrose, and are supersensitive to the acute effects of cocaine. The generally held assumption is that drugs of abuse act at the mesolimbic system that normally encodes natural reward of processes like food intake, and sexual behavior, and that both drugs of abuse and natural rewards trigger mesolimbic dopamine release, albeit to a different extent (Wise, 2002). If a common circuitry mediates any type of reward, one would expect that SERT−/−mediated changes in this reward system are similar to any type of reward. As this is not the case for cocaine vs. natural rewards in SERT−/− rats, this disparity may relate to the pharmacological effects of cocaine that may differentialy interact with the mesolimbic dopamine system. Similarly, several lines of evidence have shown that impulsive behavior and drug self-administration are positively associated (Dalley *et al.*, 2007), yet not in SERT−/− rats. In this regard, an intriguing question that remains to be answered is how cocaine affects behavioral control in SERT−/− rats. The SERT−/− rat displays a behavioral profile equivalent to increased stress-sensitivity and strong acquisition of conditioned responses, induced by either positive or negative reinforcers.

SSRIs

Interestingly, chronic SSRI treatment results in a profound reduction in SERT expression and function (Benmansour *et al.*, 1999), and increased extracellular 5-HT levels. Furthermore, SSRI-induced reduction in 5-HT_{1A} receptor function has been reported (Dawson *et al.*, 2002). Adaptations that have been observed in SERT−/− rats are strikingly similar. This may suggest that the SERT−/− rat can be considered as a model for studying the consequences of chronic SSRI treatment. However, SERT−/− rats paradoxically show anxiety- and depression-like phenotypes. Ansorge and colleagues (2004) have shown that early postnatal SSRI treatment induces rather than ameliorates anxiety- and depression-like symptoms during adulthood, which are comparable to symptoms found in SERT−/− mice. It has been hypothesized that hyperserotonemia at early stages of development can cause loss of 5-HT terminals in the brain that persists throughout subsequent development (Whitaker-Azmitia, 2005). Hence, early SSRI treatment or the constitutive loss of the SERT is expected to have profound effects on brain development (Persico *et al.*, 2001; Salichon *et al.*, 2001), which obviously differ from the impact of chronic SSRI on the mature brain (Taravosh-Lahn *et al.*, 2006). The finding that prenatal exposure to chronic fluoxetine increases cocaine sensitivity in adult rats (Forcelli and Heinrichs, 2007), together with the cocaine hypersensitivity found in SERT−/− rats (Homberg *et al.*, manuscript submitted), supports this developmental hyperserotonemia hypothesis. Otherwise, chronic SSRI treatment decreases aggressive (Fuller, 1996; Olivier, 2004) and sexual behavior (de Jong *et al.*, 2005) in rats, phenotypes that are also observed in SERT−/− rats (Homberg *et al.*, 2007c, and unpublished observations). Apparently, not all SERT−/− related behavioral phenotypes oppose those resulting from chronic SSRI treatment during adulthood. Although highly speculative, it is possible that some effects of chronic SSRI treatment relate directly to SERT inhibition and increased extraneuronal 5-HT levels, while others depend on associated compensatory adaptations.

CONCLUSION

Although the ENU-driven target-selected mutagenesis approach to generate knock-out rats could be associated theoretically with unknown mutations additional to the premature stopcodon in the SERT gene, the SERT−/− rat has proven to exhibit both expected and novel phenotypes that may contribute to the further understanding of the function of SERT and its role in diseases. Furthermore, the SERT−/− rat models several important endophenotypes, and can be used as such. While research on SERT−/− mice has already revealed several novel 5-HT-mediated phenotypes and processes, the SERT−/− rat allows complementary in-depth research through its greater accessibility of behavioral and neurochemical techniques. The SERT−/− rat has only recently been generated (Smits *et al.*, 2006), and based on the output the knock-out rat has already provided, we expect that this mutant will become a very valuable research tool in neuroscience research and beyond.

REFERENCES

Abel K, Waikar M, Pedro B, Hemsley D, Geyer M (1998). Repeated testing of prepulse inhibition and habituation of the startle reflex: a study in healthy human controls. *J Psychopharmacol* **12**: 330–7.

Adamec R, Burton P, Blundell J, Murphy D L, Holmes A (2006). Vulnerability to mild predator stress in serotonin transporter knockout mice. *Behav Brain Res* **170**: 126–40.

Altamura C, Dell'Acqua M L, Moessner R, Murphy D L, Lesch K P, Persico A M (2007). Altered neocortical cell density and layer thickness in serotonin transporter knockout mice: a quantitation study. *Cereb Cortex* **17**: 1394–401.

Ansorge M S, Zhou M, Lira A, Hen R, Gingrich J A (2004). Early-life blockade of the 5-HT transporter alters emotional behavior in adult mice. *Science* **306**: 879–81.

Asberg M, Thoren P, Traskman L, Bertilsson L, Ringberger V (1976a). "Serotonin depression" – a biochemical subgroup within the affective disorders? *Science* **191**: 478–80.

Asberg M, Träskman L, Thorén P (1976b). 5-HIAA in the cerebrospinal fluid. A biochemical suicide predictor? *Arch Gen Psychiatry* **33**: 1193–97.

Baker K E, Parker R (2004). Nonsense-mediated mRNA decay: terminating erroneous gene expression. *Curr Opin Cell Biol* **16**: 293–9.

Bengel D, Murphy D L, Andrews A M, *et al.* (1998). Altered brain serotonin homeostasis and locomotor insensitivity to 3,4-methylenedioxymethamphetamine ("Ecstasy") in serotonin transporter-deficient mice. *Mol Pharmacol* **53**: 649–55.

Benmansour S, Cecchi M, Morilak D A, *et al.* (1999). Effects of chronic antidepressant treatments on serotonin transporter function, density and mRNA level. *J Neuroscience* **19**: 10 494–501.

Bentley A, MacLennan B, Calvo J, Dearolf C R (2000). Targeted recovery of mutations in *Drosophila*. *Genetics* **156**: 1169–73.

Bill D J, Knight M, Forster E A, Fletcher A (1991). Direct evidence for an important species difference in the mechanism of 8-OH-DPAT-induced hypothermia. *Br J Pharmacol* **103**: 1857–64.

Birrell J M, Brown V J (2000). Medial frontal cortex mediates perceptual attention set shifting in the rat. *J Neurosci* **20**: 4320–4.

Blier P, de Montigny C, Chaput Y (1990). A role for the serotonin system in the mechanism of action of antidepressant treatments: preclinical evidence. *J Clin Psychiatry* **51**: 14–20.

Blier P, Seletti B, Gilbert F, Young S N, Benkelfat C (2002). Serotonin 1A receptor activation and hypothermia in humans: lack of evidence for a presynaptic mediation. *Neuropsychopharmacology* **27**: 301–08.

Bolles R C, Woods P J (1964). The ontogeny of behavior in the albino rat. *Anim Behav* **12**: 427–41.

Boulougouris V, Dalley J W, Robbins T W (2007). Effects of orbitofrontal, infralimbic, and prelimbic cortical lesions on serial spatial reversal learning in the rat. *Behav Brain Res* **179**: 219–28.

Bouwknecht J A, Hijzen T H, van der G J, Maes R A, Olivier B (2000). Stress-induced hyperthermia in mice: effects of flesinoxan on heart rate and body temperature. *Eur J Pharmacol* **400**: 59–66.

Boyce-Rustay J M, Wiedholz L M, Millstein R A, *et al.* (2006). Ethanol-related behaviors in serotonin transporter knockout mice. *Alcohol Clin Exp Res* **30**: 1957–65.

Braff D L, Geyer M A (1990). Sensorimotor gating and schizophrenia. Human and animal model studies. *Arch Gen Psychiatry* **47**: 181–8.

Briley M, Moret C (1993). Neurobiological mechanisms involved in antidepressant therapies. *Clin Neuropharmacol* **16**: 387–400.

Cannon T D, Zorrilla L E, Shtasel D, *et al.* (1994). Neuropsychological functioning in siblings discordant for schizophrenia and healthy volunteers. *Arch Gen Psychiatry* **51**: 651–61.

Capecchi M R (1989a). Altering the genome by homologous recombination. *Science* **244**: 1288–92.

Capecchi M R (1989b). The new mouse genetics: altering the genome by gene targeting. *Trends Genet* **5**: 70–6.

Carey R J, DePalma G, Damianopoulos E, Muller C P, Huston J P (2004). The 5-HT$_{1A}$ receptor and behavioral stimulation in the rat: effects of 8-OHDPAT on spontaneous and cocaine-induced behavior. *Psychopharmacology* **177**: 46–54.

Carey R J, DePalma G, Damianopoulos E, Shanahan A, Muller C P, Huston J P (2005). Evidence that the 5-HT1A autoreceptor is an important pharmacological target for the modulation of cocaine behavioral stimulant effects. *Brain Res* **1034**: 162–71.

Carli M, Robbins T W, Evenden J L, Everitt B J (1983). Effects of lesions to ascending noradrenergic neurons on performance of a 5-choice serial reaction time task in rats – implications for theories of dorsal noradrenergic bundle function based on selective attention and arousal. *Behav Brain Res* **9**: 361–80.

Carli M, Samanin R (1992). Serotonin2 receptor agonists and serotonergic anorectic drugs affect rats' performance differentially in a five-choice serial reaction time task. *Psychopharmacology* **106**: 228–34.

Carlsson M, Carlsson A (1988). A regional study of sex differences in rat brain serotonin. *Prog Neuropsychopharmacol Biol Psychiatry* **12**: 53–61.

Carroll J C, Boyce-Rustay J M, Millstein R, *et al.* (2007). Effects of mild early life stress on abnormal emotion-related behaviors in 5-HTT knockout mice. *Behav Genet* **37**: 214–22.

Carroll M E, Lac S T, Ascencio M, Kragh R (1990). Fluoxetine reduces intravenous cocaine self-administration in rats. *Pharmacol Biochem Behav* **35**: 237–44.

Chon H, Gaillard C A, van der Meijden B B, *et al.* (2004). Broadly altered gene expression in blood leukocytes in essential hypertension is absent during treatment. *Hypertension* **43**: 947–51.

Chudasama Y, Passetti F, Rhodes S E, Lopian D, Desai A, Robbins T W (2003). Dissociable aspects of performance on the 5-choice serial reaction time task following lesions of the dorsal anterior cingulate, infralimbic and orbitofrontal cortex in the rat: differential effects on selectivity, impulsivity and compulsivity. *Behav Brain Res* **146**: 105–19.

Clarke H F, Dalley J W, Crofts H S, Robbins T W, Roberts A C (2004). Cognitive inflexibility after prefrontal serotonin depletion. *Science* **304**: 878–80.

Clarke H F, Walker S C, Crofts H S, Robbins T W, Roberts A C (2005). Prefrontal serotonin depletion affects reversal learning but not attentional set shifting. *J Neurosci* **12**: 532–8.

Connor T J, Kelliher P, Shen Y, Harkin A, Kelly J P, Leonard B E (2000). Effect of subchronic antidepressant treatments on behavioral, neurochemical, and endocrine changes in the forced-swim test. *Pharmacol Biochem Behav* **65**: 591–7.

Coppen A, Eccleston E, Craft I, Bye P (1973). Letter: Total and free plasma-tryptophan concentration and oral contraception. *Lancet* **2**: 1498.

Cowen P J, Parry-Billings M, Newsholme E A (1989). Decreased plasma tryptophan levels in major depression. *J Affect Disord* **16**: 27–31.

Cryan J F, Kelliher P, Kelly J P, Leonard B E (1999). Comparative effects of serotonergic agonists with varying efficacy at the 5-HT(1A) receptor on core body temperature: modification by the selective 5-HT(1A) receptor antagonist WAY 100635. *J Psychopharmacol* **13**: 278–83.

Dalley J W, Cardinal R N, Robbins T W (2004). Prefrontal executive and cognitive functions in rodents: neural and neurochemical substrates. *Neurosci Biobehav Rev* **28**: 771–84.

Dalley J W, Fryer T D, Brichard L, *et al.* (2007). Nucleus accumbens D2/3 receptors predict trait impulsivity and cocaine reinforcement. *Science* **315**: 1267–70.

Daws L C, Montañez S, Munn J L, *et al.* (2006). Ethanol inhibits clearance of brain serotonin by a serotonin transporter-independent mechanism. *J Neurosci* **26**: 6431–8.

Dawson L A, Nguyen H Q, Smith D L, Schechter L E (2002). Effect of chronic fluoxetine and WAY-100635 treatment on serotonergic neurotransmission in the frontal cortex. *J Psychopharmacol* **16**: 145–52.

De Boer S F, Lesourd M, Mocaer E, Koolhaas J M (2000). Somatodendritic 5-HT1A autoreceptors mediate the antiaggressive actions of 5-HT1A receptor agonists in rats: an ethopharmacological study with S-15535, Alenspirone and WAY-100635. *Neuropsychopharmacology* **23**: 20–33.

De Bruin J P C, Feenstra M G P, Broersen L M, *et al.* (2000). Role of the prefrontal cortex of the rat in learning and decision making: effects of transient inactivation. *Prog Brain Res* **126**: 103–13.

de Jong T R, Pattij T, Veening J G, Waldinger M D, Cools A R, Olivier B (2005). Effects of chronic selective serotonin reuptake inhibitors on 8-OH-DPAT-induced facilitation of ejaculation in rats: comparison of fluvoxamine and paroxetine. *Psychopharmacology* **179**: 509–15.

de Visser L, van den Bos R, Kuurman W W, Kas M J, Spruijt B M (2006). Novel approach to the behavioral characterization of inbred mice: automated home cage observations. *Genes Brain Behav* **5**: 458–66.

Dekeyne A, Brocco M, Adhumeau A, Gobert A, Millan M J (2000). The selective serotonin (5-HT)1A receptor ligand, S-15535, displays anxiolytic-like effects in the social interaction and Vogel models and suppresses dialysate levels of 5-HT in the dorsal hippocampus of freely moving rats. A comparison with other anxiolytic agents. *Psychopharmacology* **152**: 55–66.

Dominguez R, Cruz-Morales S E, Carvalho M C, Xavier M, Brandao M L (2003). Sex differences in serotonergic activity in dorsal and median raphe nucleus. *Physiol Behav* **80**: 203–10.

Dragan W Ł, Oniszczenko W (2006). Association of a functional polymorphism in the serotonin transporter gene with personality traits in females in a Polish population. *Neuropsychobiology* **54**: 45–50.

Drevets W C, Frank E, Price J C, *et al.* (1999). PET imaging of serotonin 1A receptor binding in depression. *Biol Psychiatry* **46**: 1375–87.

Edwards D H, Kravitz E A (1997). Serotonin, social status and aggression. *Curr Opin Neurobiol* **7**: 812–9.

Fabre V, Beaufour C, Evrard A, *et al.* (2000). Altered expression and functions of serotonin 5-HT1A and 5-HT1B receptors in knock-out mice lacking the 5-HT transporter. *Eur J Neurosci* **12**: 2299–310.

Fairbanks L A, Melega W P, Jorgensen M J, Kaplan J R, McGuire M T (2001). Social impulsivity inversely associated with CSF 5-HIAA and fluoxetine exposure in vervet monkeys. *Neuropsychopharmacology* **24**: 370–8.

Ferrari P F, Palanza P, Parmigiani S, de Almeida R M, Miczek K A (2005). Serotonin and aggressive behavior in rodents and nonhuman primates: predispositions and plasticity. *Eur J Pharmacol* **526**: 259–73.

Forcelli P A, Heinrichs S C (2007). Teratogenic effects of maternal antidepressant exposure on neural substrates of drug-seeking behavior in offspring. *Addict Biol* **13**: 52–62.

Fox M A, Andrews A M, Wendland J R, Lesch K P, Holmes A, Murphy D L (2007). A pharmacological analysis of mice with a targeted disruption of the serotonin transporter. *Psychopharmacology* **195**: 147–66.

Fuller R W (1996). The influence of fluoxetine on aggressive behavior. *Neuropsychopharmacology* **14** (2): 77–81.

Gerra G, Zaimovic A, Timpano M, Zambelli U, Delsignore R, Brambilla F (2000). Neuroendocrine correlates of temperamental traits in humans. *Psychoneuroendorinology* **25**: 479–96.

Geyer M A, Krebs-Thomson K, Braff D L, Swerdlow N R (2001). Pharmacological studies of prepulse inhibition models of sensorimotor gating deficits in schizophrenic patients: a decade in review. *Psychopharmacology* **156**: 117–54.

Geyer M A, Tapson G S (1988). Habituation of tactile startle is altered by drugs acting on serotonin-2 receptors. *Neuropsychopharmacology* **1**: 135–47.

Gibbs R A, Weinstock G M, Metzker M L, *et al.* (2004). Genome sequence of the Brown Norway rat yields insight into mammalian evolution. *Nature* **428**: 493–521.

Goodwin G M, De Souza R J, Green A R (1985). Presynaptic serotonin receptor-mediated response in mice attenuated by antidepressant drugs and electroconvulsive shock. *Nature* **317**: 531–3.

Goodwin G M, De Souza R J, Green A R, Heal D J (1987). The pharmacology of the behavioral and hypothermic responses of rats to 8-hydroxy-2-(di-*n*-propylamino)tetralin (8-OH-DPAT). *Psychopharmacology* **91**: 506–11.

Gorman J M (2006). Gender differences in depression and response to psychotropic medication. *Gend Med* **3**: 93–109.

Griffith R R, Bigelow G E, Henningfield J E (1980). Similarities in animal and human drug-taking behavior. In Mello NK, editor. *Advances in substance abuse* Vol. 1. Greenwich, CT: JAI Press, pp. 1–90.

Haberstick B C, Smolen A, Hewitt J K (2006). Family-based association test of the 5HTTLPR and aggressive behavior in a general population sample of children. *Biol Psychiatry* **59**: 36–43.

Haleem D J, Kennett G A, Curzon G (1990). Hippocampal 5-hydroxytryptamine synthesis is greater in female rats than in males and more decreased by the 5-HT1A agonist 8-OH-DPAT. *J Neural Transm Gen Sect* **79**: 93–101.

Harison A A, Everitt B J, Robbins T W (1997). Central 5-HT depletion enhances impulsive responding without affecting the accuracy of attentional performance: interactions with dopaminergiz mechanisms. *Psychopharmacology* **133**: 329–42.

Heikkila R E, Orlansky H, Cohen G (1975). Studies on the distinction between uptake inhibition and release of [^{3}H]dopamine in rat brain tissue slices. *Biochem Pharmacol* **24**: 847–52.

Heinz A, Jones D W, Mazzanti C, *et al.* (2000). A relationship between serotonin transporter genotype and in vivo protein expression and alcohol neurotoxicity. *Biol Psychiatry* **47**: 643–9.

Higley J D, Linnoila M (1997). Low central nervous system serotonergic activity is traitlike and correlates with impulsive behavior. A nonhuman primate model investigating genetic and environmental influences on neurotransmission. *Ann NY Acad Sci USA* **836**: 39–56.

Higgins G A, Bradbury A J, Jones B J, Oakley N R (1988). Behavioral and biochemical consequences following activation of 5HT1-like and GABA receptors in the dorsal raphe nucleus of the rat. *Neuropharmacology* **27**: 993–1001.

Hillegaart V (1991). Effects of local application of 5-HT and 8-OH-DPAT into the dorsal and median raphe nuclei on core temperature in the rat. *Psychopharmacology* **103**: 291–6.

Hodos W (1961). Progressive ratio as a measure of reward strength. *Science* **134**: 943–4.

Hogg S (1996). A review of the validity and variability of the elevated plus-maze as an animal model of anxiety. *Pharmacol Biochem Behav* **54**: 21–30.

Hol T, Van den Berg C, Van Ree J M, Spruijt B M (1999). Isolation during the play period in infancy decreases adult social interactions in rats. *Behav Brain Res* **100**: 91–7.

Holmes A, Li Q, Murphy D L, Gold E, Crawley J N (2003a). Abnormal anxiety-related behavior in serotonin transporter null mutant mice: the influence of genetic background. *Genes Brain Behav* **2**: 365–80.

Holmes A, Murphy D L, Crawley J N (2002a). Reduced aggression in mice lacking the serotonin transporter. *Psychopharmacology* **161**: 160–7.

Holmes A, Murphy D L, Crawley J N (2003b). Abnormal behavioral phenotypes of serotonin transporter knockout mice: parallels with human anxiety and depression. *Biol Psychiatry* **54**: 953–9.

Holmes A, Yang R J, Murphy D L, Crawley J N (2002b). Evaluation of antidepressant-related behavioral responses in mice lacking the serotonin transporter. *Neuropsychopharmacology* **27**: 914–23.

Homberg J R, Arends B, Wardeh G, Raasø H S, Schoffelmeer A N M, De Vries T J (2004). Individual differences in the effects of serotonergic anxiolytic drugs on the motivation to self-administer cocaine. *Neuroscience* **128**: 121–30.

Homberg J R, Braam B, Ellenbroek B, Cuppen E, Joles J A (2006). Blood pressure in mutant rats lacking the 5-hydroxytryptamine (5-HT) transporter. *Hypertension* **48**: e115–6.

Homberg J R, Olivier J D A, Smits B M G, *et al.* (2007a). Characterization of the serotonin transporter knockout rat: a selective change in the functioning of the serotonergic system. *Neuroscience* **146**: 1662–76.

Homberg J R, Pattij T, Janssen M C W, *et al.* (2007c). Serotonin transporter deficiency in rats improves inhibitory control but not behavioral flexibility. *Eur J Neurosci* **26**: 2066–73.

Homberg J R, Schiepers O J G, Schoffelmeer A N M, Cuppen E, Vanderschuren L J M J (2007b). Acute and constitutive increases in central serotonin levels reduce social play behavior in periadolescent rats. *Psychopharmacology* **195**: 175–82.

Jans L A, Riedel W J, Markus C R, Blokland A (2007). Serotonergic vulnerability and depression: assumptions, experimental evidence and implications. *Mol Psychiatry* **12**: 522–43.

Jansen G, Hazendonk E, Thijssen K L, Plasterk R H (1997). Reverse genetics by chemical mutagenesis in *Caenorhabditis elegans*. *Nat Genet* **17**: 119–21.

Kalueff A V, Fox M A, Gallagher P S, Murphy D L (2007a). Hypolocomotion, anxiety and serotonin syndrome-like behavior contribute to the complex phenotype of serotonin transporter knockout mice. *Genes Brain Behav* **6**: 389–400.

Kalueff A V, Gallagher P S, Murphy D L (2006). Are serotonin transporter knockout mice 'depressed'?: hypoactivity but no anhedonia. *Neuroreport* **17**: 1347–51.

Kalueff A V, Jensen C L, Murphy D L (2007b). Locomotory patterns, spatiotemporal organization of exploration and spatial memory in serotonin transporter knockout mice. *Brain Res* **1169**: 87–97.

Kelaï S, Aïssi F, Lesch K P, Cohen-Salmon C, Hamon M, Lanfumey L (2003). Alcohol intake after serotonin transporter inactivation in mice. *Alcohol Alcohol* **38**: 386–9.

Kim D K, Tolliver T J, Huang S J, *et al.* (2005). Altered serotonin synthesis, turnover and dynamic regulation in multiple brain regions of mice lacking the serotonin transporter. *Neuropharmacology* **49**: 798–810.

Koob G F (1992). Drugs of abuse: anatomy, pharmacology and function of reward pathways. *Trends Pharmacol Sci* **13**: 177–84.

Kranzler H, Lappalainen J, Nellissery M, Gelernter J (2002). Association study of alcoholism subtypes with a functional promoter polymorphism in the serotonin transporter protein gene. *Alcohol Clin Exp Res* **26**: 1330–5.

Larson E T, Summers C H (2001). Serotonin reverses dominant social status. *Behav Brain Res* **121**: 95–102.

Lauder J M (1990). Ontogeny of the serotonin system in the rat: serotonin as a developmental signal. *Ann NY Acad Sci* **600**: 297–313.

Leibowitz S F, Alexander J T (1998). Hypothalamic serotonin in control of eating behavior, meal size, and body weight. *Biol Psychiatry* **44**: 851–64.

LeMarquand D, Pihl R O, Benkelfat C (1994). Serotonin and alcohol intake, abuse, and dependence: findings of animal studies. *Biol Psychiatry* **36**: 395–421.

Linnoila M, Virkkunen M, Scheinin M, Nuutile A, Rimon R, Goodwin F K (1983). Low cerebrospinal-fluid 5-hydroxyindoleacetic acid concentration differentiates impulsive from non-impulsive violent behavior. *Life Sci* **33**: 2609–14.

Lira A, Zhou M, Castanon N, *et al.* (2003). Altered depression-related behaviors and functional changes in the dorsal raphe nucleus of serotonin transporter-deficient mice. *Biol Psychiatry* **54**: 960–71.

Mann J J, Huang Y Y, Underwood M D, *et al.* (2000). A serotonin transporter gene promoter polymorphism. (5-HTTLPR) and prefrontal cortical binding in major depression and suicide. *Arch Gen Psychiatry* **57**: 729–38.

Masaki D, Yokoyama C, Kinoshita S, *et al.* (2006). Relationship between limbic and cortical 5-HT neurotransmission and acquisition and reversal learning in a go/no-go task in rats. *Psychopharmacology* **189**: 249–58.

Maurel S, De Vry J, Schreiber R (1999). Comparison of the effects of the selective serotonin-reuptake inhibitors fluoxetine, paroxetine, citalopram and fluvoxamine in alcohol-preferring cAA rats. *Alcohol* **17**: 195–201.

Martin K F, Phillips I, Hearson M, Prow M R, Heal D J (1992). Characterization of 8-OH-DPAT-induced hypothermia in mice as a 5-HT1A autoreceptor response and its evaluation as a model to selectively identify antidepressants. *Br J Pharmacol* **107**: 15–21.

Mathews T A, Fedele D E, Coppelli F M, Avila A M, Murphy D L, Andrews A M (2004). Gene dose-dependent alterations in extraneuronal serotonin but not dopamine in mice with reduced serotonin transporter expression. *J Neurosci Methods* **140**: 169–81.

McBride W J, Murphy J M, Gatto G J, *et al.* (1993). CNS mechanisms of alcohol administration. *Alcohol Alcohol* **2**: 463–7.

McCallum C M, Comai L, Greene E A, Henikoff S (2000). Targeted screening for induced mutations. *Nat Biotechnol* **18**: 455–7.

Millan M J, Rivet J M, Canton H, *et al.* (1993a). S 15535: a highly selective benzodioxopiperazine 5-HT1A receptor ligand which acts as an agonist and an antagonist at presynaptic and postsynaptic sites respectively. *Eur J Pharmacol* **230**: 99–102.

Millan M J, Rivet J M, Canton H, le Marmouille-Girardon S, Gobert A (1993b). Induction of hypothermia as a model of 5-hydroxytryptamine1A receptor-mediated activity in the rat: a pharmacological characterization of the actions of novel agonists and antagonists. *J Pharmacol Exp Ther* **264**: 1364–76.

Montañez S, Owens W A, Gould G G, Murphy D L, Daws L C (2003). Exaggerated effect of fluvoxamine in heterozygote serotonin transporter knockout mice. *J Neurochem* **86**: 210–9.

Muir J L, Everitt B J, Robbins T W (1996). The cerebral cortex of the rat and visual attentional function: dissociable effects of mediofrontal, cingulate, anterior dorsolateral, and parietal cortex lesions on a five-choice serial reaction time task. *Cereb Cortex* **6**: 470–81.

Murphy F C, Smith K A, Cowen P J, Robbins T W, Sahakian B J (2002). The effects of tryptophan depletion on cognitive and affective processing in healthy volunteers. *Psychopharmacology* **163**: 42–53.

Muscat R, Papp M, Willner P (1992). Reversal of stress-induced anhedonia by the atypical antidepressants, fluoxetine and maprotiline. *Psychopharmacology* **109**: 433–8.

Myers D P, Renaut S D, Collier M J (2004). The Morris maze as a test of learning and memory in rats – a case study demonstrating the value of re-testing the same set of animals. *Toxicology* **202**: 132–3.

Naranjo C A, Kadlec K E, Sanhueza P, Woodley-Remus D, Sellers E M (1990). Fluoxetine differentially alters alcohol intake and other consummatory behaviors in problem drinkers. *Clin Pharmacol Ther* **47**: 490–8.

New A S, Buchsbaum M S, Hazlett E A, *et al.* (2004). Fluoxetine increases relative metabolic rate in prefrontal cortex in impulsive aggression. *Psychopharmacology* **176**: 451–8.

Newman-Tancredi A, Rivet J, Chaput C, Touzard M, Verriele L, Millan M J (1999). The 5HT(1A) receptor ligand, S-15535, antagonises G-protein activation: a [35S] GTPgammaS and [3H]S-15535 autoradiography study. *Eur J Pharmacol* **384**: 111–21.

Ni W, Lookingland K, Watts S W (2006). Arterial 5-hydroxytryptamine transporter function is impaired in deoxycorticosterone acetate and *N*{omega}-nitro-L-arginine but not spontaneously hypertensive rats. *Hypertension* **48**: 134–40.

Nishizawa S, Benkelfat C, Young S N, *et al.* (1997). Differences between males and females in rates of serotonin synthesis in human brain. *Proc Natl Acad Sci USA* **94**: 5308–13.

Olivier B (2004). Serotonin and aggression. *Ann NY Acad Sci* **1036**: 382–92.

Olivier B, Chan J S, Pattij T, *et al.* (2006). Psychopharmacology of male rat sexual behavior: modeling human sexual dysfunctions? *Int J Impot Res* **18** (suppl. 1): S14–23.

Olivier J D A, van der Hart M G C, van Swelm R P L, *et al.* (2008). A study in male and female serotonin transporter knockout rats: an animal model for anxiety and depression disorders. *Neuroscience* **152**: 573–84.

Olivier B, Zethof T J, Ronken E, van der Heyden J A (1998). Anxiolytic effects of flesinoxan in the stress-induced hyperthermia paradigm in singly-housed mice are 5-HT1A receptor mediated. *Eur J Pharmacol* **342**: 177–82.

Owens M J, Nemeroff C B (1998). The serotonin transporter and depression. *Depression Anxiety* **8**: 5–12.

Paine T A, Jackman S L, Olmstead M C (2002). Cocaine-induced anxiety: alleviation by diazepam, but not buspirone, dimenhydrinate or diphenhydramine. *Behav Pharmacol* **13**: 511–23.

Passetti F, Dalley J W, Robbins T W (2003). Double dissociation of serotonergic and dopaminergic mechanisms on attentional performance using a rodent five-choice reaction time task. *Psychopharmacology* **165**: 136–45.

Pellis S M, Pasztor T J (1999). The developmental onset of a rudimentary form of play fighting in C57 mice. *Dev Psychobiol* **34**: 175–82.

Peltier R, Schenk S (1993). Effects of serotonergic manipulations on cocaine self-administration in rats. *Psychopharmacology* **110**: 390–4.

Perry J A, Wang T L, Welham T J, *et al.* (2003). A TILLING reverse genetics tool and a web-accessible collection of mutants of the legume Lotus japonicus. *Plant Physiol* **131**: 866–71.

Persico A M, Mengual E, Moessner R, *et al.* (2001). Barrel pattern formation requires serotonin uptake by thalamocortical afferents, and not vesicular monoamine release. *J Neurosci* **21**: 6862–73.

Pierce R C, Kumaresan V (2006). The mesolimbic dopamine system: the final common pathway for the reinforcing effect of drugs of abuse? *Neurosci Biobehav Rev* **30**: 215–38.

Poole T B, Fish J (1975). An investigation of playful behavior in *Rattus norvegicus* and *Mus musculus* (Mammalia). *J Zool* **175**: 61–71.

Popova L K (2006). From genes to aggressive behavior: the role of serotonergic system. *Bioessays* **28**: 495–503.

Prickaerts J, Raaijmakers W, Blokland A (1996). Effects of myocardial infarction and captopril therapy on anxiety-related behaviors in the rat. *Physiol Behav* **60**: 43–50.

Prut L, Belzung C (2003). The open field as a paradigm to measure the effects of drugs on anxiety-like behaviors: a review. *Eur J Pharmacol* **463**: 3–33.

Reith M E, Sershen H, Lajtha A (1980). Saturable [^{3}H]cocaine binding in central nervous system of mouse. *Life Sci* **27**: 1055–62.

Richardson N R, Roberts D C S (1996). Fluoxetine pretreatment reduces breaking points on a progressive ratio schedule reinforced by intravenous cocaine self-administration in the rat. *Life Sci* **49**: 833–840.

Robbins T W (2005). Chemistry of the mind: neurochemical modulation of prefrontal cortical function. *J Comp Neurol* **493**: 140–6.

Rogers R D, Blackshaw A J, Middleton H C, *et al.* (1999). Tryptophan depletion impairs stimulus-reward learning while methylphenidate disrupts attentional control in healthy young adults: implications for the monaminergic basis of impulsive behavior. *Psychopharmacology* **146**: 482–91.

Rogers D C, Fisher E M, Brown S D, Peters J, Hunter A J, Martin J E (1997). Behavioral and functional analysis of mouse phenotype: SHIRPA, a proposed protocol for comprehensive phenotype assessment. *Mamm Genome* **8**: 711–3.

Salichon N, Gaspar P, Upton A L (2001). Excessive activation of serotonin (5-HT) 1B receptors disrupts the formation of sensory maps in monoamine oxidase a and 5-HT transporter knock-out mice. *J Neurosci* **21**: 884–96.

Sargent P A, Kjaer K H, Bench C J, *et al.* (2000). Brain serotonin1A receptor binding measured by positron emission tomography with [11C]WAY-100635: effects of depression and antidepressant treatment. *Arch Gen Psychiatry* **57**: 174–80.

Saykin A J, Shtasel D, Gur R E, *et al.* (1994). Neuropsychological deficits in neuroleptic naive patients with first-episode schizophrenia. *Arch Gen Psychiatry* **51**: 124–31.

Seibell P J, Demarest J, Rhoads D E (2003). 5-HT1A receptor activity disrupts spontaneous alternation behavior in rats. *Pharmacol Biochem Behav* **74**: 559–64.

Serretti A, Mandelli L, Lorenzi C, *et al.* (2006). Temperament and character in mood disorders: influence of DRD4, SERTPR, TPH and MAO-A polymorphisms. *Neuropsychobiology* **53**: 9–16.

Shen H W, Hagino Y, Kobayashi H, *et al.* (2004). Regional differences in extracellular dopamine and serotonin assessed by in vivo microdialysis in mice lacking dopamine and/or serotonin transporters. *Neuropsychopharmacology* **29**: 1790–9.

Shephard R A, Broadhurst P L (1982). Hyponeophagia and arousal in rats: effects of diazepam, 5-methoxy-*N*,*N*-dimethyltryptamine, D-amphetamine and food deprivation. *Psychopharmacology* **78**: 368–72.

Simpson K L, Fisher T M, Waterhouse B D, Lin R C (1998). Projection patterns from the raphe nuclear complex to the ependymal wall of the ventricular system in the rat. *J Comp Neurol* **399**: 61–72.

Smits B M G, Cuppen E (2005). Rat genetics: the next episode. *Trends Genetics* **22**: 232–40.

Smits B M G, Mudde J, Plasterk R H A, Cuppen E (2004). Target-selected mutagenesis of the rat. *Genomics* **83**: 332–4.

Smits B M, Mudde J B, van de Belt J, *et al.* (2006). Generation of gene knockouts and mutant models in the laboratory rat by ENU-driven target-selected mutagenesis. *Pharmacogenet Genomics* **16**: 159–69.

Sora I, Hall F S, Andrews A M, *et al.* (2001). Molecular mechanisms of cocaine reward: combined dopamine and serotonin transporter knockouts eliminate cocaine place preference. *Proc Natl Acad Sci USA* **98**: 5300–05.

Sora I, Wichems C, Takahashi N, *et al.* (1998). Cocaine reward models: conditioned place preference can be established in dopamine- and in serotonin-transporter knockout mice. *Proc Natl Acad Sci USA* **13**: 7699–704.

Taravosh-Lahn K, Bastida C, Delville Y (2006). Differential responsiveness to fluoxetine during puberty. *Behav Neurosci* **120**: 1084–92.

Till B J, Reynolds S H, Weil C, *et al.* (2004). Discovery of induced point mutations in maize genes by TILLING. *BMC Plant Biol* **28**: 4–12.

Van den Berg C L, Hol T, Van Ree J M, Spruijt B M, Everts H, Koolhaas J M (1999). Play is indispensable for an adequate development of coping with social challenges in the rat. *Dev Psychobiol* **34**: 129–38.

Vanderschuren L J M J, Niesink R J M, van Ree J M (1997). The neurobiology of social play behavior in rats. *Neurosci Biobehav Rev* **21**: 309–26.

Vizi E S, Zsilla G, Caron M G, Kiss J P (2004). Uptake and release of norepinephrine by serotonergic terminals in norepinephrine transporter knock-out mice:

implications for the action of selective serotonin reuptake inhibitors. *J Neurosci* **24**: 7888–94.
Walsh S L, Cunningham K A (1997). Serotonergic mechanisms involved in the discriminative stimulus, reinforcing and subjective effects of cocaine. *Psychopharmacology* **130**: 41–58.
Watts S W (2005). 5-HT in systemic hypertension: foe, friend or fantasy? *Clin Sci (Lond.)* **108**: 399–412. Review. PMID: 15831089.
Watts A G, Stanley H F (1984). Indoleamines in the hypothalamus and area of the midbrain raphe nuclei of male and female rats throughout postnatal development. *Neuroendocrinology* **38**: 461–6.
Wellman C L, Izquierdo A, Garrett J E, *et al.* (2007). Impaired stress-coping and fear extinction and abnormal corticolimbic morphology in serotonin transporter knock-out mice. *J Neurosci* **27**: 684–91.
Whitaker-Azmitia P M (2005). Behavioral and cellular consequences of increasing serotonergic activity during brain development: a role in autism? *Int J Dev Neurosci* **23**: 75–83.
Wichems C H, Andrews A M, Heils A, Li Q, Lesch K P, Murphy D L (1998). Spontaneous behavior differences and altered responses to psychomotor stimulants in mice lacking the serotonin transporter. *28th Annual Meeting of the Society for Neuroscience.*
Willner P, Towell A, Sampson D, Sophokleous S, Muscat R (1987). Reduction of sucrose preference by chronic unpredictable mild stress, and its restoration by a tricyclic antidepressant. *Psychopharmacology* **93**: 358–64.
Winstanley C A, Chadusama Y, Dalley J W, Theobald D E, Glennon J C, Robbins T W (2003). Intra-prefrontal 8-OHDPAT and M100907 improve visuospatial attention and decrease impulsivity on the five-choice serial reaction time task in rats. *Psychopharmacology* **167**: 304–14.
Winstanley C A, Dalley J W, Theobald D E, Robbins T W (2004). Fractionating impulsivity: contrasting effects of central 5-HT depletion on different measures of impulsive behavior. *Neuropsychopharmacology* **7**: 1331–43.
Winstanley C A, Eagle D M, Robbins T W (2006). Behavioral models of impulsivity in relation to ADHD: translation between clinical and preclinical studies. *Clin Psychol Rev* **26**: 379–95.
Wise R A (2002). Brain reward circuitry: insights from unsensed incentives. *Neuron* **36**: 229–40.
Yamada J, Sugimoto Y, Horisaka K (1988). The behavioral effects of 8-hydroxy-2-(di-*N*-propylamino)tetralin (8-OH-DPAT) in mice. *Eur J Pharmacol* **154**: 299–304.
Zan Y, Haag J D, Chen K S, *et al.* (2003). Production of knockout rats using ENU mutagenesis and a yeast-based screening assay. *Nat Biotech* **21**: 645–51.
Zhao S, Edwards J, Carroll J, *et al.* (2006). Insertion mutation at the C-terminus of the serotonin transporter disrupts brain serotonin function and emotion-related behaviors in mice. *Neuroscience* **140**: 321–34.
Zhou F C, Lesch K P, Murphy D L (2002). Serotonin uptake into dopamine neurons via dopamine transporters: a compensatory alternative. *Brain Res* **942**: 109–19.

LIPA CICIN-SAIN AND BRANIMIR JERNEJ

7

Wistar–Zagreb 5HT rats: a rodent model with constitutional upregulation/downregulation of serotonin transporter

ABSTRACT

By selective breeding for the extreme values of platelet serotonin level (PSL), two sublines of rats with constitutional hyperserotonemia/hyposerotonemia were developed. The velocity of platelet serotonin uptake (PSU), the main determinant of PSL, was used as a further, more specific selection criterion. Directed breeding for its extremes resulted in two sublines of rats with constitutional upregulation/downregulation of platelet 5HT transporter activity, and showed consequent alterations of entire 5HT homeostasis. These sublines, termed Wistar–Zagreb 5HT (WZ-5HT) rats, constitute a genetic rodent model described in this chapter. Besides changes in peripheral 5HT homeostasis, high-5HT and low-5HT sublines of WZ-5HT rats also demonstrate changes in central serotonergic mechanisms. Under physiological conditions, neurochemical differences in the 5HT system between sublines were almost undetectable, but they became evident upon specific pharmacologic challenge as shown by brain microdialysis study. Differential behavioral phenotypes of 5HT sublines in response to various environmental challenges provide further evidence for differences in their brain functioning. Thus, high-5HT rats exhibit enhanced anxiety-like behaviors while depressive-like behavior and higher alcohol intake co-occur in low-5HT rats. Observed functional and behavioral differences between sublines of WZ-5HT rats strongly indicate that brain serotonergic activity was increased in rats from the high-5HT subline as compared to low-5HT rats. The WZ-5HT rat model may represent an integrative model for serotonin and serotonin transporter research,

Experimental Models in Serotonin Transporter Research, eds. A. V. Kalueff and J. L. LaPorte. Published by Cambridge University Press.

incorporating changes at the genomic/genetic and phenotypic (neurodevelopmental, structural, biochemical, behavioral, etc.) levels, and encompassing both central and peripheral 5HT functioning.

INTRODUCTION

The involvement of serotonin (5-hydroxytryptamine, 5HT) in central and peripheral (patho)physiological functions has been evidenced during past decades, but complete understanding of the relation between 5HT system activity and the broad diversity of 5HT effects is still missing.

Animal models, enabling experimental manipulations of brain structures, represent important tools in searching for the role of 5HT in the expression of specific phenotypes. By manipulation of genes encoding the main regulatory 5HT synaptic proteins – transporter, receptors, and metabolic enzymes – several models, mostly murine (transgenic, knock-out, antisense oligonucleotides, and, most recently, RNA-interfering models) have been generated and phenotypes of these animals have been characterized extensively (for review see [1–6]). In addition to sophisticated molecular-genetic techniques, classical genetic approaches are successfully used in studying the contribution of 5HT signaling to mammal physiology and behavior, such as studies on inbred rodent strains [7, 8] or animals selected for a particular phenotype; for example, differences in emotional reactivity, depression-related behaviors, learning ability, differential response to serotonergic or cholinergic agents, etc. [9–12 and references therein].

In designing these breeding models, an individual animal reactivity may serve as a criterion for selective breeding, followed by testing of developed sublines for possible alterations in 5HT system functioning. In an attempt to obtain a model with a constitutive alteration of the 5HT system itself, we have applied an inverse approach – selective breeding of animals for 5HT parameters and then searching selected sublines for physiological and behavioral consequences of breeding. For this purpose, we took advantage of the expression of serotonin transporter (5HTT, SERT), the main controller of free (extracellular) 5HT concentration in both brain and periphery, on readily accessible blood platelets. This unique peculiarity of the mammalian serotonergic system, as compared with other monoamine transmitters, serves as a basis for using platelets as a model for serotonergic neurons, which was suggested as long ago as 40 years [13, 14]. These small, anucleated fragments of megakaryocytic cytoplasm, differing from neurons in physiology, morphology, embryology, functional role, etc., possess their own serotonin system consisting of vesicles with 5HT densely packed in conjunction with divalent cations and ATP molecules (dense granula), high-affinity membrane 5HT transporter, vesicular monoamine transporter (VMAT2), 5HT receptor (2A subtype) on the plasma membrane, and 5HT-degrading enzyme, monoamine oxidase (MAO-B subtype in humans) in the mitochondrial membrane. Biochemical and pharmacological characteristics of these proteins – transporter, receptor, and enzyme – were found to be very similar to those of analogous 5HT proteins in serotonergic neurons, forming the basis of the mentioned platelet model in neurobiology. The subsequent demonstration of the structural and genetic identity of neuronal and platelet 5HT-related proteins [15–17] additionally supported validity of the platelet model. In biological psychiatry, platelet 5HT elements have been studied, with more or less success, as potential trait markers, disease state markers, and pharmacodynamic indicators in the course of treatment with 5HT-related drugs [18–21].

In contrast to humans, collection of larger platelet samples from the rat has been regularly associated with sacrifice of the animal, which considerably hampered experimental studies. We have developed a method for repetitive measuring of platelet serotonin level (PSL) and kinetics of platelet serotonin uptake (PSU) simultaneously in a sample (1 ml) of rat blood [22, 23] and described the fundamental physiology of these two platelet 5HT parameters: frequency distributions, sex and age influences, and individual stability over time in a large population of rats of Wistar origin [24–26]. The possibility of ex vivo monitoring of PSL and PSU, as well as findings of stability of their values in the individual animal [24, 26], which clearly indicated their heritability, enabled selective breeding for the extreme values of the above-mentioned platelet 5HT parameters and permitted development of rat sublines with constitutionally altered 5HT system.

DEVELOPMENT OF WISTAR–ZAGREB 5HT (WZ-5HT) SUBLINES

Selective breeding for divergence in platelet 5HT parameters, primarily for extremes in PSL values, has been initiated from a large original outbred population of Wistar rats from the breeding colony of the Rudjer Boskovic Institute, in which approximately 2.5-fold natural variation between extremes of PSL was found [24]. The breeding strategy has been described elsewhere [27, 28]. In brief, males and females with the highest and the lowest PSL, respectively, were mated to generate

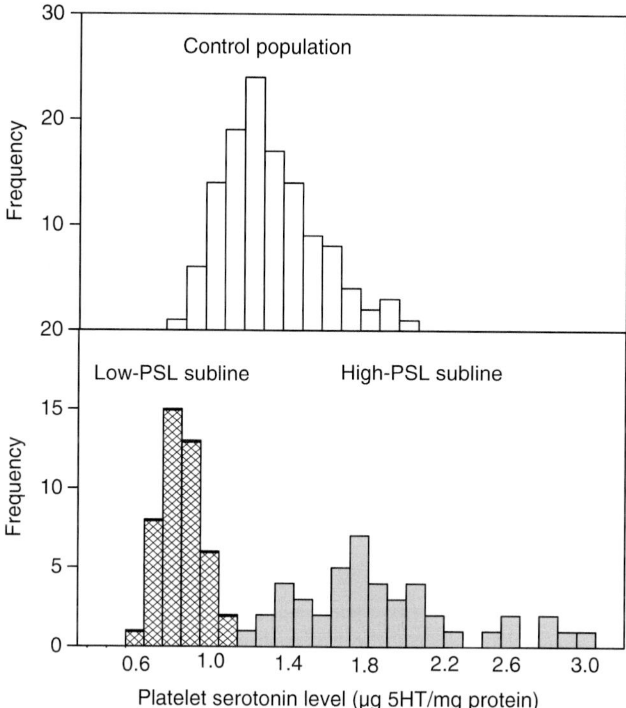

Figure 7.1 Frequency distribution histogram of individual platelet serotonin level (PSL) in control population of rats and in sublines genetically selected for low and high values of this trait (F8 generation) (adapted from [24, 27, 28]).

high and low sublines. For each subline, 12–16 litters were grown at each generation and determination of PSL was performed in offspring when they reached about 100 g of body weight. In selecting breeders for the next generation, mating of brother × sister was avoided as well as mating of animals with extreme platelet counts. A shift in mean PSL values appeared as early as in the F2 generation, while divergence of selected populations was completed by the F8 generation, with mean values stabilized at about 70% (low-PSL subline, hyposerotonemic) and 150% (high-PSL subline, hyperserotonemic) of the mean PSL value of control/unselected population [27, 28] (Figures 7.1 and 7.4a), i.e. the range of PSL values was approximately doubled by directed breeding. Morphometrical analysis performed on electron micrographs of platelets from both sublines revealed that the number of their 5HT storage vesicles (dense granula) has changed proportionally to the 5HT level (Fig. 7.3). This indicates that the volume of platelet 5HT storage vesicles

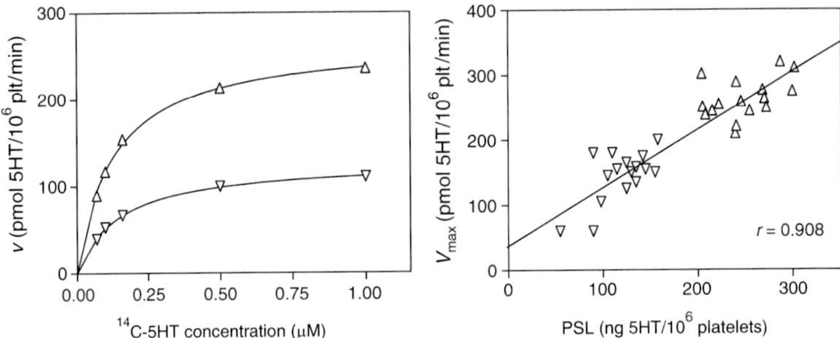

Figure 7.2 Representative saturation curve of serotonin (5HT) transport into platelets of rats from high-5HT and low-5HT sublines. Velocities (v) in control animals were in between (not presented) (left). Individual correlation of values of platelet serotonin level (PSL) and maximal velocity (V_{max}) of platelet serotonin uptake in animals from both sublines, $r =$ correlation coefficient (right).

itself is somehow predetermined, and that platelets modify their 5HT storage capacity by changing the number, but not the volume, of dense granula (counterpart of synaptic 5HT vesicles).

With regard to individual extremes in PSL values, directed selection resulted in more than a fourfold difference in this parameter (Fig. 7.1). From generation F8 on, a frequency distribution of PSL showed a different pattern between sublines. In the low-PSL subline, distribution was narrow and of Gaussian shape, while in the high-PSL subline, the histogram was multimodal, indicating differences in the inheritance pattern between sublines [27, 28].

Platelets, in contrast to neurons, lack the enzymatic potential for serotonin synthesis. Their 5HT content is a result of the transporter-mediated uptake of the amine from the surrounding plasma, so the activity of membrane 5HT transporter (5HTT) appeared as the most probable candidate underlying obtained inherited differences in PSL. Indeed, comparative full-kinetic analysis of ^{14}C-5HT uptake into platelets of animals from selected sublines revealed significant differences in its maximal velocity (V_{max}), reflecting different numbers of 5HT transporter sites on their membranes [29] (Figures 7.2, 7.3). Correlation coefficients between PSL and velocity of PSU were regularly higher than 0.90. On the other hand, the affinity (K_m values) of the transporter was similar in both sublines and not influenced by selective breeding.

Further molecular-genetic studies demonstrated analogous differences in two other platelet 5HTT parameters: transporter protein, measured by Western blot [30], and transporter mRNA, measured by either

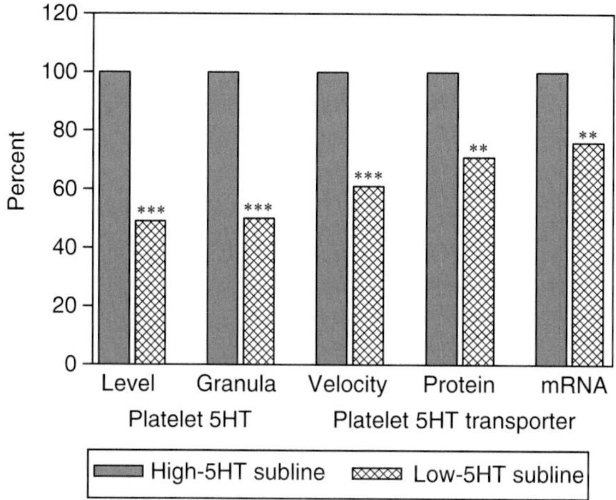

Figure 7.3 Relation among platelet 5HT measures in rats from low-5HT and high-5HT sublines (taken as 100%). High-5HT rats: platelet 5HT level: 2.12 ng 5HT/10^6 platelets; number of dense granules: 192/1000 platelets; velocity of 5HT transporter: 2.45 pmol 5HT/10^6 platelets/min; 5HTT protein: intensity of bands (relative units); 5HTT mRNA: intensity of bands in relation to cyclophylin (relative units); $^{**}p<0.01$, $^{***}p<0.001$ (adapted from [27–32]).

Northern blot or semi-quantitative RT-PCR method [31, 32]. Values of platelet 5HT-related measures were 30–50% lower in animals from the low-PSL subline, depending on the parameter measured (Figure 7.3). It was concluded that selective breeding for the extreme values of 5HT content in platelets leads to a parallel divergence of platelet membrane 5HT transporter protein.

In line with these results, development of a more specific genetic rat model, based on selection of animals for the extremes of PSU activity, was initiated [29], and this model was termed Wistar–Zagreb 5HT (WZ-5HT) rats. The breeding procedure was essentially the same as described for sublines selected on the basis of PSL values, but after first screening of offspring for PSL in each breeding generation, their PSU velocities were measured and used as the main criterion for selecting breeders for the next generation. Again, bidirectional changes in mean values of PSU velocity were produced, paralleled with consequent differences in mean values of PSL.

In comparison to the selection of animals for divergence in PSL, two major differences emerged as a result of selection for PSU velocity. First, the progress of separation of sublines was faster, completed practically in the F5 generation; and second, distribution histograms of 5HT parameters were similar and approximately normal in both sublines. A final divergence of the mean platelet 5HT parameters between sublines was somewhat higher for PSL than for the PSU (2 to 2.5-fold and 1.5 to 2.0-fold, respectively) with no overlap between sublines in distribution of PSL values and with little overlap in distribution of PSU values. This indicates that factors other than PSU may have contributed, to some extent, to the 5HT content in platelets (e.g. the activity of tryptophan hydroxylase, a rate-limiting enzyme for 5HT synthesis). Namely, higher synthesis and higher release of 5HT from the gastrointestinal tract into blood plasma could contribute to PSL according to the scavenging function of platelets for free serotonin in plasma [33, 34].

As the selection procedure progressed, the number of pups liveborn became smaller, and there was reduction in fertility and a rise in the occurrence of deaths during early postnatal life. This could be the consequence of inbreeding depression, but given the role played by 5HT in mammalian reproduction [35, 36], it may also have been related to altered 5HT functioning/homeostasis. However, no systematic pattern of these events could be observed across sublines. In parallel with selected sublines, a non-selected (control) line was periodically grown in order to monitor progress of selection as well as natural fluctuations in the population from which selection was started.

CHARACTERIZATION OF WISTAR–ZAGREB 5HT RAT SUBLINES

As a result of bidirectional selective breeding for extreme values of PSU velocity (and consequently PSL), two discrete rat sublines were obtained with differentially affected 5HT homeostasis. These sublines, characterized by high or low velocity of PSU and high or low PSL, were termed the high-5HT and low-5HT sublines, respectively. In this report, a large part of the neurochemical and behavioral outcomes in these rat sublines are summarized; figures are compiled from our published results, preliminary reports, and unpublished data.

Peripheral 5HT

Besides being present in platelets, 5HT is also present in most peripheral organs where it mediates the neural and local control of their functioning [34]. Dysregulation of 5HT transporter is thought to be associated specifically with cardiovascular and gastrointestinal disorders [37–40]. Several aspects of the 5HT system have been investigated in WZ-5HT sublines in searching for consequences of selective breeding on peripheral 5HT homeostasis.

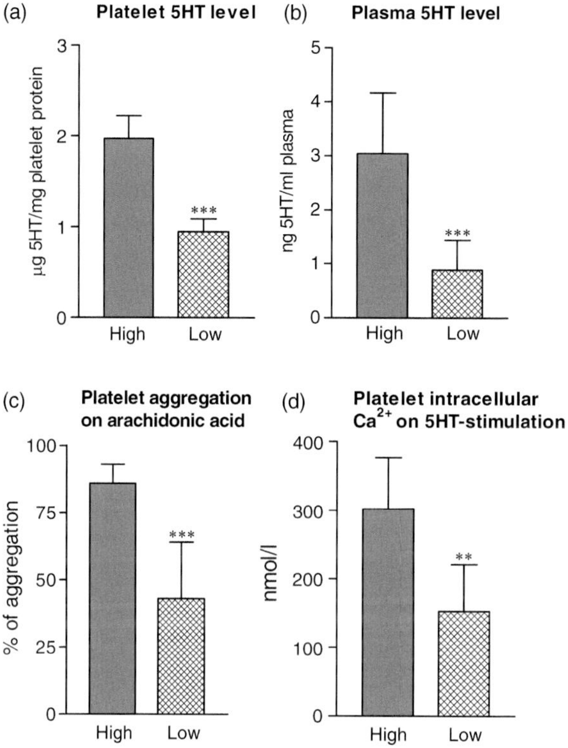

Figure 7.4 Comparison of blood/platelet measures in animals from high-5HT and low-5HT sublines. (a) Platelet 5HT measured fluorimetrically; (b) Plasma-free 5HT measured by HPLC; (c) aggregation measured 2nd minute after addition of arachidonic acid (compare to Figure 7.6); (d) platelet $[Ca^{2+}]_i$ on stimulation with 5 μM 5HT. Mean ± SD, N per subline: (a–b) 9; c–d) 6–7. $^{**}p<0.01$, $^{***}p<0.001$. See text for additional explanation (adapted from [29, 51, 54]).

Tissue 5HT content, measured in several peripheral organs (lungs, spleen, heart, small intestine, cecum, colon, etc.) by ion-exchange chromatography-fluorimetry [41], showed higher values in animals from the high-5HT subline as compared to low-5HT animals. The magnitude of differences was dependent on the organ examined and ranged from 10–25% in distinct parts of the gastrointestinal tract through 35% in lungs (having unusually large interindividual variations) to an almost 50% difference in the spleen (probably related to the high content of platelets in this organ).

Intriguingly, extracellular 5HT concentration, measured in platelet-free plasma, was also significantly higher in high-5HT animals (Figure 7.4b). The same results were obtained by using different analytical methods (HPLC-ED and RIA) and in plasma samples of animals from two consecutive breeding generations, but they still should be taken with some caution. Namely, the concentration of 5HT in plasma is lower in magnitude than in platelets [33, 42], and, in spite of all methodological attentiveness, activation of highly reactive platelets and consequent release of some 5HT could occur during blood processing. The level of biologically active 5HT in blood plasma results from the tightly regulated equilibrium between its synthesis/release from the gut and inactivation by uptake and enzymatic degradation (lungs, platelets, liver) [33, 34]. The capacity for cleaning plasma from 5HT is approximately twofold larger in platelets (and presumably, and much more importantly, in lungs) from high-5HT rats, so at first glance a lower plasma 5HT concentration might be expected in this subline. The mechanisms leading in the end to the increased level of free 5HT in rats with higher activity of platelet 5HTT is unclear thus far.

Regardless of the mechanisms underlying alterations in peripheral 5HT homeostasis, WZ-5HT sublines may represent a model for studying the role of 5HT in physiology and in somatic disorders, similarly to 5HTT-deficient or transgenic mice models [43, 44]. In addition, animals from the high-5HT subline displaying hyperserotoninemia could contribute to a better understanding of this phenomenon in clinical conditions such as autism [45].

Pharmacodynamic response

Administration of 5HT-related drugs elicited a markedly different response of platelet 5HT parameters: PSL and velocity of PSU, between sublines.

1. The increase in PSL following parenteral treatment of rats with 5HT itself, or with its metabolic precursor, 5-hydroxytryptophan (5HTP), was more pronounced in rats with higher activity of 5HTT [46] (Figure 7.5a). Similarly, hypofunctioning of membrane 5HT transporter in low-5HT animals was reflected by attenuated response of their PSL to selective serotonin reuptake inhibitors (SSRIs) fluvoxamine and fluoxetine [46] (Figure 7.5b). On the other hand, no differences in PSL response between 5HT sublines were observed following administration of reserpine, a drug that does not interfere with membrane 5HT reuptake.
2. Similarly to the effect on PSL, serotonin reuptake inhibitors had differential effects on transmembrane 5HT transport

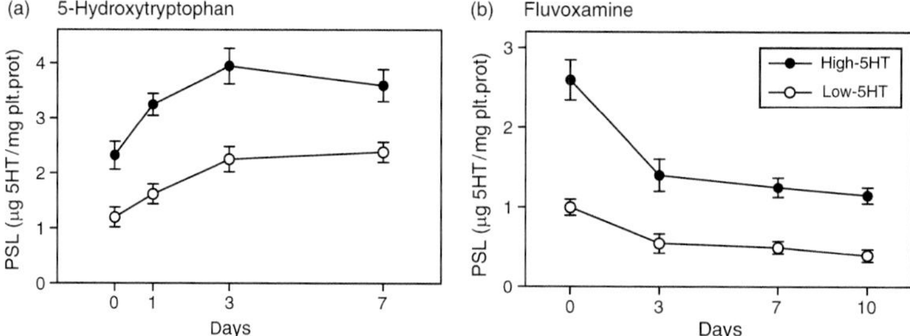

Figure 7.5 Platelet serotonin level (PSL) in animals from high-5HT and low-5HT sublines in the course of treatment with (a) 5-hydroxytryptophan (30 mg/kg/day, 7 days) and (b) fluvoxamine (20 mg/kg/day, 10 days). Daily i.p. injections were given through 7 or 10 days; PSL was measured 24 h after injections indicated on the x axis. Basal (pretreatment) PSL values are presented at day 0. Mean $\pm$ SD, $N = 6$ (adapted from [46]).

between sublines. In platelets of high-5HT rats, the decrease in 5HT uptake rate was more pronounced during treatment with fluvoxamine, as compared to platelets of low-5HT animals [46]. The observed proportionality of the PSU response to the SSRI treatment to the basal (constitutional) PSU values of the animal may be indicative of analogous central pharmacodynamic effects of SSRIs, and support the claim for personalized approaches to SSRI treatments in humans that was suggested by pharmacogenomic studies [47–50].

Platelet aggregation and intracellular calcium

Platelet response reaction in WZ-5HT sublines was studied by measuring in vitro aggregation of platelets on induction by arachidonic acid. Clear differences between sublines were demonstrated. Platelets from high-5HT animals underwent a stronger and faster aggregation response as compared to the later start, slower rise, and lower percent of aggregated platelets in the low-5HT animals [51] (Figures 7.4c, 7.6). Because of increased 5HT content in platelets of high-5HT animals, these results accord well with the suggested role of 5HT as a potent amplifier of the platelet aggregation response [52]. The mechanism of amplification is mediated by 5HT-2A receptors on the platelet membrane, whose activation results in the increase of cytosolic free calcium levels.

A study on measuring intracellular Ca^{2+} concentration in fura-2-loaded platelets revealed significantly higher resting intracellular Ca^{2+}

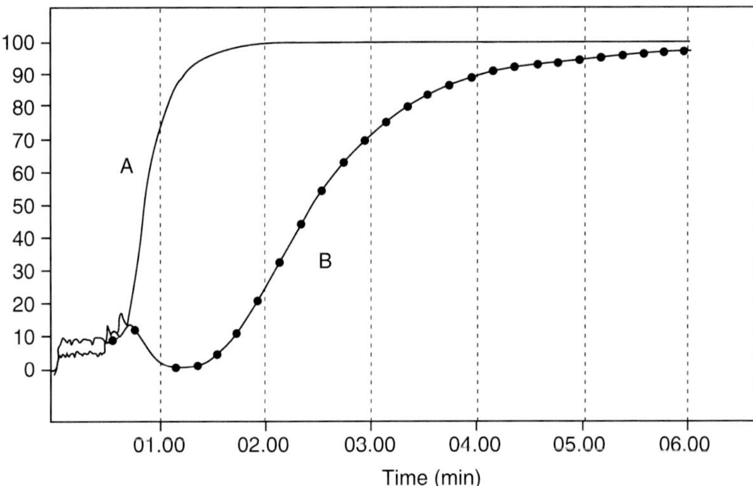

Figure 7.6 Aggregation curves of platelets from high-5HT (A) and low-5HT (B) rat recorded in the course of 5 min period after addition of arachidonic acid to the platelet sample. A typical synchronous aggregometric tracing is shown (compare to Figure 7.4c) (adapted from [51]).

in platelets of animals from the high-5HT subline [53]. Additionally, stimulation of platelets by 5HT in vitro resulted in a significantly enhanced rise in intracellular calcium levels in high-5HT rats [54] (Figure 7.4d). These results provide evidence for functional differences in platelet response reaction between 5HT sublines that may include alteration of intracellular signaling through 5HT-2A receptors and/or calcium signalization. Given the role which platelets have in cardiovascular disorders, specifically atherosclerosis [55, 56], rats with constitutive differences in platelet response may be useful for better understanding clinical pathologies such as myocardial infarction or stroke.

Central 5HT

As mentioned earlier, platelet 5HTT is structurally identical to its neuronal counterpart and encoded by the same gene [17]. Although this does not necessarily implicate functional parallelism between periphery and brain, we hypothesized that selective breeding for extremes of platelet 5HTT activity might result in some correspondence in 5HT neurons. Indeed, neurochemical and behavioral studies provide evidence that selection for peripheral 5HT parameters induced alterations in brain 5HT homeostasis as well.

Physiological conditions

5HT transporter analysis

Neuronal 5HTT has been explored for alterations between 5HT sublines regarding transporter functionality, density of binding sites, and gene expression.

1. Kinetics of [^{14}C]-5HT uptake by synaptosomes prepared from the frontal cortex revealed similar saturation curves with no alterations in either V_{max} or K_m values [57]. The absence of differences in brain 5HT uptake rate between sublines is substantially contrasted to findings in platelets [31], indicating different regulation of 5HTT activity in the periphery and brain. Our studies were performed by the use of a common radiochemical method, and the possibility that this method was not sensitive enough to detect small changes in brain 5HT uptake velocity [58] should be taken into consideration (although not very likely under our experimental conditions). A radiochemical method did not reveal differences in the 5HT uptake rate between heterozygous 5HTT knock-out (5HTT+/−) and wildtype (5HTT+/+) mice [59], while high-speed chronoamperometry revealed a marked reduction in 5HTT+/− mice [60]. On the other hand, in heterozygous 5HTT+/− rats, V_{max} of 5HT uptake in hippocampal synaptosomes was reduced by only 13% [61]. In our sublines, more subtle disturbances in the 5HT system and, consequently, even smaller differences in 5HTT velocity, were expected. We have compared 5HTT activity only in frontal cortex synaptosomes so the possibility of region-dependent differences in brain 5HTT function, as shown to exist in different rat strains [7], could be considered in future research. The possibility of compensatory 5HT uptake by other monoamine transporters, as has been reported for the 5HTT knock-out mouse [1], should also be taken into consideration.
2. Multiple brain regions of 5HT sublines were explored for divergence in 5HTT protein by saturation-binding assay of [^{3}H]-citalopram [62]. Results demonstrated small (<10%) but significant region-dependent changes in density of [^{3}H]-citalopram binding sites with higher values observed in high-5HT animals in 9 of 13 brain regions investigated [62].

Assuming that [^{3}H]-citalopram binds both membrane and cytoplasmic (non-functional) transporters, the observation that citalopram binding, but not 5HT uptake, differs slightly between 5HT sublines may suggest differences in the cytoplasmic pool of 5HT transporters between sublines. Hypothetically, the total number of neuronal 5HT transporters differs between 5HT sublines, but differences in the number of functional transporters on the cell membrane appear only on stimulation (e.g. membrane depolarization (see below)). Redistribution of transporters, resulting in changes in V_{max}, with no alterations in K_m, represents a mode of presynaptic reuptake regulation [63, 64].

3. The possibility of altered 5HTT gene expression in 5HT sublines was explored by measuring mRNA transcripts for 5HTT in midbrain raphe nuclei by semi-quantitative RT-PCR.
   A tendency to higher 5HTT mRNA levels in the high-5HT rats (~15%) was observed, but the difference in the expression of 5HTT between sublines was not significant [31].

Tissue 5HT and 5HIAA concentrations

Tissue levels of 5HT and its major metabolite, 5-hydroxyindole-acetic acid (5HIAA), have been examined by the use of HPLC-ED and ion-exchange chromatography-spectrofluorimetry [41] in multiple brain regions (raphe nuclei, frontal cortex, striatum, hippocampus (Figure 7.7a), basal ganglia, amygdala, hypothalamus, and thalamus) of 5HT sublines [62, 65]. No significant differences in either 5HT or 5HIAA concentrations were observed in any of the brain regions investigated, but in general, a trend towards a reduction in 5HT and elevation of 5HIAA concentrations could be noticed in high-5HT rats, resulting in a significantly higher metabolic ratio (5HIAA/5HT) in most brain regions (~10%, $p<0.05$) (Figure 7.7b). Results were indicative of slightly increased brain 5HT turnover in animals from the high-5HT subline as compared to the low-5HT animals. Interestingly, a similar increase in tissue 5HIAA/5HT ratio has been observed in 5HTT−/− mice and rats, but the reason for this is not understood [61, 66, 67].

Metabolic enzymes

To explore potential alterations in 5HT metabolism between sublines, indicated by differential 5HT turnover, we have compared

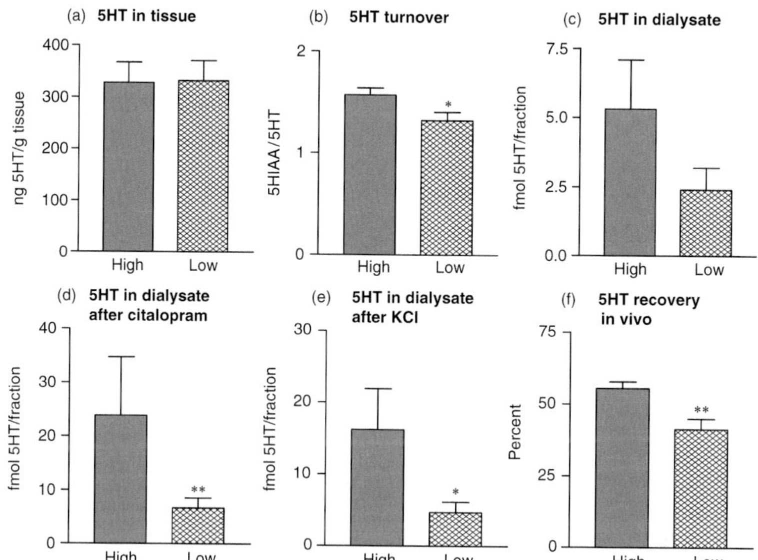

Figure 7.7 Comparison of 5HT measures in hippocampus of animals from high-5HT and low-5HT sublines. (a) Tissue 5HT; (b) Tissue 5HT metabolic rate; (c) basal dialysate 5HT in ventral hippocampus, 20-min fractions; (d) dialysate 5HT in 2nd fraction after infusion of 1 μmol/l citalopram; (e) dialysate 5HT in 1st fraction after infusion of KCl; (f) recovery of exogenous 5HT by hippocampal tissue (100 nmol 5HT/l added through dialysis probe); (a)–(b) mean ± SD, $N = 12$ per subline; (c)–(f) mean ± SEM, $N = 5$–7; $^{*}p<0.05$, $^{**}p<0.01$ (**C–F** estimated based on refs [62, 65]; see text for additional explanation).

activities/expression of their tryptophan hydroxylase (TPH), a rate-limiting enzyme for 5HT synthesis, and of monoamine oxidase (MAO), the major 5HT-degrading enzyme. 5HT is mainly oxidized by MAO-A isoenzyme, but serotonergic neurons (as well as human platelets) contain predominantly the MAO-B isoform.

1. The level of TPH in the raphe nuclei region of 5HT sublines was compared by the use of the immunochemical (Western blot) method. There were no statistically significant differences between sublines in the amount of TPH protein, although a tendency toward lower (~30%, non-significant) levels was noticed in animals from the high-5HT subline [68].
2. Full kinetic analysis of MAO-A and MAO-B isoenzymes in whole brain homogenates demonstrated no differences in either V_{max} or K_m between 5HT sublines. Further, by the use of

semi-quantitative RT-PCR, mRNA transcripts for MAO-A and MAO-B isoforms were measured in brain cortex and in raphe region of animals from 5HT sublines. With the exception of a noticed tendency toward the increase in MAO-B mRNA in the cortical region of low-5HT rats (~15%, $p<0.05$), no other differences were found.

Extraneuronal 5HT concentration

Extracellular 5HT concentration, assessed in ventral hippocampus (vHPC) by in vivo microdialysis, revealed an approximately twofold difference in baseline 5HT values between sublines [62] (Figure 7.7c). Elevated 5HT levels were observed in high-5HT rats compared to low-5HT rats, while values in control (unselected) animals were intermediate [62]. The difference in extraneuronal 5HT concentration between sublines, although large in magnitude, did not reach statistical significance (likely due to relatively small group sizes and large intergroup variations). However, pronounced divergences in neurochemical and behavioral responses between 5HT sublines, observed in subsequent studies (see below), support the existence of elevated brain 5HT activity in animals from the high-5HT subline in relation to their low-5HT counterparts. Elevated extracellular 5HT concentration in brains of high-5HT rats resembles, in some way, the situation in the periphery in that they also possess a higher extracellular pool of 5HT in the blood, although the responsible mechanisms may be quite different.

Intriguingly, animals selected for higher 5HTT activity seem to resemble 5HTT-deficient mice in having elevated basal extracellular 5HT concentrations, although this elevation in 5HTT−/− mice is comparatively much higher (~10-fold) [61, 69–71], and, as contrasted to our high-5HT subline, these mice show markedly reduced tissue 5HT and 5HIAA concentrations [66, 67]. On the other hand, heterozygous 5HTT+/− mice, which have moderately reduced 5HT uptake rate, have unchanged tissue 5HT and 5HIAA levels and no alterations in extracellular 5HT concentrations [58, 66, 70]. Further, transgenic mice having two- to threefold over-expression of 5HTT possess reduced tissue 5HT, unchanged 5HIAA, and decreased extracellular 5HT concentration [72].

(Dis)similarities in neurochemical phenotypes among mentioned models stress the complexity of 5HT regulation mechanisms, and apparently paradoxical situations such as, for instance, antidepressant clinical efficacy of both drugs that enhance 5HT reuptake (tianeptine; [73]) and drugs that inhibit 5HT reuptake (commonly used antidepressants); or another example, the information that deficiency of 5HT function is associated with an increased risk for anxiety/depression, while pharmacologic blockade of 5HTT has an anxiolytic/antidepressant effect [1, 2, 48, 74].

5HT-receptors

Differences in 5HT extraneuronal level and turnover between our sublines, although only moderate, could be expected to induce adaptive changes in the 5HT receptor systems, their signal transducing mechanisms, and/or expression of related genes, similarly to changes observed in 5HTT-deficient mice [1, 2, 71, 75, 76].

By the use of RT-PCR, we have measured mRNAs for 5HT-1A, 5HT-1B, and 5HT-2A receptors in hippocampus, striatum, and cortex, respectively, in animals from high-5HT and low-5HT sublines. No measurable alterations were observed in mRNA levels for the mentioned 5HT receptors in the brain regions investigated. Further, preliminary studies showed similar densities of 5HT-1A and 5HT-2A receptors, as measured by binding of [^{3}H]8-OH-DPAT and [^{3}H]-ketanserin, respectively, in cortical regions of 5HT sublines, and a lack of differences in cortical 5HT-2A protein amount assessed by Western blot method [77–79]. It seems, therefore, that imbalances in brain 5HT homeostasis in our genetically selected animals were not large enough to produce measurable compensatory/adaptational changes in 5HT receptor systems under physiological conditions, at least in the brain cortex. Bearing in mind that adaptational changes in 5HT receptors are region-specific and often small in magnitude, even following complete inactivation of 5HTT [71, 75, 76], the inability to detect alterations in our 5HT sublines was not so unexpected. Research on the expression of regulatory somatodendritic 5HT-1A autoreceptors as well as comparison of their functionality between sublines is in course.

At present, we have not studied the potential consequences of disturbed 5HT homeostasis in WZ-5HT rats on other brain neurotransmitter systems; for instance, the noradrenergic or dopaminergic systems, which have strong interactions with the 5HT system. However, no major changes in functioning of several non-serotonergic systems in 5HTT-deficient [3, 61, 70] or 5HTT over-expressing animals [72] have been demonstrated, which makes it unlikely that such changes are present in our model under physiological conditions.

Response to challenges

Neurochemical response

By using in vivo microdialysis, marked differences in response of 5HT neurons to specific pharmacological challenges were observed between 5HT sublines [62], confirming underlying constitutive alterations in functionality of their brain 5HT systems. Thus, an increase in extracellular 5HT concentration in ventral hippocampus (vHPC), provoked by infusion of selective reuptake inhibitor citalopram through the dialysis probe, was much more pronounced in the brains of high-5HT rats (Figure 7.7d). Similarly, K^+-evoked release of 5HT in vHPC, produced by infusion of hypertonic KCl through the dialysis probe, was also significantly higher in the same subline (Figure 7.7e).

Observed differences in drug-responsiveness between 5HT sublines may be interpreted as resulting from latent differences in activity of their 5HTT that are not detectable under physiological conditions (although adaptive changes in 5HT release cannot be ruled out as contributing to these observations).

Further evidence for differences in functionality of the brain 5HT system between 5HT sublines was obtained by estimation of in vivo recovery of exogenous 5HT added to the hippocampal tissue, which was also significantly higher in animals from the high-5HT subline [62] (Figure 7.7f). In the light of the results obtained under conditions of pharmacologically challenged 5HTT, it could be speculated that earlier described differences in basal 5HT dialysate between sublines are underestimated.

Demonstration of much stronger responsiveness of brain 5HT system under pharmacological challenges in high-5HT animals, together with elevated extracellular 5HT concentration and 5HT turnover in this subline, speak in favor of an increased serotonergic tone (i.e. hyperactivity of 5HT system) in high-5HT rats, as compared to rats from the low-5HT subline.

Behavioral responses

Given the importance of the 5HT system in integrating sensory processing, motor activities, and cognitive functions, we assumed the existence of divergent behavioral phenotypes in 5HT sublines, which was confirmed by further studies.

SEROTONIN SYNDROME

Excessive brain 5HT functioning, induced by administration of various combinations of 5HT-enhancing drugs, leads to development of distinctive, life-threatening, motor behavioral 5HT syndrome in both rodent models and in humans [80–82]. It has been observed that 5HTT knock-out mice, having elevated basal extracellular 5HT concentration, displayed spontaneous serotonin syndrome-like behavior [91].

Behaviors associated with the 5HT syndrome, induced by MAO inhibition and 5HT precursor loading (pargyline + 5HTP), were examined in animals from WZ-5HT sublines. Although not all symptoms were different between the sublines, the response of high-5HT rats was generally more pronounced compared to low-5HT animals [78]. Among behavioral/neuromuscular symptoms, the most prominent differences were observed in body tremor and hyper-reactivity scores, while regarding autonomic phenomena, marked differences were present in the elevation of body temperature [78] (Figure 7.8b). In addition, a clear difference between sublines was noticed in lethal answer to the 5HT syndrome. Although non-specific, this answer could be considered as a valuable indicator of a "final response" of the organism summarizing 5HT-induced dysregulations [78] (Figure 7.8a). In pharmacological studies, using 5HT receptor antagonists, a specific role for 5HT-2A receptors in development of both body tremor and hyperthermia has been documented [83, 84], making it possible that differences in 5HT-2A receptors contributed to the differences in the development of 5HT-syndrome between sublines. In contrast to 5HTT knock-out mice, no spontaneous serotonin syndrome-like behavior was observed in our WZ-5HT sublines.

Regardless of the underlying mechanisms, functional differences between 5HT sublines indicate that the basal serotonergic tone of the individual plays a critical role in the intensity of response/symptoms to 5HT-enhancing drugs. An increased behavioral sensitivity to these drugs has been shown also in mice with deletion of 5HTT function [82], suggesting the possibility of their use as a model for humans at greater risk for developing 5HT-syndrome [82]. Our high-5HT subline may serve a similar purpose regarding this clinical condition.

ANXIETY-RELATED PHENOTYPE

In line with the current, although oversimplified, hypothesis that increased anxiety-related behaviors are related to increased 5HT neurotransmission [5, 50, 85, 86], we hypothesized that animals from 5HT sublines could display differences in anxiety-related behaviors.

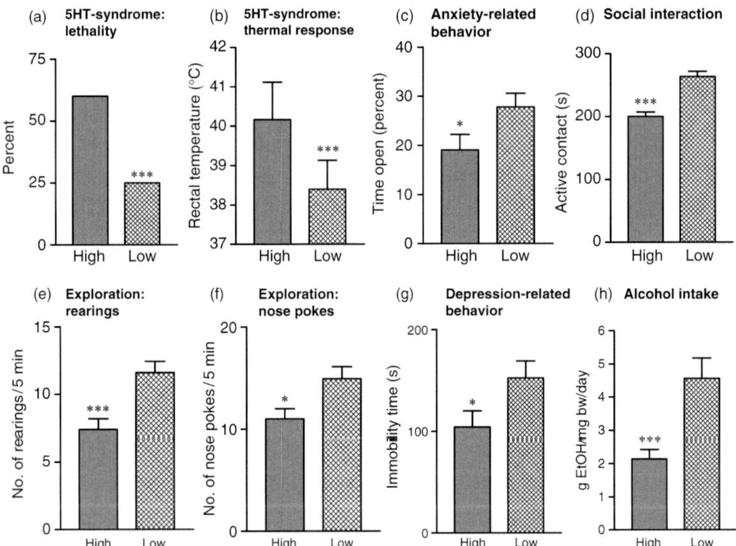

Figure 7.8 Behavioral measures in animals from high-5HT and low-5HT sublines. (a),(b) 5HT syndrome induced with 50 mg/kg pargyline + 5 mg/kg 5HTP; lethality recorded 24 h after 5HTP injections, temperature measured 90 min after 5HTP injection; (c),(e) 5-min elevated plus maze; (d) 10-min open field, 300 lx; (f) 5-min hole-board; (g) 5-min forced swimming; (h) two-bottle choice paradigm, average intake of 12% alcohol during 12 days in females; mean ± SEM, *N* per subline: (b),(g),(h) 6–7; (d),(f) 12; (a),(c),(e) 20–23; $^{*}p<0.05$, $^{***}p<0.001$. See text for additional explanation (adapted from [54, 88, 89, 108]).

Their anxiety-like phenotype was tested in several common paradigms using animals from three breeding generations. Results were partly obtained in an independent laboratory (Seville, Spain; [89]), providing additional strength to the findings.

Overall, significant differences were observed between sublines, with high-5HT animals displaying a higher level of anxiety-related behavior and lower level of exploration, which are in line with the view that avoidance and novelty seeking share common mechanisms [87]. Specifically, high-5HT rats spent less time in the open arms of the elevated plus maze (Figure 7.8c). In the social interaction test they spent less time in active contact with conspecifics [88] (Figure 7.8d) and displayed a narrower spectrum of social behaviors [88]. High-5HT animals also showed lower levels of exploratory activity across three different anxiety-related tests (zero-maze, elevated-plus maze, hole-board) [88] (Figures 7.8e, f). The most prominent difference between

5HT sublines was considerably enhanced freezing behavior in high-5HT animals when compared to their low-5HT counterparts and to control animals [89]. Since the exposure of a rat to a novel environment represents a mild stressor, there is a possibility that different emotionality in our sublines might be related to their different response to stress. On the other hand, it is unlikely that increased anxiety-related behaviors were a consequence of altered locomotion, as 5HT sublines did not differ in the number of squares entered [88] or distance traveled in the open field test.

Enhanced anxiety-related behaviors in animals from the high-5HT subline accord well with presumed over-activity of their 5HT system. Again, findings in high-5HT animals (with upregulated 5HTT) resembled, surprisingly, that of mice with deleted 5HTT gene, which consistently displayed heightened anxiety-like behaviors (and are hyperserotonergic) [2, 67, 87, 87, 90, 91]. It is also in line with the low-anxiety phenotype displayed in 5HTT-over-expressing mice [72].

DEPRESSION-RELATED PHENOTYPE

As opposed to the excessive 5HT neurotransmission in anxiety, deficient 5HT transmission has usually been associated with depression [92, 93] and enhancement of 5HT availability has been thought to underlie the therapeutic effects of conventional antidepressants [94]. However, the situation seems much more complex: thus, drugs that inhibit the 5HTT have both anxiolytic and antidepressant potential, symptoms of anxiety and depression are often comorbid and functional gene variants in the 5HTT are associated with greater risk for depression as well as anxiety disorders [50, 86, 95]. Making a distinction between anxiety- and depression-like behaviors in animal models [96] is not easy, either.

WZ-5HT rats were tested for depression-related behaviors in the forced swimming test (FST), one of the most widely used models of depression [97]. Results showed significantly increased immobility of low-5HT rats, being an indicator for a depression-like phenotype (Figure 7.8g). Three distinct types of active behavior (climbing, swimming, and diving), which are thought to be affected differently by various classes of antidepressant drugs [98, 99], were scored separately, showing that between 5HT sublines, the climbing behavior was most different.

Given that depressive behaviors are related to deficient brain 5HT transmission, increased immobility in low-5HT rats may refer to the presumed hypofunctioning of their 5HT system, while decreased immobility in high-5HT rats may reflect an antidepressant-like coping reaction mediated by increased 5HT transmission. Intriguingly, an increased level of depression-related immobility has been observed in 5HTT knock-out mice [67, 100], a finding that is opposite to what might be expected from their hyperserotonergic tonus. However, there are also situations/paradigms where 5HTT-deficient mice failed to demonstrate depression-like behaviors [101, 102], indicating that these mice may not be suitable for studying baseline depression-like behaviors. Recently, a higher depression-like state in 5HTT knock-out rats has also been suggested based on their increased immobility in FST and reduced sucrose consumption [103].

ALCOHOL PREFERENCE

An inverse relationship between brain serotonergic tone and alcohol consumption has been demonstrated repeatedly [104, 105] with accumulating evidence indicating abnormal 5HTT function in alcoholic patients and respective animal models [106].

Voluntary alcohol consumption, studied in WZ-5HT rats using a two-bottle choice paradigm, showed significant differences between sublines. Low-5HT rats demonstrated much higher alcohol preference defined in terms of both alcohol intake (g EtOH/kg/day) and percentage of total fluid consumed [107] (Figure 7.8h). Alcohol consumption in females exceeded that of males in both 5HT sublines and, in females, differences between sublines were even more pronounced [108]. The amount of alcohol consumed by low-5HT females (4–5 g/kg/day) fell near the range of alcohol intake in sublines of animals specifically bred for alcohol preference [108]. Conversely, high-5HT males avoided alcohol virtually completely in the regimen applied. Low-5HT rats also consumed a larger amount of alcohol in the forced drinking paradigm, when alcohol was given to animals as the only drinking fluid [109]. We suggest that the low-5HT subline of WZ-5HT rats could represent an additional animal model for studying inter-relations between 5HT and alcohol.

Given the inverse relationship between brain 5HT activity and alcohol consumption, the observed higher alcohol intake/preference in low-5HT animals are in line with the supposed hypoactivity of their brain 5HT system. Correspondingly, lower alcohol consumption was shown in hyperserotonergic 5HTT knock-out mice in comparison to wildtype mice [110, 111].

In the end, differential behavioral phenotypes of 5HT sublines in response to various challenges provide further evidence for differences in their brain functioning. High-5HT rats exhibit enhanced anxiety-like behaviors while depressive-like behavior and higher alcohol intake co-occur in low-5HT animals. This relationship confirms, in a novel model, that these behavioral features may result from the constitutive alterations in brain 5HT functioning. With considerable simplifications, hyperactivity of the 5HT system has been generally related to anxious behaviors [50, 85, 86] and 5HT hypoactivity has been related to the pathogenesis of depression and alcoholism [92, 93]. Thus, the pattern of behavioral divergence between 5HT sublines on challenge could be used as evidence for hyper- and hypofunctioning of brain 5HT system in high-5HT and low-5HT sublines of WZ-5HT rats, respectively. It is possible to speculate that WZ-5HT rats may be suitable to model human 5HT-ergic dysfunctions associated with 5HTT genetic polymorphisms. The fact that our rats selected for high 5HTT activity resembled in several aspects 5HTT-deficient animals was opposite to our expectations. It seems challenging to discern the full range of processes/behaviors disrupted by the selection of animals for the extreme activities of 5HTT.

Finally, in the course of developing both our models – hyperserotonemic/hyposerotonemic sublines (selection for PSL) and WZ-5HT rats (selection for PSU) – various other aspects of their reactivity were also tested. Pronounced differences in their immune reactivity were demonstrated [112, 113], preliminary studies of their learning ability [89] and pain sensitivity [114] were performed, and gender-related differences in responsiveness to challenges between sublines were studied. These results, however, fall beyond the scope of this chapter.

CONCLUDING REMARKS

By selective breeding for the extreme values of platelet serotonin level (PSL) two sublines of rats with constitutional hyperserotonemia/hyposerotonemia were developed. The velocity of platelet serotonin uptake (PSU), the main determinant of PSL, was used as a further, more specific selection criterion, and directed breeding for its extremes resulted in two sublines of rats with constitutional alteration of platelet 5HT transporter activity, and consequent alterations of entire 5HT homeostasis. The mentioned sublines, termed Wistar–Zagreb 5HT rats (WZ-5HT rats), constitute a genetic rodent model described in this chapter. Besides changes in peripheral 5HT homeostasis, high-5HT and low-5HT sublines of WZ-5HT rats also demonstrate changes in central serotonergic mechanisms.

Under basal conditions, neurochemical differences in the 5HT system between sublines were almost undetectable, indicating its large potential to resist continuous directed genetic pressure. However, upon an additional challenge (pharmacological, environmental), adaptation equilibrium is exceeded and latent differences between 5HT sublines become evident. Given the results of neuropharmacologic (in vivo microdyalisis) and behavioral studies, it could be argued that the brain serotonergic activity is increased in rats from the high-5HT subline as compared to low-5HT rats. As such, WZ-5HT rats might provide an appropriate model to address the biological and behavioral impact of altered regulation of the 5HTT gene with its main characteristics summarized as follows.

1. The model has been generated by directed breeding for naturally occurring extremes of specific biochemical phenotypes and, as such, it resembles the physiological situation more closely than models developed by genetic engineering techniques (although continuous selective pressure finally escapes the field of genuine physiology).
2. The range of divergence of phenotypic measure under selection – 5HTT activity – is only moderate when compared with the original population. However, pronounced differences in 5HTT activity exist between sublines themselves, with expected divergence in their 5HT homeostasis.
3. Dysregulation of 5HTT is constitutional, i.e. present during the ontogeny, and thus could influence developing serotonergic neurocircuitry with consequent alterations in brain 5HT system functioning.
4. Generation of the model is a stable and reproducible process as evidenced by restarting selective breeding several times during the last 15 years with essentially the same results.
5. Bidirectional selection offers the possibility of simultaneous studies on animals with virtually identical constitution, except for dysregulation (upregulation/downregulation) of a parameter under selection – 5HTT activity (although the possibility of some non-specific co-selections could not be completely excluded).
6. WZ-5HT rats represent an integrative model for 5HTT (and serotonin in general) research, incorporating changes at genomic/genetic and phenotypic (neurodevelopmental, structural, biochemical, behavioral, etc.) levels and encompassing both central and peripheral 5HT functioning.
7. An important outcome of model development is the demonstration of a close inter-relation between peripheral and

central components of the 5HT system in the rat – namely, by changing the platelet we have changed the rat brain (there is no intent to make a direct analogy to humans in this respect).

8. The WZ-5HT rat model may be relevant for investigating central/peripheral 5HT functioning in physiological, pathological, pharmacological, neurodevelopmental, etc., conditions.

Further neurochemical, behavioral, and molecular characterizations of WZ-5HT sublines are currently underway, including neurodevelopmental studies (somatosensory barrel fields), studies of the effects of dysregulated 5HT transmission on spatial memory, as well as sequencing of the 5HTT gene in search of potential polymorphic gene variants linked to the particular subline.

ACKNOWLEDGMENTS

The work presented in this chapter was supported by grants from the Croatian Ministry of Science, Education and Sport. We would like to express our thanks to all colleagues and collaborators who helped us in developing and maintaining described model during the past two decades, with specific thanks to our senior technician Mrs. Katarina Karlo.

REFERENCES

1. Lesch K P, Mossner R (2006). Inactivation of 5HT transport in mice: modelling altered 5HT homeostasis implicated in emotional dysfunction, affective disorders and somatic syndromes. *Handb Exp Pharmacol* **175**: 417–56.
2. Murphy D L, Lesch K P (2008). Targeting the murine serotonin transporter: insights into human neurobiology. *Nat Rev Neurosci* **9**: 85–96.
3. Fox M A, Andrews A M, Wendland J R, Lesch K P, Holmes A, Murphy D L (2007a). A pharmacological analysis of mice with a targeted disruption of the serotonin transporter. *Psychopharmacology* **195**: 147–66.
4. Berger M, Tecott L H (2006). Serotonin system gene knockouts. In Roth B L, editor. *The serotonin receptors: from molecular pharmacology to human therapeutics.* Totowa: Humana Press, pp. 537–75.
5. Bechtholt A, Lucki I (2006). Effects of serotonin-related gene deletion on measures of anxiety, depression and neurotransmission. In Roth B L, editor. *The serotonin receptors: from molecular pharmacology to human therapeutics.* Totowa: Humana Press, pp. 577–606.
6. Shih J C (2004). Cloning, after cloning, knock-out mice and physiological functions of MAO A and B. *Neurotoxicology* **25**: 21–30.
7. Fernandez F, Sarre S, Launay J M, *et al.* (2003). Rat strain differences in peripheral and central serotonin transporter protein expression and function. *Eur J Neurosci* **17**: 494–506.
8. Calcagno E, Cannetta A, Guzzetti S, Cervo L, Ivernizzi R W (2007). Strain differences in basal and post-citalopram extracellular 5-HT in the mouse

medial prefrontal cortex and dorsal hippocampus: relation with tryptophan hydroxylase-2 activity. *J Neurochem* **103**: 1111–20.

9. Van der Staay F J (2006). Animal models of behavioural dysfunctions: basic concepts and classifications, and an evaluation strategy. *Brain Res Rev* **52**: 131–59.
10. Singewald N (2007). Altered brain activity processing in high-anxiety rodents revealed by challenge paradigms in functional mapping. *Neurosci Biobehav Rev* **31**: 18–40.
11. Nestler E J, Gould E, Manji H, *et al.* (2002). Preclinical models: status of basic research in depression. *Biol Psychiatry* **52**: 503–28.
12. Crabbe J C (2002). Alcohol and genetics: new models. *Am J Med Genet* **114**: 969–74.
13. Pletscher A (1968). Metabolism, transfer and storage of 5HT in blood platelets. *Br J Pharmacol* **32**: 1–16.
14. Stahl S M, Meltzer H Y (1978). A kinetic and pharmacologic analysis of 5-hydroxytryptamine transport by human platelets and platelet storage granules: comparison with central serotonergic neurons. *J Pharmacol Exp Ther* **205**: 118–32.
15. Chen K, Wu H F, Shih J C (1993). The deduced amino acid sequences of human platelet and frontal cortex monoamine oxidase B are identical. *J Neurochem* **61**: 187–90.
16. Cook E H, Fletcher K E, Wainwright M, Marks N, Yan S Y, Leventhal B L (1994). Primary structure of the human platelet serotonin 5HT2A receptor: identity with the frontal cortex serotonin 5HT2A receptor. *J Neurochem* **63**: 465–9.
17. Lesch K P, Wolozin B L, Murphy D L, Riederer P (1993). Primary structure of the human platelet serotonin uptake site: identity with the brain serotonin transporter. *J Neurochem* **60**: 2319–21.
18. Pletscher A (1988). Platelets as models: use and limitations. *Experientia* **44**: 152–5.
19. Hrdina P D (1994). Platelet serotonergic markers in psychiatric disorders: use, abuse and limitations. *J Psychiatry Neurosci* **19**: 87–90.
20. Jernej B (1995). Platelet *versus* neuron: a glimpse from serotonergic perspective. *Period Biol* **97**: 183–90.
21. Camacho A, Dimsdale J E (2000). Platelets and psychiatry: lessons learned from old and new studies. *Psychosom Med* **62**: 326–36.
22. Jernej B, Cicin-Sain L, Iskric S (1988). A simple and reliable method for monitoring platelet serotonin levels in rats. *Life Sci* **43**: 1663–70.
23. Jernej B, Froebe A, Hranilovic D, Cicin-Sain L (1999a). Platelet serotonin transporter: ex vivo monitoring of kinetic parameters in the individual rat. *Neurosci Res Comm* **24**: 163–72.
24. Jernej B, Cicin-Sain L, Kveder S (1989). Physiological characteristics of platelet serotonin in rats. *Life Sci* **45**: 485–92.
25. Cicin-Sain L, Jernej B, Magnus V (1989). Platelet serotonin levels and gonadal hormones in rats. *Life Sci* **45**: 1885–92.
26. Cicin-Sain L, Froebe A, Jernej B (1998). Physiological characteristics of serotonin transporter on rat platelets. *Comp Biochem Phys A* **120**: 723–9.
27. Jernej B, Cicin-Sain L (1990). Platelet serotonin level in rats is under genetic control. *Psychiat Res* **32**: 167–74.
28. Cicin-Sain L, Perovic S, Iskric S, Jernej B (1995). Development of sublines of Wistar-derived rats with high or low platelet serotonin level. *Period Biol* **97**: 211–16.

29. Cicin-Sain L, Froebe A, Bordukalo-Niksic T, Jernej B (2005). Serotonin transporter kinetics in rats selected for extreme values of platelet serotonin level. *Life Sci* **77**: 452–61.
30. Hranilovic D, Herak-Kramberger C, Cicin-Sain L, Sabolic I, Jernej B (2001). Serotonin transporter in rat platelets: level of protein expression underlies inherited differences in uptake kinetics. *Life Sci* **69**: 59–65.
31. Bordukalo-Niksic T, Cicin-Sain L, Jernej B (2004). Expression of brain and platelet serotonin transporters in sublines of rats with constitutionally altered serotonin homeostasis. *Neurosci Lett* **369**: 44–9.
32. Jernej B, Hranilovic D, Cicin-Sain L (1999b). Serotonin transporter on rat platelets: level of mRNA underlie inherited differences in uptake kinetics. *Neurochem Int* **33**: 519–23.
33. Anderson G M, Stevenson J M, Cohen D J (1987). Steady-state model for plasma-free and platelet serotonin in man. *Life Sci* **41**: 1777–85.
34. Fozard J R (1989). *The peripheral actions of 5-hydroxytryptamine*. New York: Oxford University Press.
35. Dube F, Amireault P (2007). Local serotonergic signaling in mammalian follicles, oocytes and early embrios. *Life Sci* **81**: 1627–37.
36. Hull E M, Muschamp J W, Sato S (2004). Dopamine and serotonin: influences on male sexual behavior. *Physiol Behav* **83**: 291–307.
37. Gershon M D, Tack J (2007). The serotonin signalling system: from basic understanding to drug development for functional GI disorders. *Gastroenterology* **132**: 397–414.
38. Watts S W (2005). 5-HT in systemic hypertension: foe, friend or fantasy? *Clin Sci (Lond.)* **108**: 399–412.
39. Blakely R D (2001). Physiological genomics of antidepressant targets: keeping periphery in mind. *J Neurosci* **21**: 8319–23.
40. Murphy D L, Lerner A, Rudnick G, Lesch K P (2004). Serotonin transporter: gene, genetic disorders and pharmacogenetics. *Mol Interv* **4**: 109–23.
41. Cicin-Sain L, Oreskovic D, Perovic S, Jernej B, Iskric S (1990). Determination of serotonin in peripheral rat tissues by ion-exchange chromatography-fluorometry. Validation by high performance liquid chromatography with electrochemical detection. *Biogen Amines* **7**: 641–50.
42. Ortiz J, Artigas F (1992). Effects of monoamine uptake inhibitors on extracellular and platelet 5-hydroxytryptamine in rat blood: different effects of clomipramine and fluoxetine. *Br J Pharmacol* **105**: 941–6.
43. Mekontso-Dessap A, Brouri F, Pascal O, *et al.* (2006). Deficiency of the 5-hydroxytryptamine transporter gene leads to cardiac fibrosis and valvulopathy in mice. *Circulation* **113**: 81–9.
44. Guignabert C, Izikki M, Tu L I, *et al.* (2006). Transgenic mice overexpressing the 5-hydroxytryptamine transporter gene in smooth muscle develop pulmonary hypertension. *Circ Res* **98**: 1323–30.
45. Janusonis S, Anderson G M, Shifrovich I, Rakic P (2006). Ontogeny of brain and blood serotonin levels in 5-HT1A receptor knockout mice: potential relevance to the neurobiology of autism. *J Neurochem* **99**: 1019–31.
46. Cicin-Sain L, Froebe A, Jernej B (1996). The effect of antidepressants on platelet serotonin level and serotonin uptake in rats genetically selected for these traits. *Eur Neuropsychopharm* **6** (Suppl. 4): 76–7.
47. Binder E B, Holsboer F (2006). Pharmacogenomics and antidepressant drugs. *Ann Med* **38**: 82–94.
48. Serretti A, Benedetti F, Zanardi R, Smeraldi E (2005). The influence of serotonin transporter promoter polymorphism (SERTPR) and other

polymorphisms of the serotonin pathway on the efficacy of antidepressant treatments. *Prog Neuropsychopharmacol Biol Psychiatry* **29**: 1074–84.

49. Lesch K P, Gutknecht L (2005). Pharmacogenetics of the serotonin transporter. *Prog Neuropsychopharmacol Biol Psychiatry* **29**: 1062–73.
50. Lesch K P, Mossner R (1998). Genetically driven variation in serotonin uptake: is there a link to affective spectrum, neurodevelopmental and neurodegenerative disorders. *Biol Psychiatry* **44**: 179–92.
51. Jernej B, Cicin-Sain L, Banovic M (1994). Platelet aggregation in rats genetically selected for high or low platelet serotonin levels. *Can J Physiol Pharmacol* **72** (Suppl. 1): 10.
52. De Clerck F, de Chaffoy de Courcelles D (1990). Serotonergic amplification in platelet function: mechanisms and in vivo relevance. In *Progress in pharmacology and clinical pharmacology 7/4*. Stuttgart: Gustav Fischer Verlag, pp. 51–9.
53. Froebe A, Cicin-Sain L, Jernej B (1997). Intracellular calcium in platelets of rats with genetically altered serotonin system. *Period Biol* **99** (Suppl. 1): 85.
54. Froebe A (2006). *Serotonin-2A receptor and its signaling: studies in rats with altered serotonergic homeostasis*. PhD Thesis, University of Zagreb, pp. 1–83.
55. Vanhoutte P M (1985). *Serotonin and the cardiovascular system*. New York: Raven Press.
56. Vorchheimer D A, Becker R (2006). Platelets in atherothrombosis. *Mayo Clin Proc* **81**: 59–68.
57. Hegedis K (2001). *Serotonin transporter: kinetic studies in rat cerebral cortex*. MSc Thesis, University of Zagreb, pp. 1–61.
58. Perez X A, Bianco L E, Andrews A M (2006). Filtration disrupts synaptosomes during radiochemical analysis of serotonin uptake: comparison with chronoamperometry in SERT knockout mice. *J Neurosci Methods* **154**: 245–55.
59. Bengel D, Murphy D L, Andrews A, *et al.* (1998). Altered brain serotonin homeostasis and locomotor insensitivity to 3,4-methylendioxymethamphetamine ("ecstasy") in serotonin transporter-deficient mice. *Mol Pharmacol* **53**: 649–55.
60. Perez X A, Andrews A M (2005). Chronoamperometry to determine differential reductions in uptake in brain synaptosomes from serotonin transporter knockout mice. *Anal Chem* **77**: 818–26.
61. Homberg J R, Olivier J D A, Smits B M G, *et al.* (2007). Characterization of the serotonin transporter knockout rat: a selective change in the functioning of the serotonergic system. *Neuroscience* **146**: 1662–76.
62. Romero L, Jernej B, Bel N, Cicin-Sain L, Cortes R, Artigas F (1998). Basal and stimulated extracellular serotonin concentration in the brain of rats with altered serotonin uptake. *Synapse* **28**: 313–21.
63. Jayanthi L D, Ramamoorthy S (2005). Regulation of monoamine transporters: influence of psychostimulants and therapeutic antidepressants. *Am Ass Pharmaceut Sci J* **7**: E728–38.
64. Zahniser N R, Doolen S (2001). Chronic and acute regulation of Na^+/Cl^--dependent neurotransmitter transporters: drugs, substrates, presynaptic receptors, and signaling systems. *Pharmacol Ther* **92**: 21–55.
65. Bokulic Z, Cicin-Sain L, Jernej B (2003). Wistar–Zagreb 5HT rats: study of serotonergic activity in brain regions. *Neurol Croat* **52** (Suppl.): 91.
66. Kim D K, Tolliver T J, Huang S J, *et al.* (2005). Altered serotonin synthesis, turnover and dynamic regulation in multiple brain regions of mice lacking the serotonin transporter. *Neuropharmacology* **49**: 798–810.
67. Zhao S, Edwards J, Carroll J, *et al.* (2006). Insertion mutation at the C-terminus of the serotonin transporter disrupts brain serotonin function and emotion-related behaviors in mice. *Neuroscience* **140**: 321–34.

68. Stefulj J (2005). *Tryptophan hydroxylase: polymorphism and expression of the gene in altered serotonergic homeostasis.* PhD Thesis, University of Zagreb, pp. 1–76.
69. Montanez S, Owens W A, Gould G G, Murphy D L, Daws L C (2003). Exaggerated effect of fluvoxamine in heterozygote serotonin transporter knockout mice. *J Neurochem* **86**: 210–9.
70. Mathews T A, Fedele D E, Coppelli F M, Avila A M, Murphy D L, Andrews A M (2004). Gene dose-dependent alterations in extraneuronal serotonin but not dopamine in mice with reduced serotonin transporter expression. *J Neurosci Methods* **140**: 169–81.
71. Fabre V, Beaufour C, Evrard A, *et al.* (2000). Altered expression and function of serotonin 5-HT1A and 5-HT1B receptors in knock-out mice lacking the 5HT transporter. *Eur J Neurosci* **12**: 2299–310.
72. Jennings K A, Loder M K, Sheward W J, *et al.* (2006). Increased expression of the 5HT transporter confers a low-anxiety phenotype linked to decreased 5HT transmission. *J Neurosci* **26**: 8955–64.
73. Wagstaff A J, Ormrod D, Spencer C M (2001). Tianeptine: a review of its use in depressive disorders. *CNS Drugs* **15**: 231–59.
74. Hariri A R, Holmes A (2006). Genetics of emotional regulation: the role of the serotonin transporter in neuronal function. *Trends Cogn Sci* **10**: 182–91.
75. Li Q, Wichems C H, Ma L, Van de Kar L D, Garcia F, Murphy D L (2003). Brain region-specific alterations of 5-HT2A and 5-HT2C receptors in serotonin transporter knockout mice. *J Neurochem* **84**: 1256–65.
76. Rioux A, Fabre V, Lesch K P, *et al.* (1999). Adaptive changes of serotonin 5-HT2A receptors in mice lacking the serotonin transporter. *Neurosci Lett* **262**: 113–6.
77. Bordukalo-Niksic T, Mokrovic G, Jernej B, Cicin-Sain L (2007). Expression of 5HT-1A and 5HT-1B receptor genes in brains of Wistar–Zagreb 5HT rats. *Coll Antropol* **31**: 37–41.
78. Bordukalo-Niksic T (2003). *Gene expression of 5HT-synaptic elements in brain of rats with altered serotonin homeostasis.* MSc Thesis, University of Zagreb, pp. 1–73.
79. Froebe A, Cicin-Sain L, Bordukalo-Niksic T, Jernej B (2007). Serotonin-2A receptors and its signal transduction in brains and platelets of Wistar–Zagreb 5HT rats. *Neurol Croat* **56** (Suppl. 2): 7.
80. Isbister G K, Buckley N A (2005). The pathophysiology of serotonin toxicity in animals and humans: implications for diagnosis and treatment. *Clin Neuropharmacol* **28**: 205–14.
81. Kalueff A V, LaPorte J, Murphy D L (2007b). Perspectives on genetic animal models of serotonin toxicity. *Neurochem Int* **52**: 649–58.
82. Fox M A, Jensen C L, Gallagher P S, Murphy D L (2007b). Receptor mediation of exaggerated response to serotonin-enhancing drugs in serotonin transporter (SERT)-deficient mice. *Neuropharmacology* **53**: 643–56.
83. Van Oekelen D, Megens A, Meert T, Luyten W H, Leysen J E (2002). Role of 5HT2 receptors in the tryptamine-induced 5HT syndrome in rats. *Behav Pharmacol* **13**: 313–8.
84. Nisijima K, Yoshino T, Yui K, Katoh S (2001). Potent serotonin (5-HT)(2A) receptor antagonists completely prevent the development of hyperthermia in an animal model of the 5-HT syndrome. *Brain Res* **890**: 23–31.
85. Briley M, Chopin P (1991). Serotonin in anxiety: evidence from animal models. In Sandler M, Coppen A, Harnett S, editors. *5-Hydroxytryptamine in psychiatry: a spectrum of ideas.* New York: Oxford University Press, pp. 177–97.
86. Lesch K P, Zeng Y, Reif A, Gutknecht L (2003). Anxiety-related traits in mice with modified genes of the serotonergic pathway. *Eur J Phamacol* **480**: 185–204.

87. Holmes A, Li Q, Murphy D L, Gold E, Crawley J N (2003). Abnormal anxiety related behavior in serotonin transporter null mutant mice: the influence of genetic background. *Genes Brain Behav* **2**: 365–80.
88. Hranilovic D, Cicin-Sain L, Bordukalo-Niksic T, Jernej B (2005). Rats with constitutionally upregulated/downregulated platelet 5HT transporter: differences in anxiety-related behavior. *Behav Brain Res* **165**: 271–7.
89. Quevedo G, Moscoso O, Prado-Moreno A, Cicin-Sain L, Jernej B, Delgado-Garcia J M (2002). Behavioral and molecular studies in rats over-expressing and under-expressing serotonin transporter. *COST B10: Brain Damage Repair*, 11th Committee Meeting, Dublin, Abstract book, p. 15.
90. Ansorge M S, Zhou M, Lira A, Hen R, Gingrich J A (2004). Early-life blockade of the 5HT transporter alters emotional behavior in adult mice. *Science* **306**: 879–81.
91. Kalueff A V, Fox M A, Gallagher P S, Murphy D L (2007a). Hypolocomotion, anxiety and serotonin syndrome-like behavior contribute to the complex phenotype of serotonin transporter knockout mice. *Gen Brain Behav* **6**: 389–400.
92. Mann J (1999). Role of serotonergic system in the pathogenesis of major depression and suicidal behavior. *Neuropsychopharmacology* **21**: 99S–105S.
93. Ordway G A, Klimek V, Mann J J (2002). Neurocircuitry of mood disorders. In Davis K L, Charney D, Coyle J T, Nemeroff C, editors. *Neuropsychopharmacology – the fifth generation of progress*. Philadelphia: Lippincott, Williams and Wilkins, pp. 1051–64.
94. Blier P, de Montigny C (1994). Current advances and trends in the treatment of depression. *Trends Pharmacol Sci* **15**: 220–6.
95. Ressler K J, Nemeroff C B (2000). Role of serotonergic and noradrenergic systems in the pathophysiology of depression and anxiety disorders. *Depress Anxiety* **12**: 2–19.
96. Kalueff A V, Tuohimaa P (2004). Experimental modelling of anxiety and depression. *Acta Neurobiol Exp* **64**: 439–48.
97. Cryan J F, Markou A, Lucki I (2002). Assessing antidepressant activity in rodents: recent developments and future needs. *Trends Pharmacol Sci* **23**: 238–45.
98. Detke M J, Rickels M, Lucki I (1995). Active behaviors in the rat forced swimming test differentially produced by serotonergic and noradrenergic antidepressants. *Psychopharmacology* **121**: 66–72.
99. Reneric J P, Bouvard M, Stinus L (2002). In the rat forced swimming test, chronic but not subacute administration of dual 5-HT/NA antidepressant treatments, may produce greater effects than selective drugs. *Behav Brain Res* **136**: 521–32.
100. Lira A, Zhou M, Castanon N, *et al.* (2003). Altered depression-related behaviors and functional changes in the dorsal raphe nucleus of serotonin transporter deficient mice. *Biol Psychiatry* **54**: 960–71.
101. Holmes A, Yang R J, Murphy D L, Crawley J N (2002). Evaluation of antidepressant-related behavioral responses in mice lacking the serotonin transporter. *Neuropsychopharmacology* **27**: 914–23.
102. Kalueff A V, Gallagher P S, Murphy D L (2006). Are serotonin transporter knockout mice depressed? Hypoactivity but no anhedonia. *Neuroreport* **17**: 1347–51.
103. Olivier J D A, Van der Hart M G C, Van Swelm R P L, *et al.* (2008). A study in male and female 5HT transporter knockout rats: an animal model for anxiety and depression disorders. *Neuroscience* **152**: 573–84.

104. LeMarquand D, Phil R O, Benkelfat C (1994b). Serotonin and alcohol intake, abuse and dependence: findings of animal studies. *Biol Psychiatry* **36**: 395–421.
105. LeMarquand D, Phil R O, Benkelfat C (1994a). Serotonin and alcohol intake, abuse and dependence: clinical evidence. *Biol Psychiatry* **36**: 326–37.
106. Lesch K P (2005). Alcohol dependence and gene × environment interaction in emotion regulation: is serotonin the link? *Eur J Pharmacol* **526**: 113–24.
107. Cicin-Sain L, Bordukalo-Niksic T, Jernej B (2004). Wistar–Zagreb 5HT rats: a new animal model of alcoholism. *Alcoholism* **40** (Suppl. 3): 92–3.
108. McBride W J, Li T K (1998). Animal models of alcoholism: neurobiology of high alcohol-drinking behavior in rodents. *Crit Rev Neurobiol* **12**: 339–69.
109. Mokrovic G, Cicin-Sain L (2006). Chronic ethanol intake and brain monoamine oxidase A and B in rats with constitutionally altered serotonin homeostasis. 5th Forum of European Neuroscience, Vienna, book of abstracts, A165.19.
110. Kelai S, Aissi F, Lesch K P, Cohen-Salmon C, Hamon M, Lanfumey L (2003). Alcohol intake after serotonin transporter inactivation in mice. *Alcohol Alcohol* **38**: 386–9.
111. Boyce-Rustay J M, Wiedholz L M, Millstein R A, *et al.* (2006). Ethanol-related behaviors in serotonin transporter knockout mice. *Alcohol Clin Exp Res* **30**: 1957–65.
112. Gabrilovac J, Cicin-Sain L, Osmak M, Jernej B (1992). Alteration of NK- and ADCC-activities in rats genetically selected for low or high platelet serotonin level. *J Neuroimmunol* **37**: 213–22.
113. Poljak-Blazi M, Jernej B, Cicin-Sain L, Boranic M (1990). Immunological response of rats selected for high or low platelet serotonin content. *Period Biol* **92**: 189–90.
114. Djurkovic M, Tvrdeic A, Cicin-Sain L, Jernej B, Birus I (2004). Pain sensitivity in Wistar and Wistar–Zagreb 5HT rats: the effect of habituation to experimental conditions. Fourth Croatian Congress of Pharmacology, Split, book of abstracts, p. 78.

F. SCOTT HALL, ICHIRO SORA, MARIA T. G. PERONA AND GEORGE R. UHL

8

The role of the serotonin transporter in reward mechanisms

ABSTRACT

In recent years, gene knock-out studies have greatly expanded understanding of the molecular basis of drug reward and drug addiction. One of the consequences of these studies has been to produce a more pluralistic view of the underlying neurochemical mechanisms that mediate drug reward after the development of a strongly dopamine-centered view in the 1980s. This is not to say that dopamine does not have a central role in drug reward and drug addiction, but rather a fuller examination of these mechanisms involves the complex neurocircuitry of which dopamine systems are a part. This view is not new, but has been expressed from a variety of perspectives. Gene knock-out studies have indicated a particular approach to examining the nature of interactions between different parts of this circuitry. This chapter will focus on the role of serotonin, and in particular the serotonin transporter (SERT), in drug reward. This more pluralistic perspective became apparent in gene knock-out studies of the rewarding effects of drugs of abuse which demonstrated that deletion of the dopamine transporter (DAT) did not eliminate the rewarding effects of cocaine, and subsequent findings that implicated a critical role of SERT in a variety of circumstances. These studies also validated the central role of dopamine in drug reward, and consequently the role of SERT must be considered largely from the point of view of interactions with dopamine systems. These discoveries also indicate that variation in genes such as SERT, may contribute to individual differences in response to

Experimental Models in Serotonin Transporter Research, eds. A. V. Kalueff and J. L. LaPorte. Published by Cambridge University Press.

drugs of abuse as part of a polygenic and heterogeneous genetic basis of addiction.

INTRODUCTION

When knock-out mice were first produced for genes thought to be relevant to addiction, or at least to the initial actions of drugs of abuse, the presumption was that certain drug targets were more important than others (e.g. DAT). Thus, despite the fact that stimulant drugs, such as cocaine, act upon multiple monoamine systems, it was thought that the rewarding effects were determined almost exclusively by effects on dopamine systems. These initial presumptions were based upon a large scientific literature that used pharmacological and lesion methods to specify the particular neurotransmitter systems and brain regions that were involved in the actions of drugs of abuse (for a summary of this view, see Wise and Bozarth, 1987). Initial studies of the DAT knock-out mouse produced findings completely consistent with these initial expectations, including a profound hyperactivity under baseline conditions and elimination of cocaine-induced locomotor stimulant effects (Giros *et al.*, 1996). In part because locomotor stimulant effects were supposed to be an index of rewarding effects, these findings were taken to indicate reduced rewarding effects of cocaine, and thus the use of the phrase "indifference to cocaine" in that initial publication. However, it was subsequently found that cocaine reward was not eliminated in DAT knock-out mice when reward was specifically examined in a conditioned place preference (CPP) paradigm (Sora *et al.*, 1998), or a self-administration paradigm (Rocha *et al.*, 1998a). The natural conclusion would be that other targets of cocaine were normally involved in the rewarding effects of cocaine, or at least could mediate the rewarding effects of cocaine under some conditions, such as when the dopamine transporter is completely absent: the two most likely candidates were SERT and the norepinephrine transporter (NET).

THE ROLE OF SERT IN COCAINE REWARD

The first publication demonstrating that cocaine reward was unaffected by DAT gene knock-out (KO) also included the investigation of cocaine CPP in SERT KO mice (Sora *et al.*, 1998). Based on the hypothesis that either SERT or the norepinephrine transporter must mediate cocaine reward in DAT knock-out mice, it was expected that elimination of one or both of these genes might produce a reduction in cocaine CPP.

However, this was not the case, and in fact, cocaine CPP was found to be increased in both SERT KO (Sora *et al.*, 1998) and NET KO (Xu *et al.*, 2000) mice. There are several possible interpretations of these findings, but the most straightforward is that SERT mediates some of the aversive effects of cocaine, so that its removal results in a net increase in the rewarding effects of cocaine (Uhl *et al.*, 2002), an idea supported by the observation that the combination of SERT and NET gene deletion greatly elevates cocaine CPP (Hall *et al.*, 2002). None the less, the hypothesis was put forward that SERT was involved in the rewarding effects of cocaine as well; the basic premise being that if deletion of one cocaine target did not eliminate the rewarding effects of cocaine, then elimination of multiple targets would do so. Thus, combined deletion of DAT and SERT were examined in the CPP paradigm and, under these conditions, it was found that combined deletion did in fact eliminate the rewarding effects of cocaine (Sora *et al.*, 2001), indicating that SERT also had a critical role in the rewarding effects of cocaine. In order to further elucidate the interacting roles of dopamine and serotonin function in cocaine reward, the effects of these knock-outs alone and in combination were examined on serotonin and dopamine release using in vivo microdialysis (Shen *et al.*, 2004). In this study it was found that SERT KO increased basal extracellular levels of 5-HT in the dorsal striatum, nucleus accumbens (NAC), and prefrontal cortex, while DAT KO elevated basal extracellular levels of DA in the striatum and NAC, but not the prefrontal cortex. These basal differences made examination of cocaine effects on DA release difficult, but when these baseline differences were taken into account the effects of cocaine were found to vary substantially with region. Cocaine continued to increase DA in the dorsal striatum of DAT KO mice, but was eliminated in combined DAT–SERT double knock-out mice, in a pattern similar to that observed in the cocaine CPP study described above. In the NAC, DAT KO alone was sufficient to eliminate cocaine-induced increases in DAT, while SERT KO was without effect. In the prefrontal cortex, the effects of cocaine on dopamine release were not affected by either knock-out. Although SERT KO reduced the ability of cocaine to release 5-HT in the dorsal striatum, it was only eliminated in DAT–SERT double knock-out mice, and a similar pattern was observed in the NAC, while SERT KO alone eliminated 5-HT release in the prefrontal cortex. These data demonstrate interactive consequences of DAT and SERT deletion on both dopamine and serotonin release in a highly regionally dependent manner, but it must be noted that previous, less-extensive studies have not necessarily replicated all aspects of this pattern of effects.

For instance, other studies have found cocaine-induced DA increases in the NAC of DAT KO mice (Mateo *et al.*, 2004), and no increases in DA after cocaine when the probe region included both ventral and dorsal striatal regions (Rocha *et al.*, 1998a).

Obviously only limited conclusions can be drawn from the small number of studies that have addressed these problems to date, particularly given the apparent discrepancies between studies. It would be quite likely that specific anatomical loci and interactions between dopamine and serotonin systems underlie the interactive effects of DAT and SERT knock-outs on drug reward. Several approaches are being undertaken to address these issues, including local drug infusions. For instance, the study by Shen and colleagues (2004) also indicated that the basis of cocaine responses might very well be different in DAT KO and SERT KO mice compared to wildtype mice. Local infusion of cocaine in the striatum did not increase DA release in DAT KO mice, and produced a greatly diminished effect on 5-HT in SERT KO mice, while the converse was largely without effect, indicating that the locus of striatal changes in cocaine-induced elevations in DA and 5-HT are fundamentally changed in DAT and SERT knock-out mice, respectively. The lack of effect of locally applied cocaine was confirmed in another study (Mateo *et al.*, 2004). This may indicate that increases in NAC dopamine levels induced by peripheral cocaine administration act in DA cell body regions, rather than on terminals, perhaps through the effects of cocaine on other neurotransmitter systems on SERT in DAT knock-out mice. There is some evidence to this effect. Selective blockade of the serotonin transporter by fluoxetine produces novel rewarding effects in the CPP paradigm in DAT KO mice (Hall *et al.*, 2002; Mateo *et al.*, 2004), and increases dopamine release in the dorsal striatum (Mateo *et al.*, 2004; Shen *et al.*, 2004). Furthermore, local application of cocaine or fluoxetine into the ventral tegmental area (VTA) increases dopamine release in the NAC (Mateo *et al.*, 2004), indicating that changes in response to cocaine in this structure underlies the different mechanism producing dopamine release in DAT KO mice. It is interesting to note that the effect of VTA cocaine in wildtype (WT) mice in that study appeared to be inhibitory, perhaps associated with the greater VTA release of DA observed in those mice. This was not observed in WT mice after fluoxetine, which had no effect on either NAC or VTA dopamine release, while fluoxetine substantially released DA in the VTA in DAT KO mice. These data indicate that the ventral tegmental area is a key region underlying the effects of cocaine in DAT KO mice. This is obviously not the only brain region that may underlie unusual mechanisms that are not typically observed in WT mice. For instance, similar to the effects of fluoxetine in DAT KO mice, the selective DAT blocker GBR12909 produced elevations in 5-HT levels in SERT KO mice that are not observed in WT mice (Shen *et al.*, 2004). (+)-3,4-Methylenedioxy-methamphetamine (MDMA) releases dopamine in the nucleus accumbens, but not the prefrontal cortex, of SERT KO mice (Trigo *et al.*, 2007), which might also indicate a differential release mechanism in SERT KO mice that is not mediated by direct effects on SERT.

Further supporting the role of SERT in drug reward, at least under certain conditions, are findings from the dopamine-deficient mouse, in which tyrosine hydroxylase has been inactivated only in dopamine neurons (Zhou and Palmiter, 1995). This transgenic manipulation resulted in near total elimination of tissue dopamine, with no effect on norepinephrine. Cocaine CPP is relatively normal in these mice, with just a slight reduction at higher doses (Hnasko *et al.*, 2007). These authors developed additional evidence that cocaine was producing rewarding effects in these mice via inhibition of the serotonin transporter, in an interesting parallel to the findings discussed above for DAT KO mice. Similar to observations in DAT KO mice, fluoxetine also had rewarding effects in dopamine-deficient mice (an effect not observed in WT mice). Furthermore, the 5-HT1 receptor antagonist methiothepin blocked the rewarding effects of both cocaine and fluoxetine in these mice, indicating that one of the 5-HT1 receptor subtypes may be involved in these effects, and perhaps also the changes observed in DAT KO mice given some of the similarities noted above. Dopamine-deficient mice demonstrate a second instance in which profound alterations in dopamine systems reveal the importance of SERT for the rewarding effects of cocaine and some interesting directions of research that may help elaborate the specific anatomical loci and serotonin receptor subtypes that underlie these alternate types of dopamine/serotonin interactions. There are likely to be a number of potentially important interactions, as described in the next sections.

SEROTONIN RECEPTOR SUBTYPES

Collectively, these findings from transgenic mice implicate a role of serotonin, and SERT, in both cocaine reward and cocaine aversion, but how can the various findings in SERT KO mice be reconciled? Serotonin is a very complex neurotransmitter system with a great variety of receptor subtypes expressed in diverse brain regions (for review see Fink and Gothert, 2007). Even when just considering interactions with dopamine systems, numerous serotonin receptors are known to affect dopaminergic function, including the 5-HT1A, 5-HT1B, 5-HT2A, 5-HT2C, 5-HT3, 5-HT4, and 5-HT6 receptors. In many early studies, pharmacological agents acting at these receptors were not particularly selective, but subsequent studies with selective agents have confirmed the involvement of these receptors (thus, for brevity, it is not noted below when selective or non-selective agonists were used).

5-HT1A agonists increased basal and stimulated activity of dopaminergic neurons (Arborelius *et al.*, 1993; Lejeune and Millan, 1998) and increased the release of dopamine in the nucleus accumbens (Lejeune and Millan, 1998). 5-HT1A antagonists reduce DA cell firing, and in particular, burst firing (Minabe *et al.*, 2003). Under some conditions, the effects of 5-HT1A manipulations are limited to mesolimbic neurons or produce different effects in mesolimbic and nigrostriatal neurons (Arborelius *et al.*, 1993; Minabe *et al.*, 2003). The mechanisms of 5-HT1A effects are not entirely certain, but may involve a combination of effects based on increased autoreceptor function, producing an overall decrease in serotonergic neurotransmission, and direct postsynaptic effects as demonstrated by excitatory effects of 5-HT1A agonists injected directly into the VTA and SNC (substantia nigra compacta) (Arborelius *et al.*, 1993). Indirect effects, such as activation of excitatory cortical projections to the VTA, may also be involved (Diaz-Mataix *et al.*, 2005, 2006).

Stimulation of the 5-HT1B receptor in either the nucleus accumbens or the ventral tegmental area increases dopamine release in the nucleus accumbens (Yan and Yan, 2001). In the VTA, activation of 5-HT1B receptors disinhibits midbrain dopaminergic neurons by inhibiting GABA afferents (Johnson *et al.*, 1992). 5-HT1B agonists also potentiate the effects of cocaine on dopamine release (O'Dell and Parsons, 2004; Parsons *et al.*, 1999), in part by increasing the ability of cocaine to inhibit VTA GABA levels (O'Dell and Parsons, 2004), which may also increase DA cell firing (Yan *et al.*, 2004). Additionally, 5-HT administration directly into the nucleus accumbens increases DA release, and this effect is potentiated by 5-HT1B agonists (Hallbus *et al.*, 1997). 5-HT1B receptors also affect other parts of the limbic system, including the hippocampus and prefrontal cortex, that may also modulate dopamine function (Boulenguez *et al.*, 1996, 1998; Iyer and Bradberry, 1996).

Selective 5-HT2A antagonists attenuate stimulated dopamine release in the nucleus accumbens, striatum, and medial prefrontal cortex (De Deurwaerdere and Spampinato, 1999; Pehek *et al.*, 2001; Porras *et al.*, 2002b), while 5-HT2A agonists increase basal DA release or potentiate stimulated DA release (Gobert and Millan, 1999; Ichikawa and Meltzer, 1995; Lucas and Spampinato, 2000; Yan, 2000; Yan *et al.*, 2000). 5-HT2C receptors have often been shown to have opposite effects to 5-HT2A receptors. Antagonism of the 5-HT2C receptor increases basal dopamine release in the striatum, nucleus accumbens, and frontal cortex (De Deurwaerdere and Spampinato, 1999; Di Giovanni *et al.*, 1999; Gobert *et al.*, 2000), stimulates dopamine release (Navailles *et al.*, 2004) and both basal and burst firing of dopamine neurons (Di Giovanni *et al.*, 1999). Conversely, 5-HT2C agonists decrease dopamine cell firing and release (Di Giovanni *et al.*, 2000; Di Matteo *et al.*, 2000; Gobert *et al.*, 2000; Pierucci *et al.*, 2004). Interestingly, it appears that some 5-HT2C effects, such as on burst firing, are limited to mesolimbic dopamine neurons under some conditions (Di Giovanni *et al.*, 1999, 2000).

Systemic or local administration of 5-HT3 receptor antagonists block elevations in dopamine release produced by a variety of drugs, including cocaine, amphetamine, morphine, and ethanol (Campbell and McBride, 1995; Imperato and Angelucci, 1989; Kankaanpaa *et al.*, 1996, 2002; McNeish *et al.*, 1993; Wozniak *et al.*, 1990; Yoshimoto *et al.*, 1992), as well as dorsal raphe stimulation (De Deurwaerdere *et al.*, 1998), while 5-HT3 agonists increase DA release (Chen *et al.*, 1991; Liu *et al.*, 2006a, 2006b; Santiago *et al.*, 1995). Elevations in prefrontal cortex dopamine produced by selective serotonin uptake inhibitors are also 5-HT3-mediated (Tanda *et al.*, 1995). Most of these effects are thought to be mediated by actions on dopamine terminals, although there has also been some suggestion the 5-HT3 can affect midbrain dopaminergic activity as well (Mylecharane, 1996). 5-HT4 antagonism blocks the increase in DA release produced by 5-HT (Bonhomme *et al.*, 1995; De Deurwaerdere *et al.*, 1997; Thorre *et al.*, 1998), as well as the increases produced by cocaine, amphetamine, and morphine (Porras *et al.*, 2002a; Pozzi *et al.*, 1995), while 5-HT4 agonists increase DA release (Steward *et al.*, 1996). In contrast to some other 5-HT receptors mentioned previously, the 5-HT4 receptor subtype may affect the nigrostriatal dopamine system to a greater degree than the mesolimbic dopamine system (Lucas *et al.*, 2001). Antagonists of the 5-HT6 receptor have also been shown to increase dopamine release in the prefrontal cortex (Lacroix *et al.*, 2004).

In summary, selective activation of the majority of 5-HT receptors has been shown to increase dopaminergic function, although some subtypes reduce dopaminergic function. The precise effects vary substantially, depending on the state of DA activity, the particular brain region examined, and whether the manipulation involves dopamine terminals or cell bodies. Despite this fact, direct serotonin application to dopaminergic neurons produces substantial inhibitory responses as well as excitatory responses (Cameron *et al.*, 1997; Gongora-Alfaro *et al.*, 1997; Pessia *et al.*, 1994), the particular proportion varying from study to study. Similarly, dorsal raphe stimulation causes both inhibitory and excitatory responses in dopaminergic cells (Dray *et al.*, 1978). Importantly for the present discussion, the ratio of excitatory to inhibitory responses can be altered by manipulations such as 5-HT depletion (Gervais and Rouillard, 2000). Generally, elevated serotonin function produced by selective serotonin reuptake inhibition, which would be expected to indirectly affect all serotonin receptor subtypes, reduces dopamine cell firing (Di Mascio *et al.*, 1998). Cocaine partially inhibits dopaminergic neurons, and although this is largely attributable to autoreceptor inhibition (Einhorn *et al.*, 1988), serotonin release also contributes to this inhibition (Brodie and Bunney, 1996).

Returning to consideration of the role of SERT in drug reward, it would seem obvious that the consequences of SERT deletion in knock-out mice would depend upon the relative expression of serotonin receptor subtypes. The effects produced by elevations in extracellular serotonin consequent to SERT blockade would be highly dependent on the particular receptors activated. Pharmacological studies have identified numerous drug reward modulating effects of serotonergic manipulations mediated by the 5-HT1A receptor (Tomkins *et al.*, 1994a, 1994b; Wilson *et al.*, 1998), the 5-HT1B receptor (Fletcher and Korth, 1999; Harrison *et al.*, 1999; Maurel *et al.*, 1999; Parsons *et al.*, 1998; Tomkins and O'Neill, 2000; Wilson *et al.*, 1998), the 5-HT2C receptor (Fletcher *et al.*, 2002; Grottick *et al.*, 2000), the 5-HT3 receptor (Fadda *et al.*, 1991; Higgins *et al.*, 1992; Kostowski *et al.*, 1993; Rompre *et al.*, 1995; Tomkins *et al.*, 1995), and the 5-HT4 receptor (Bisaga *et al.*, 1993), although in many cases the specific consequences of serotonergic stimulation of particular receptors have been in dispute. In part this was due to initial lack of specific 5-HT agonists and antagonists, but this also may reflect differential involvement of 5-HT receptor subtypes in the rewarding effects of particular drugs of abuse. For example, in the case of the 5-HT1B receptor, agonists have been suggested to reduce the rewarding effects of ethanol (Maurel *et al.*, 1999; Tomkins and O'Neill, 2000), brain stimulation reward (Harrison *et al.*, 1999), and amphetamine (Fletcher and Korth, 1999), but to enhance cocaine reward (Parsons *et al.*, 1998). This might reflect differential involvement of that receptor in the rewarding effects of drugs acting via different mechanisms, but discrepancies between studies have been observed for individual drugs in 5-HT1B knock-out mice in which the rewarding effects of ethanol have been reported to be reduced (Risinger *et al.*, 1996) or unchanged

(Risinger *et al.*, 1999), and the rewarding effects of cocaine increased (Rocha *et al.*, 1998b) or decreased (Belzung *et al.*, 2000). Several factors might contribute to these different findings; at the very least, these data indicate that serotonergic activity can modulate drug reward, both positively and negatively. This modulation is highly dependent on the specific receptors activated, the rewarding substance that is studied, the brain regions affected, and perhaps other factors, such as genetic background and developmental experiences.

Returning to the question of the particular serotonin receptor subtypes that may be altered in DAT KO mice, much remains to be done. Initial observations indicated that there were no substantial changes in 5-HT1A or 5-HT1B receptor densities in a number of dopamine cell body and terminal regions (Sora *et al.*, 2001). The numerous other serotonin receptor subtypes have not been examined extensively, although there do not appear to be changes in receptor mRNA in several brain regions (Li, Hall and Uhl, unpublished observations). Much more has been done in SERT KO mice, although not necessarily in areas that would be highly relevant to dopamine/serotonin interactions; none the less, these findings are discussed in some detail below.

COMPENSATORY ALTERATIONS IN SEROTONIN FUNCTION IN SERT KO MICE

One way to interpret the different effects of SERT gene knock-out on drug reward is to consider the effects of combination of SERT KO with other gene knock-outs as a special case of gene background. To begin this discussion, let us first consider the effects of SERT knock-out itself on serotonin receptors, pharmacological responses, and neurochemical function. This literature has been reviewed in great detail elsewhere (Fox *et al.*, 2007a), so only a brief summary will be presented here. SERT KO produces substantial elevations in extracellular serotonin (Mathews *et al.*, 2004; Shen *et al.*, 2004), resulting in a variety of compensatory changes. These include a marked reduction in tissue serotonin concentrations in the brain (Bengel *et al.*, 1998; Zhao *et al.*, 2006) and a near absence of cortical serotonin assessed immunocytochemically (Persico *et al.*, 2001). Serotonin concentrations are also reduced dramatically in the pituitary and adrenal glands (Tjurmina *et al.*, 2002) and other peripheral tissues (Kim *et al.*, 2005). Reductions in tissue 5-HT concentrations occur despite substantially enhanced 5-HT synthesis (Kim *et al.*, 2005). In addition, that study indicated that regional and sex-dependent alterations in the ability to upregulate synthesis may relate to the degree of reduction of tissue serotonin concentrations. These differences may also relate to region-specific changes in postsynaptic function discussed below.

There is a pronounced desensitization of 5-HT1A receptors in SERT KO mice (Fabre *et al.*, 2000; Holmes *et al.*, 2003; Li *et al.*, 1999, 2000) resulting from a reduction in somatic 5-HT1A receptor binding, as well as terminal 5-HT1A receptor binding in some regions associated with reduced behavioral and neuroendocrine responses to 5-HT1A agonists. Note, however, that these effects are regionally dependent and vary with sex (Fabre *et al.*, 2000; Li *et al.*, 2000); it must also be noted that some of the differences between the last two studies may be the result of differing genetic backgrounds used in the two studies (C57BL/6J vs. CD1−129svev). In any case, reductions in 5-HT1A levels in the dorsal raphe are consistently observed and 5-HT1A mediated inhibition of dorsal raphe cell firing is reduced both in vitro (Mannoury la Cour *et al.*, 2001), and in vivo (Gobbi *et al.*, 2001). This last study also found reduced postsynaptic 5-HT1A function in SERT KO mice (Gobbi *et al.*, 2001), along with other changes in serotonin neuronal function, including a reduction in basal firing rate. This was confirmed in another study which also found a dramatic reduction in serotonergic cell number (Lira *et al.*, 2003).

Other postsynaptic receptors are also affected by SERT KO, but in a highly regionally dependent manner that is not explained solely by a global response to elevated extracellular serotonin. This includes changes in both 5-HT2A and 5-HT2C receptors (Li *et al.*, 2003; Rioux *et al.*, 1999). In the most comprehensive study (Li *et al.*, 2003), increased density of 5-HT2A receptors was observed in subregions of the hypothalamus and septum, while reduced density of 5-HT2A receptors were observed in subregions of the striatum, notably the ventral striatum. For the 5-HT2C receptor, increased levels were observed in the amygdala. It must be noted that no changes were observed in most brain regions, and the changes that were observed appeared to be unrelated to changes in mRNA levels. Unfortunately, these autoradiographic methods were not sensitive enough to measure receptor levels in regions with low overall density, including many regions that would be of interest in the present discussion. However, in the study by Rioux *et al.* (1999), reduced levels of 5-HT2A receptors were observed in the substantia nigra. Importantly, an examination of 5-HT2A/2C activation of phospholipase A2, which induces activation of diverse brain regions in WT mice including the dorsal and ventral striatum, found no activation in SERT−/− mice in any region of the brain and a marked attenuation of DOI-induced head twitches (Qu *et al.*, 2005).

Reduced locomotor responses have also been observed to a 5-HT1A/1B agonist in SERT KO mice (Holmes *et al.*, 2002a). This might be thought to be associated with the previously mentioned reductions in 5-HT1A receptors, but reductions of 5-HT1B receptors in the substantia nigra have also been observed in SERT KO mice (Fabre *et al.*, 2000) where they would be more likely to affect motor function. Like changes in other receptors, changes in 5-HT1B receptors were also highly regionally dependent. In addition, in the substantia nigra, the ability of a 5-HT1B antagonist to enhance serotonin release was eliminated in SERT KO mice, consistent with the reduction in 5-HT1B receptors observed in these mice (Fabre *et al.*, 2000).

As can be seen from this short summary, the consequences of SERT deletion on postsynaptic receptor function are highly dependent on which receptor subtype, and which brain region, is under consideration. Thus, it is likely that the particular consequences of SERT knock-out are determined by the balance of changes in any particular brain region, resulting in not just the increase or decrease of particular pharmacological responses, but also in fundamental changes in some types of responses, which are furthermore dependent on other factors, such as genetic background and the presence of other genetic manipulations. For example, although methamphetamine-induced hyperthermia was unaffected by SERT knock-out alone, in DAT KO mice heterozygous SERT deletion reduced methamphetamine-induced hyperthermia, and produced an initial hypothermia that was not observed in wildtype or single knock-out mice (Numachi *et al.*, 2007). Homozygous SERT deletion in DAT−/− mice eliminated methamphetamine-induced hyperthermia, producing only a pronounced hypothermia. The basis of these changes has yet to be elicited fully, but the paradoxical hypothermia does not involve actions at the norepinephrine transporter. An alternative would be that changes in the ratios of serotonin receptor subtypes in regions involved in temperature regulation underlie this hypothermia. This does not involve 5-HT1A-mediated hypothermia, which is eliminated in SERT KO mice (Li *et al.*, 1999), so it must involve other mechanisms that have yet to be elucidated.

In summary, it would appear that the functions of 5-HT1A, 5-HT1B, and 5-HT2A receptors are reduced in SERT KO mice, albeit in a regionally dependent manner. The pharmacological evidence discussed in the previous section would seem to suggest that these effects would most likely be associated with reduced dopamine function and perhaps reduced rewarding effects of cocaine. However, these may not be the most relevant changes in serotonin function with regard to interactions with dopamine function or drug reward. In particular, the changes in 5-HT1A and 5-HT1B function may reflect the generally elevated and prolonged release of serotonin in SERT KO mice, which would have greater effects at other receptor subtypes. It may just be this alteration in the balance of serotonin receptor activation that underlies increased rewarding effects of cocaine in SERT KO mice.

BEHAVIORAL CHANGES IN SERT KO MICE

The pattern of changes in presynaptic and postsynaptic serotonin function in SERT KO mice is paralleled by changes in behavior that have long been associated with serotonin function, including behavior related to anxiety, depression, and aggression. Studies in SERT KO mice have included two types of approaches. In the first approach, SERT gene knock-out was produced by homologous recombination disrupting the N-terminus (Bengel *et al.*, 1998; Lira *et al.*, 2003), including the start codon in Exon 2. In the second approach, SERT deletion was produced by random insertion of a viral vector (gene trapping), resulting in a C-terminus deletion (Zhao *et al.*, 2006). Both of these approaches should be expected to produce equivalent effects. Of perhaps greatest importance is background strain. In particular, the original SERT KO strain (Bengel *et al.*, 1998) has been placed on several genetic backgrounds for comparison, which have not always produced identical results.

There is some evidence that SERT KO mice express a baseline depressive phenotype. SERT KO mice on a 129S6 background exhibit increased immobility in the forced swim test, but the opposite profile in the tail suspension test (Holmes *et al.*, 2002b; Lira *et al.*, 2003). However, SERT KO mice on a C57BL/6J background exhibited no baseline differences in those models (Holmes *et al.*, 2002b), although other studies have found increased immobility in both tests (Carroll *et al.*, 2007; Zhao *et al.*, 2006). Importantly, other studies in C57BL/6J SERT KO mice found no baseline differences but increased immobility emerged with repeated testing (Wellman *et al.*, 2007; Zhao *et al.*, 2006), suggesting a predisposition to stress in SERT KO mice. Consistent with this idea, 129S6 SERT KO mice exhibited behavior in a shock escape paradigm (Lira *et al.*, 2003), similar to what is observed after exposure to chronic inescapable stress (e.g. learned helplessness). C57BL/6J SERT KO mice did not have impairments in fear conditioning or extinction, but did have an impairment of extinction recall (Wellman *et al.*, 2007). SERT KO mice did not have a depressive phenotype, anhedonia, in a sucrose consumption test (Kalueff *et al.*, 2006), prompting those authors to suggest that results from other models may be confounded by differences in motor function in SERT KO mice. However, given the previous indications that SERT KO mice may be differentially sensitive to stress, it would be interesting to examine sucrose responses after stress.

These findings from behavioral studies are supported by studies demonstrating that SERT KO mice have an exaggerated adrenomedullary epinephrine release in response to stress (Armando *et al.*, 2003; Tjurmina *et al.*, 2002), reduced adrenal levels of epinephrine and norepinephrine after stressors (Armando *et al.*, 2003), elimination of stress-induced increases in tyrosine hydroxylase mRNA (Armando *et al.*, 2003), and potentiated responses to a mild predator stress (Adamec *et al.*, 2006). Collectively, these data indicate that SERT KO mice do have a depressive phenotype, or at least the propensity for a depressive phenotype that can be evoked by stressful experiences or is more likely to be evident in the context of particular genetic backgrounds. The relationship of this depressive phenotype to addictive phenotypes, particularly in relation to enhanced stress responses, has yet to be investigated, but would certainly be an interesting direction for future research.

Even more consistent differences in anxiety function have been found in SERT KO mice, although genetic background is again a critical factor. C57BL/6J SERT KO mice have increased anxiety in a number of standard anxiety paradigms (Armando *et al.*, 2003; Carroll *et al.*, 2007; Holmes *et al.*, 2003; Kalueff *et al.*, 2007a; Zhao *et al.*, 2006), while 129S6 SERT KO exhibit no differences in these tests (Holmes *et al.*, 2003; Lira *et al.*, 2003). However, this may not be a true interaction with background strain, but might rather be the result of ceiling effects resulting from elevated anxiety in the 129S6 background strain. 129S6 SERT KO mice do have an increased feeding latency in a novelty suppressed feeding paradigm (Lira *et al.*, 2003). The effects of SERT KO in many circumstances, such as the open field, may also result from other behavioral changes, including hypolocomotion and altered spatiotemporal organization of exploration (Kalueff *et al.*, 2007b), although hypoactivity appears to be highly task-dependent and largely normal motor and sensory ability is observed in most circumstances (Kalueff *et al.*, 2007b). Hypoactivity may also have impacted upon behavioral tests that identified reduced aggression in SERT KO mice (Holmes *et al.*, 2002a), but this is unlikely to account for all of the observations.

This pattern of behavioral effects in SERT KO mice is not necessarily what would be expected from elevated serotonin function per se. Indeed, they are the opposite of that which would be expected from elevated serotonin function in adult mice. Thus, it is likely that these changes result from some of the adaptations in serotonin function discussed in previous sections. In this context it is interesting to note that neonatal treatment with the SERT blocker fluoxetine produces effects similar to those observed in SERT KO mice in many of these paradigms (Ansorge *et al.*, 2004). Further evidence for such changes can also be seen in spontaneous behavior similar to the "serotonin syndrome", including Straub tail, tics, tremor, and backward gait (Kalueff *et al.*, 2007a). SERT KO mice also have an exaggerated response to serotonergic agents that induce the serotonin syndrome (Fox *et al.*, 2007b), which appear to be specifically mediated by postsynaptic 5-HT1A receptors.

It probably should not be supposed that differences in behavior in SERT knock-out mice result only from changes in serotonin neurotransmission. A variety of changes in other cellular and anatomical processes have also been observed, including differences in cerebrocortical thickness (Altamura *et al.*, 2007). SERT KO mice have reduced thickness of layer IV, an effect that is again somewhat dependent on genetic background. Reduced programmed cell death is also found in diverse brain structures, including the striatum (Persico *et al.*, 2003). The effect on cortical layer IV thickness appears to be a neurodevelopmental consequence of SERT deletion resulting in alterations in thalamocortical inputs and cortical morphology, including the failure of barrel field development (Persico *et al.*, 2001). A portion of this developmental alteration is the result of elevated 5-HT1B receptor stimulation during development (Salichon *et al.*, 2001). Differences are also seen at the cellular level; pyramidal neurons in the infralimbic cortex show differences in dendritic arborization and pyramidal neurons in the basolateral amygdala have increased synaptic spine density in SERT KO mice (Wellman *et al.*, 2007).

The interactive genetic effects of SERT KO apparent by varying genetic background can also be seen when the knock-out is combined with deletion of other genes (for a detailed review see Murphy *et al.*, 2003). Interaction with other monoamine transporters has already been discussed, which may further involve other monoamine system genes, including serotonin receptors. Other effects of SERT KO have also been shown to have important interactive effects with other gene knock-outs. The abnormal development of thalamocortical maps in SERT KO mice can be partially reversed by combination with a 5-HT1B knock-out (Salichon *et al.*, 2001). Several effects of SERT KO are exacerbated when the SERT KO is combined with a heterozygous deletion for the brain-derived neurotrophic factor gene (Ren-Patterson *et al.*, 2005), although many of these effects are highly sex-dependent (Ren-Patterson *et al.*, 2006). The interaction between SERT and BDNF knock-out has not been examined for drug reward, but it is interesting to note that BDNF knock-out has opposite effects on cocaine reward to that observed in SERT KO mice (Hall *et al.*, 2003).

In addition to the anatomical differences noted above, some other changes observed in SERT KO mice are also distinctly abnormal, including accumulation of 5-HT in dopaminergic neurons in the ventral tegmental area and substantia nigra (Zhou *et al.*, 2002). This occult reuptake of serotonin can also be produced by administration of SERT blockers, and serotonin has been subsequently shown to be released from dopamine neurons under these conditions (Zhou *et al.*, 2005). The importance of these unusual effects is uncertain, however.

REWARDING EFFECTS OF OTHER ADDICTIVE DRUGS

As discussed above, cocaine reward has been examined several times in SERT KO mice, and the effects are shown to be substantially dependent on the genetic context, in particular the presence of other gene knock-outs. The effects of genetic background, which was determined to be so important in determining emotion-related behavioral consequences of SERT KO, have not been examined for drug reward. Furthermore, given the diverse effects of serotonin manipulations on different types of abused substances, it would be important to examine the effects of SERT KO on multiple classes of abused drugs, but unfortunately, the effects of few other drug classes have been examined.

Not surprisingly, the locomotor stimulant effects of MDMA were abolished in SERT KO mice, although the locomotor stimulant effects of D-amphetamine were unaffected (Bengel *et al.*, 1998). It must be noted that only a single high dose of each drug was examined. However, as exemplified by findings in DAT KO mice (Sora *et al.*, 1998), locomotor stimulant and rewarding effects of drugs of abuse are often divergent in genetic models. In this case, however, MDMA self-administration is also eliminated in SERT KO mice (Trigo *et al.*, 2007). Further emphasizing the important interactions between dopamine and serotonin systems that underlie the effects of these drugs, MDMA reduced locomotor activity in DAT KO mice in contrast to the normal stimulant effects that were observed in WT mice (Powell *et al.*, 2004). Indeed, under some circumstances, the locomotor hyperactivity observed in DAT KO mice is reduced not only by typical stimulant drugs (cocaine, amphetamine, and methylphenidate), but drugs that selectively enhance serotonin function (fluoxetine, quipazine, 5-hydroxytryptophan, and L-tryptophan; Gainetdinov *et al.*, 1999). The precise nature of these effects is open to question, in particular the initial description as "calming", but regardless of the nature of these effects they certainly demonstrate two important points: (1) important dopaminergic phenotypes involve interactions between serotonin and dopamine systems; and (2) profound changes in serotonergic function have occurred in DAT KO mice that emphasize the role of serotonin systems in the actions of drugs such as cocaine in these mice.

Given the extensive evidence for the involvement of serotonin systems in the effects of ethanol and in alcoholism, SERT KO would be expected to also have effects on the rewarding effects of ethanol. Thus, it is not surprising that voluntary ethanol consumption is reduced in SERT KO mice (Kelai *et al.*, 2003). Although decreased ethanol consumption was observed at high ethanol concentrations (15–20%), another study found slightly reduced consumption in SERT KO mice, but only at low ethanol concentrations (5–7%; Boyce-Rustay *et al.*, 2006). The effects of SERT KO were examined for several other ethanol-mediated effects in this study. The sedative effects of ethanol administration were enhanced in SERT KO mice, but several other effects were unaltered. More importantly, there was no difference in ethanol CPP, although only one dose was examined (2 mg/kg), so it remains possible that there may also be a dose-dependent change in CPP. Ethanol has diverse neurochemical effects, but some of these differences may be directly related to potentiated ethanol-induced inhibition of serotonin clearance in SERT−/− mice (Daws *et al.*, 2006).

The paucity of research on drugs of abuse other than cocaine in SERT knock-out mice makes this an area of important future investigation, particularly given findings in humans implicating SERT in addiction to a number of classes of drugs. The literature in humans also indicates that consideration of drug reward alone may not be sufficient, as variation in SERT may affect specific phenotypes such as compulsive craving (Bleich, 2007). As discussed below, many effects of SERT KO on drug reward may be indirect, relating to self-medication, for anxiety and depression. In addition, it will be important to gain further understanding of the role of changes in serotonin function consequent to differences in other genes, either as the result of gene knock-out or a function of genetic background, that influence drug reward. In many instances, including the unusual effects of SERT inhibition in DAT KO mice, it can be seen that SERT plays a pivotal role that influences the consequences of serotonergic stimulation.

The research summarized above indicates that SERT may play an important role in drug reward and potentially in addiction. This is not a possibility that has been investigated thoroughly, except in regard to alcoholism, although there has been substantial research into the potential role of SERT in depression and anxiety (for review see Hariri and Holmes, 2006). Of particular interest for the models discussed above, a common allelic variant of the human SERT gene has been identified, and the "short" allelic variant of this polymorphism is associated with reduced SERT expression in the brain (Heinz *et al.*, 2000) and with both depression and anxiety (Caspi *et al.*, 2003; Lesch *et al.*, 1996). For direct comparison to the transgenic models discussed above, it would then seem to be of critical importance which phenotypes result from heterozygous SERT knock-out, which reduces SERT expression by 50%, and would thus be comparable to the changes in SERT expression observed in humans with the "short" SERT allelic variant. However, this may not be sufficient, as illustrated by the substantial interactive genetic effects observed in transgenic studies. Variations in SERT expression must be considered in the context of other genetic, and perhaps environmental, effects to gain a full understanding of the role of SERT, and perhaps to prevent being misled by false negative findings. In this regard, it is important to note that the effect of the SERT polymorphism discussed above interacted meaningfully with the number of stressful life events to determine the ultimate depressive phenotype (Caspi *et al.*, 2003), just as depressive phenotypes were not necessarily observed in SERT KO mice unless those mice were subjected to repeated stressors (Wellman *et al.*, 2007). None the less, there is substantial evidence for an association between SERT allelic variants and alcoholism (see discussion in Lesch, 2005). Those authors further emphasize important interactive effects between SERT genotype and experience, and also potential interactions with other predisposing genes. For instance, an interaction has recently been demonstrated between allelic variant in the SERT and monoamine oxidase A genes in alcoholism (Herman *et al.*, 2005). Given the wealth of data from animal models, it will be important to extend these findings in humans to other drugs of abuse, and to consider a broader range of interacting factors, including genetic factors, and to better specify in both the human and animal studies the underlying endophenotypes that predispose animals to greater consumption of drugs of abuse and humans to addiction.

CONCLUSIONS

Studies in SERT KO mice, and of SERT function consequent to the knock-out of other genes, have implicated SERT in drug reward.

Much of this research has concentrated on a limited number of addictive substances (primarily cocaine) and a limited number of phenotypes (primarily conditioned place preference). It will be important to determine to what extent these effects generalize across substances, and to what extent they result from changes in specific phenotypes rather than from general changes in drug reward. Human genetic studies indicate both that SERT is likely to affect responses to a variety of addictive drugs and that it may produce changes in specific phenotypes. The comparison between allelic variation in humans and genetic models should be made more explicit. In this regard, it is important to examine the effects of heterozygous knock-outs to the extent that they reflect the range of variation in gene expression observed in humans. In this respect, one of the usual criticisms of gene knock-outs should be considered a strength, rather than a weakness: observations of changes resulting from a knock-out may result either from reduced expression in adult animals or developmental changes. In this case, the effects of changes in SERT expression in humans may be due to developmental effects so that observations in SERT KO mice may actually have greater validity. Obviously this possibility needs further investigation in both animal models and humans in relation to addictive phenotypes.

ACKNOWLEDGMENTS

This research was supported by the Intramural Research Program of the National Institute on Drug Abuse (NIH/DHHS).

REFERENCES

Adamec R, Burton P, Blundell J, Murphy D L, Holmes A (2006). Vulnerability to mild predator stress in serotonin transporter knockout mice. *Behav Brain Res* **170**: 126–40.

Altamura C, Dell'Acqua M L, Moessner R, Murphy D L, Lesch K P, Persico A M (2007). Altered neocortical cell density and layer thickness in serotonin transporter knockout mice: a quantitation study. *Cereb Cortex* **17**: 1394–401.

Ansorge M S, Zhou M, Lira A, Hen R, Gingrich J A (2004). Early-life blockade of the 5-HT transporter alters emotional behavior in adult mice. *Science* **306**: 879–81.

Arborelius L, Chergui K, Murase S, *et al.* (1993). The 5-HT1A receptor selective ligands, (*R*)-8-OH-DPAT and (*S*)-UH-301, differentially affect the activity of midbrain dopamine neurons. *Naunyn Schmiedebergs Arch Pharmacol* **347**: 353–62.

Armando I, Tjurmina O A, Li Q, Murphy D L, Saavedra J M (2003). The serotonin transporter is required for stress-evoked increases in adrenal catecholamine synthesis and angiotensin II AT(2) receptor expression. *Neuroendocrinology* **78**: 217–25.

Belzung C, Scearce-Levie K, Barreau S, Hen R (2000). Absence of cocaine-induced place conditioning in serotonin 1B receptor knock-out mice. *Pharmacol Biochem Behav* **66**: 221–5.

Bengel D, Murphy D L, Andrews A M, *et al.* (1998). Altered brain serotonin homeostasis and locomotor insensitivity to 3,4-methylenedioxymethamphetamine ("Ecstasy") in serotonin transporter-deficient mice. *Mol Pharmacol* **53**: 649–55.

Bisaga A, Sikora J, Kostowski W (1993). The effect of drugs interacting with serotonergic 5HT3 and 5HT4 receptors on morphine place conditioning. *Pol J Pharmacol* **45**: 513–9.

Bleich S, Bönsch D, Rauh J, Bayerlein K, Fiszer R, Frieling H, Hillemacher T (2007). Association of the long allele of the 5-HTTLPR polymorphism with compulsive craving in alcohol dependence. *Alcohol Alcohol* **42**: 509–12.

Bonhomme N, De Deurwaerdere P, Le Moal M, Spampinato U (1995). Evidence for 5-HT4 receptor subtype involvement in the enhancement of striatal dopamine release induced by serotonin: a microdialysis study in the halothane-anesthetized rat. *Neuropharmacology* **34**: 269–79.

Boulenguez P, Peters S L, Mitchell S N, Chauveau J, Gray J A, Joseph M H (1998). Dopamine release in the nucleus accumbens and latent inhibition in the rat following microinjections of a 5-HT1B agonist into the dorsal subiculum: implications for schizophrenia. *J Psychopharmacol* **12**: 258–67.

Boulenguez P, Rawlins J N, Chauveau J, Joseph M H, Mitchell S N, Gray J A (1996). Modulation of dopamine release in the nucleus accumbens by 5-HT1B agonists: involvement of the hippocampo-accumbens pathway. *Neuropharmacology* **35**: 1521–9.

Boyce-Rustay J M, Wiedholz L M, Millstein R A, *et al.* (2006). Ethanol-related behaviors in serotonin transporter knockout mice. *Alcohol Clin Exp Res* **30**: 1957–65.

Brodie M S, Bunney E B (1996). Serotonin potentiates dopamine inhibition of ventral tegmental area neurons in vitro. *J Neurophysiol* **76**: 2077–82.

Cameron D L, Wessendorf M W, Williams J T (1997). A subset of ventral tegmental area neurons is inhibited by dopamine, 5-hydroxytryptamine and opioids. *Neuroscience* **77**: 155–66.

Campbell A D, McBride W J (1995). Serotonin-3 receptor and ethanol-stimulated dopamine release in the nucleus accumbens. *Pharmacol Biochem Behav* **51**: 835–42.

Carroll J C, Boyce-Rustay J M, Millstein R, *et al.* (2007). Effects of mild early life stress on abnormal emotion-related behaviors in 5-HTT knockout mice. *Behav Genet* **37**: 214–22.

Caspi A, Sugden K, Moffitt T E, *et al.* (2003). Influence of life stress on depression: moderation by a polymorphism in the 5-HTT gene. *Science* **301**: 386–9.

Chen J P, van Praag H M, Gardner E L (1991). Activation of 5-HT3 receptor by 1-phenylbiguanide increases dopamine release in the rat nucleus accumbens. *Brain Res* **543**: 354–7.

Daws L C, Montanez S, Munn J L, *et al.* (2006). Ethanol inhibits clearance of brain serotonin by a serotonin transporter-independent mechanism. *J Neurosci* **26**: 6431–8.

De Deurwaerdere P, L'Hirondel M, Bonhomme N, Lucas G, Cheramy A, Spampinato U (1997). Serotonin stimulation of 5-HT4 receptors indirectly enhances in vivo dopamine release in the rat striatum. *J Neurochem* **68**: 195–203.

De Deurwaerdere P, Spampinato U (1999). Role of serotonin(2A) and serotonin(2B/2C) receptor subtypes in the control of accumbal and striatal dopamine release elicited in vivo by dorsal raphe nucleus electrical stimulation. *J Neurochem* **73**: 1033–42.

De Deurwaerdere P, Stinus L, Spampinato U (1998). Opposite change of in vivo dopamine release in the rat nucleus accumbens and striatum that follows electrical stimulation of dorsal raphe nucleus: role of 5-HT3 receptors. *J Neurosci* **18**: 6528–38.

Di Giovanni G, De Deurwaerdere P, Di Mascio M, Di Matteo V, Esposito E, Spampinato U (1999). Selective blockade of serotonin-2C/2B receptors enhances mesolimbic and mesostriatal dopaminergic function: a combined in vivo electrophysiological and microdialysis study. *Neuroscience* **91**: 587–97.

Di Giovanni G, Di Matteo V, Di Mascio M, Esposito E (2000). Preferential modulation of mesolimbic vs. nigrostriatal dopaminergic function by serotonin(2C/2B) receptor agonists: a combined in vivo electrophysiological and microdialysis study. *Synapse* **35**: 53–61.

Di Mascio M, Di Giovanni G, Di Matteo V, Prisco S, Esposito E (1998). Selective serotonin reuptake inhibitors reduce the spontaneous activity of dopaminergic neurons in the ventral tegmental area. *Brain Res Bull* **46**: 547–54.

Di Matteo V, Di Giovanni G, Di Mascio M, Esposito E (2000). Biochemical and electrophysiological evidence that RO 60–0175 inhibits mesolimbic dopaminergic function through serotonin(2C) receptors. *Brain Res* **865**: 85–90.

Diaz-Mataix L, Artigas F, Celada P (2006). Activation of pyramidal cells in rat medial prefrontal cortex projecting to ventral tegmental area by a 5-HT1A receptor agonist. *Eur Neuropsychopharmacol* **16**: 288–96.

Diaz-Mataix L, Scorza M C, Bortolozzi A, Toth M, Celada P, Artigas F (2005). Involvement of 5-HT1A receptors in prefrontal cortex in the modulation of dopaminergic activity: role in atypical antipsychotic action. *J Neurosci* **25**: 10 831–43.

Dray A, Davies J, Oakley N R, Tongroach P, Vellucci S (1978). The dorsal and medial raphe projections to the substantia nigra in the rat: electrophysiological, biochemical and behavioural observations. *Brain Res* **151**: 431–42.

Einhorn L C, Johansen P A, White F J (1988). Electrophysiological effects of cocaine in the mesoaccumbens dopamine system: studies in the ventral tegmental area. *J Neurosci* **8**: 100–12.

Fabre V, Beaufour C, Evrard A, *et al.* (2000). Altered expression and functions of serotonin 5-HT1A and 5-HT1B receptors in knock-out mice lacking the 5-HT transporter. *Eur J Neurosci* **12**: 2299–310.

Fadda F, Garau B, Marchei F, Colombo G, Gessa G L (1991). MDL 72222, a selective 5-HT3 receptor antagonist, suppresses voluntary ethanol consumption in alcohol-preferring rats. *Alcohol Alcohol* **26**: 107–10.

Fink K B, Gothert M (2007). 5-HT receptor regulation of neurotransmitter release. *Pharmacol Rev* **59**: 360–417.

Fletcher P J, Grottick A J, Higgins G A (2002). Differential effects of the 5-HT(2A) receptor antagonist M100907 and the 5-HT(2C) receptor antagonist SB242084 on cocaine-induced locomotor activity, cocaine self-administration and cocaine-induced reinstatement of responding. *Neuropsychopharmacology* **27**: 576–86.

Fletcher P J, Korth K M (1999). Activation of 5-HT1B receptors in the nucleus accumbens reduces amphetamine-induced enhancement of responding for conditioned reward. *Psychopharmacology (Berl.)* **142**: 165–74.

Fox M A, Andrews A M, Wendland J R, Lesch K P, Holmes A, Murphy D L (2007a). A pharmacological analysis of mice with a targeted disruption of the serotonin transporter. *Psychopharmacology (Berl.)* **195**: 147–66.

Fox M A, Jensen C L, Gallagher P S, Murphy D L (2007b). Receptor mediation of exaggerated responses to serotonin-enhancing drugs in serotonin transporter (SERT)-deficient mice. *Neuropharmacology* **53**: 643–56.

Gainetdinov R R, Wetsel W C, Jones S R, Levin E D, Jaber M, Caron M G (1999). Role of serotonin in the paradoxical calming effect of psychostimulants on hyperactivity. *Science* **283**: 397–401.

Gervais J, Rouillard C (2000). Dorsal raphe stimulation differentially modulates dopaminergic neurons in the ventral tegmental area and substantia nigra. *Synapse* **35**: 281–91.

Giros B, Jaber M, Jones S R, Wightman R M, Caron M G (1996). Hyperlocomotion and indifference to cocaine and amphetamine in mice lacking the dopamine transporter. *Nature* **379**: 606–12.

Gobbi G, Murphy D L, Lesch K, Blier P (2001). Modifications of the serotonergic system in mice lacking serotonin transporters: an in vivo electrophysiological study. *J Pharmacol Exp Ther* **296**: 987–95.

Gobert A, Millan M J (1999). Serotonin (5-HT)2A receptor activation enhances dialysate levels of dopamine and noradrenaline, but not 5-HT, in the frontal cortex of freely-moving rats. *Neuropharmacology* **38**: 315–7.

Gobert A, Rivet J M, Lejeune F, *et al.* (2000). Serotonin(2C) receptors tonically suppress the activity of mesocortical dopaminergic and adrenergic, but not serotonergic, pathways: a combined dialysis and electrophysiological analysis in the rat. *Synapse* **36**: 205–21.

Gongora-Alfaro J L, Hernandez-Lopez S, Flores-Hernandez J, Galarraga E (1997). Firing frequency modulation of substantia nigra reticulata neurons by 5-hydroxytryptamine. *Neurosci Res* **29**: 225–31.

Grottick A J, Fletcher P J, Higgins G A (2000). Studies to investigate the role of 5-HT(2C) receptors on cocaine- and food-maintained behavior. *J Pharmacol Exp Ther* **295**: 1183–91.

Hall F S, Drgonova J, Goeb M, Uhl G R (2003). Reduced behavioral effects of cocaine in heterozygous brain-derived neurotrophic factor (BDNF) knockout mice. *Neuropsychopharmacology* **28**: 1485–90.

Hall F S, Li X F, Sora I, *et al.* (2002). Cocaine mechanisms: enhanced cocaine, fluoxetine and nisoxetine place preferences following monoamine transporter deletions. *Neuroscience* **115**: 153–61.

Hallbus M, Magnusson T, Magnusson O (1997). Influence of 5-HT1B/1D receptors on dopamine release in the guinea pig nucleus accumbens: a microdialysis study. *Neurosci Lett* **225**: 57–60.

Hariri A R, Holmes A (2006). Genetics of emotional regulation: the role of the serotonin transporter in neural function. *Trends Cogn Sci* **10**: 182–91.

Harrison A A, Parsons L H, Koob G F, Markou A (1999). RU 24969, a 5-HT1A/1B agonist, elevates brain stimulation reward thresholds: an effect reversed by GR 127935, a 5-HT1B/1D antagonist. *Psychopharmacology (Berl.)* **141**: 242–50.

Heinz A, Jones D W, Mazzanti C, *et al.* (2000). A relationship between serotonin transporter genotype and in vivo protein expression and alcohol neurotoxicity. *Biol Psychiatry* **47**: 643–9.

Herman A I, Kaiss K M, Ma R, *et al.* (2005). Serotonin transporter promoter polymorphism and monoamine oxidase type A VNTR allelic variants together influence alcohol binge drinking risk in young women. *Am J Med Genet B Neuropsychiatr Genet* **133**: 74–8.

Higgins G A, Joharchi N, Nguyen P, Sellers E M (1992). Effect of the 5-HT3 receptor antagonists, MDL72222 and ondansetron on morphine place conditioning. *Psychopharmacology* **106**: 315–20.

Hnasko T S, Sotak B N, Palmiter R D (2007). Cocaine-conditioned place preference by dopamine-deficient mice is mediated by serotonin. *J Neurosci* **27**: 12 484–8.

Holmes A, Lit Q, Murphy D L, Gold E, Crawley J N (2003). Abnormal anxiety-related behavior in serotonin transporter null mutant mice: the influence of genetic background. *Genes Brain Behav* **2**: 365–80.

Holmes A, Murphy D L, Crawley J N (2002a). Reduced aggression in mice lacking the serotonin transporter. *Psychopharmacology (Berl.)* **161**: 160–7.

Holmes A, Yang R J, Murphy D L, Crawley J N (2002b). Evaluation of antidepressant-related behavioral responses in mice lacking the serotonin transporter. *Neuropsychopharmacology* **27**: 914–23.

Ichikawa J, Meltzer H Y (1995). DOI, a 5-HT2A/2C receptor agonist, potentiates amphetamine-induced dopamine release in rat striatum. *Brain Res* **698**: 204–8.

Imperato A, Angelucci L (1989). 5-HT3 receptors control dopamine release in the nucleus accumbens of freely moving rats. *Neurosci Lett* **101**: 214–7.

Iyer R N, Bradberry C W (1996). Serotonin-mediated increase in prefrontal cortex dopamine release: pharmacological characterization. *J Pharmacol Exp Ther* **277**: 40–7.

Johnson S W, Mercuri N B, North R A (1992). 5-Hydroxytryptamine1B receptors block the GABAB synaptic potential in rat dopamine neurons. *J Neurosci* **12**: 2000–6.

Kalueff A V, Fox M A, Gallagher P S, Murphy D L (2007a). Hypolocomotion, anxiety and serotonin syndrome-like behavior contribute to the complex phenotype of serotonin transporter knockout mice. *Genes Brain Behav* **6**: 389–400.

Kalueff A V, Gallagher P S, Murphy D L (2006). Are serotonin transporter knockout mice 'depressed'? Hypoactivity but no anhedonia. *Neuroreport* **17**: 1347–51.

Kalueff A V, Jensen C L, Murphy D L (2007b). Locomotory patterns, spatiotemporal organization of exploration and spatial memory in serotonin transporter knockout mice. *Brain Res* **1169**: 87–97.

Kankaanpaa A, Lillsunde P, Ruotsalainen M, Ahtee L, Seppala T (1996). 5-HT3 receptor antagonist MDL 72222 dose-dependently attenuates cocaine- and amphetamine-induced elevations of extracellular dopamine in the nucleus accumbens and the dorsal striatum. *Pharmacol Toxicol* **78**: 317–21.

Kankaanpaa A, Meririnne E, Seppala T (2002). 5-HT3 receptor antagonist MDL 72222 attenuates cocaine- and mazindol-, but not methylphenidate-induced neurochemical and behavioral effects in the rat. *Psychopharmacology (Berl.)* **159**: 341–50.

Kelai S, Aissi F, Lesch K P, Cohen-Salmon C, Hamon M, Lanfumey L (2003). Alcohol intake after serotonin transporter inactivation in mice. *Alcohol Alcohol* **38**: 386–9.

Kim D K, Tolliver T J, Huang S J, *et al.* (2005). Altered serotonin synthesis, turnover and dynamic regulation in multiple brain regions of mice lacking the serotonin transporter. *Neuropharmacology* **49**: 798–810.

Kostowski W, Dyr W, Krzascik P (1993). The abilities of 5-HT3 receptor antagonist ICS 205-930 to inhibit alcohol preference and withdrawal seizures in rats. *Alcohol* **10**: 369–73.

Lacroix L P, Dawson L A, Hagan J J, Heidbreder C A (2004). 5-HT6 receptor antagonist SB-271046 enhances extracellular levels of monoamines in the rat medial prefrontal cortex. *Synapse* **51**: 158–64.

Lejeune F, Millan M J (1998). Induction of burst firing in ventral tegmental area dopaminergic neurons by activation of serotonin (5-HT)1A receptors: WAY 100,635-reversible actions of the highly selective ligands, flesinoxan and S 15535. *Synapse* **30**: 172–80.

Lesch K P (2005). Alcohol dependence and gene x environment interaction in emotion regulation: is serotonin the link? *Eur J Pharmacol* **526**: 113–24.

Lesch K P, Bengel D, Heils A, *et al.* (1996). Association of anxiety-related traits with a polymorphism in the serotonin transporter gene regulatory region. *Science* **274**: 1527–31.

Li Q, Wichems C, Heils A, Lesch K P, Murphy D L (2000). Reduction in the density and expression, but not G-protein coupling, of serotonin receptors (5-HT1A) in 5-HT transporter knock-out mice: gender and brain region differences. *J Neurosci* **20**: 7888–95.

Li Q, Wichems C, Heils A, Van De Kar L D, Lesch K P, Murphy D L (1999). Reduction of 5-hydroxytryptamine (5-HT)(1A)-mediated temperature and neuroendocrine responses and 5-HT(1A) binding sites in 5-HT transporter knockout mice. *J Pharmacol Exp Ther* **291**: 999–1007.

Li Q, Wichems C H, Ma L, Van de Kar L D, Garcia F, Murphy D L (2003). Brain region-specific alterations of 5-HT2A and 5-HT2C receptors in serotonin transporter knockout mice. *J Neurochem* **84**: 1256–65.

Lira A, Zhou M, Castanon N, *et al.* (2003). Altered depression-related behaviors and functional changes in the dorsal raphe nucleus of serotonin transporter-deficient mice. *Biol Psychiatry* **54**: 960–71.

Liu W, Thielen R J, McBride W J (2006a). Effects of repeated daily treatments with a 5-HT3 receptor antagonist on dopamine neurotransmission and functional activity of 5-HT3 receptors within the nucleus accumbens of Wistar rats. *Pharmacol Biochem Behav* **84**: 370–7.

Liu W, Thielen R J, Rodd Z A, McBride W J (2006b). Activation of serotonin-3 receptors increases dopamine release within the ventral tegmental area of Wistar and alcohol-preferring (P) rats. *Alcohol* **40**: 167–76.

Lucas G, Di Matteo V, De Deurwaerdere P, *et al.* (2001). Neurochemical and electrophysiological evidence that 5-HT4 receptors exert a state-dependent facilitatory control in vivo on nigrostriatal, but not mesoaccumbal, dopaminergic function. *Eur J Neurosci* **13**: 889–98.

Lucas G, Spampinato U (2000). Role of striatal serotonin2A and serotonin2C receptor subtypes in the control of in vivo dopamine outflow in the rat striatum. *J Neurochem* **74**: 693–701.

Mannoury la Cour C, Boni C, Hanoun N, Lesch K P, Hamon M, Lanfumey L (2001). Functional consequences of 5-HT transporter gene disruption on 5-HT(1a) receptor-mediated regulation of dorsal raphe and hippocampal cell activity. *J Neurosci* **21**: 2178–85.

Mateo Y, Budygin E A, John C E, Jones S R (2004). Role of serotonin in cocaine effects in mice with reduced dopamine transporter function. *Proc Natl Acad Sci USA* **101**: 372–7.

Mathews T A, Fedele D E, Coppelli F M, Avila A M, Murphy D L, Andrews A M (2004). Gene dose-dependent alterations in extraneuronal serotonin but not dopamine in mice with reduced serotonin transporter expression. *J Neurosci Methods* **140**: 169–81.

Maurel S, De Vry J, De Beun R, Schreiber R (1999). 5-HT2A and 5-HT2C/5-HT1B receptors are differentially involved in alcohol preference and consummatory behavior in cAA rats. *Pharmacol Biochem Behav* **62**: 89–96.

McNeish C S, Svingos A L, Hitzemann R, Strecker R E (1993). The 5-HT3 antagonist zacopride attenuates cocaine-induced increases in extracellular dopamine in rat nucleus accumbens. *Pharmacol Biochem Behav* **45**: 759–63.

Minabe Y, Schechter L, Hashimoto K, Shirayama Y, Ashby CR, Jr. (2003). Acute and chronic administration of the selective 5-HT1A receptor antagonist WAY-405 significantly alters the activity of midbrain dopamine neurons in rats: an in vivo electrophysiological study. *Synapse* **50**: 181–90.

Murphy D L, Uhl G R, Holmes A, *et al.* (2003). Experimental gene interaction studies with SERT mutant mice as models for human polygenic and epistatic traits and disorders. *Genes Brain Behav* **2**: 350–64.

Mylecharane E J (1996). Ventral tegmental area 5-HT receptors: mesolimbic dopamine release and behavioural studies. *Behav Brain Res* **73**: 1–5.

Navailles S, De Deurwaerdere P, Porras G, Spampinato U (2004). In vivo evidence that 5-HT2C receptor antagonist but not agonist modulates cocaine-induced dopamine outflow in the rat nucleus accumbens and striatum. *Neuropsychopharmacology* **29**: 319–26.

Numachi Y, Ohara A, Yamashita M, *et al.* (2007). Methamphetamine-induced hyperthermia and lethal toxicity: role of the dopamine and serotonin transporters. *Eur J Pharmacol* **572**: 120–8.

O'Dell L E, Parsons L H (2004). Serotonin1B receptors in the ventral tegmental area modulate cocaine-induced increases in nucleus accumbens dopamine levels. *J Pharmacol Exp Ther* **311**: 711–9.

Parsons L H, Koob G F, Weiss F (1999). RU 24969, a 5-HT1B/1A receptor agonist, potentiates cocaine-induced increases in nucleus accumbens dopamine. *Synapse* **32**: 132–5.

Parsons L H, Weiss F, Koob G F (1998). Serotonin1B receptor stimulation enhances cocaine reinforcement. *J Neurosci* **18**: 10 078–89.

Pehek E A, McFarlane H G, Maguschak K, Price B, Pluto C P (2001). M100,907, a selective 5-HT(2A) antagonist, attenuates dopamine release in the rat medial prefrontal cortex. *Brain Res* **888**: 51–9.

Persico A M, Baldi A, Dell'Acqua M L, *et al.* (2003). Reduced programmed cell death in brains of serotonin transporter knockout mice. *Neuroreport* **14**: 341–4.

Persico A M, Mengual E, Moessner R, *et al.* (2001). Barrel pattern formation requires serotonin uptake by thalamocortical afferents, and not vesicular monoamine release. *J Neurosci* **21**: 6862–73.

Pessia M, Jiang Z G, North R A, Johnson S W (1994). Actions of 5-hydroxytryptamine on ventral tegmental area neurons of the rat in vitro. *Brain Res* **654**: 324–30.

Pierucci M, Di Matteo V, Esposito E (2004). Stimulation of serotonin2C receptors blocks the hyperactivation of midbrain dopamine neurons induced by nicotine administration. *J Pharmacol Exp Ther* **309**: 109–18.

Porras G, Di Matteo V, De Deurwaerdere P, Esposito E, Spampinato U (2002). Central serotonin4 receptors selectively regulate the impulse-dependent exocytosis of dopamine in the rat striatum: in vivo studies with morphine, amphetamine and cocaine. *Neuropharmacology* **43**: 1099–109.

Porras G, Di Matteo V, Fracasso C, *et al.* (2002). 5-HT2A and 5-HT2C/2B receptor subtypes modulate dopamine release induced in vivo by amphetamine and morphine in both the rat nucleus accumbens and striatum. *Neuropsychopharmacology* **26**: 311–24.

Powell S B, Lehmann-Masten V D, Paulus M P, Gainetdinov R R, Caron M G, Geyer M A (2004). MDMA "ecstasy" alters hyperactive and perseverative behaviors in dopamine transporter knockout mice. *Psychopharmacology (Berl.)* **173**: 310–7.

Pozzi L, Trabace L, Invernizzi R, Samanin R (1995). Intranigral GR-113808, a selective 5-HT4 receptor antagonist, attenuates morphine-stimulated dopamine release in the rat striatum. *Brain Res* **692**: 265–8.

Qu Y, Villacreses N, Murphy D L, Rapoport S I (2005). 5-HT2A/2C receptor signaling via phospholipase A2 and arachidonic acid is attenuated in mice lacking the serotonin reuptake transporter. *Psychopharmacology (Berl.)* **180**: 12–20.

Ren-Patterson R F, Cochran L W, Holmes A, Lesch K P, Lu B, Murphy D L (2006). Gender-dependent modulation of brain monoamines and anxiety-like behaviors in mice with genetic serotonin transporter and BDNF deficiencies. *Cell Mol Neurobiol* **26**: 755–80.

Ren-Patterson R F, Cochran L W, Holmes A, *et al.* (2005). Loss of brain-derived neurotrophic factor gene allele exacerbates brain monoamine deficiencies and increases stress abnormalities of serotonin transporter knockout mice. *J Neurosci Res* **79**: 756–71.

Rioux A, Fabre V, Lesch K P, *et al.* (1999). Adaptive changes of serotonin 5-HT2A receptors in mice lacking the serotonin transporter. *Neurosci Lett* **262**: 113–6.

Risinger F O, Bormann N M, Oakes R A (1996). Reduced sensitivity to ethanol reward, but not ethanol aversion, in mice lacking 5-HT1B receptors. *Alcohol Clin Exp Res* **20**: 1401–5.

Risinger F O, Doan A M, Vickrey A C (1999). Oral operant ethanol self-administration in 5-HT1b knockout mice. *Behav Brain Res* **102**: 211–5.

Rocha B A, Fumagalli F, Gainetdinov R R, *et al.* (1998a). Cocaine self-administration in dopamine-transporter knockout mice. *Nat Neurosci* **1**: 132–7.

Rocha B A, Scearce-Levie K, Lucas J J, *et al.* (1998b). Increased vulnerability to cocaine in mice lacking the serotonin-1B receptor. *Nature* **393**: 175–8.

Rompre P P, Injoyan R, Hagan J J (1995). Effects of granisetron, a 5-HT3 receptor antagonist, on morphine-induced potentiation of brain stimulation reward. *Eur J Pharmacol* **287**: 263–9.

Salichon N, Gaspar P, Upton A L, *et al.* (2001). Excessive activation of serotonin (5-HT) 1B receptors disrupts the formation of sensory maps in monoamine oxidase a and 5-HT transporter knock-out mice. *J Neurosci* **21**: 884–96.

Santiago M, Machado A, Cano J (1995). 5-HT3 receptor agonist induced carrier-mediated release of dopamine in rat striatum in vivo. *Br J Pharmacol* **116**: 1545–50.

Shen H W, Hagino Y, Kobayashi H, *et al.* (2004). Regional differences in extracellular dopamine and serotonin assessed by in vivo microdialysis in mice lacking dopamine and/or serotonin transporters. *Neuropsychopharmacology* **29**: 1790–9.

Sora I, Hall F S, Andrews A M, *et al.* (2001). Molecular mechanisms of cocaine reward: combined dopamine and serotonin transporter knockouts eliminate cocaine place preference. *Proc Natl Acad Sci USA* **98**: 5300–5.

Sora I, Wichems C, Takahashi N, *et al.* (1998). Cocaine reward models: conditioned place preference can be established in dopamine- and in serotonin-transporter knockout mice. *Proc Natl Acad Sci USA* **95**: 7699–704.

Steward L J, Ge J, Stowe R L, *et al.* (1996). Ability of 5-HT4 receptor ligands to modulate rat striatal dopamine release in vitro and in vivo. *Br J Pharmacol* **117**: 55–62.

Tanda G, Frau R, Di Chiara G (1995). Local 5HT3 receptors mediate fluoxetine but not desipramine-induced increase of extracellular dopamine in the prefrontal cortex. *Psychopharmacology (Berl.)* **119**: 15–9.

Thorre K, Ebinger G, Michotte Y (1998). 5-HT4 receptor involvement in the serotonin-enhanced dopamine efflux from the substantia nigra of the freely moving rat: a microdialysis study. *Brain Res* **796**: 117–24.

Tjurmina O A, Armando I, Saavedra J M, Goldstein D S, Murphy D L (2002). Exaggerated adrenomedullary response to immobilization in mice with targeted disruption of the serotonin transporter gene. *Endocrinology* **143**: 4520–6.

Tomkins D M, Higgins G A, Sellers E M (1994a). Low doses of the 5-HT1A agonist 8-hydroxy-2-(di-*n*-propylamino)-tetralin (8-OH DPAT) increase ethanol intake. *Psychopharmacology (Berl.)* **115**: 173–9.

Tomkins D M, Le A D, Sellers E M (1995). Effect of the 5-HT3 antagonist ondansetron on voluntary ethanol intake in rats and mice maintained on a limited access procedure. *Psychopharmacology (Berl.)* **117**: 479–85.

Tomkins D M, O'Neill M F (2000). Effect of 5-HT(1B) receptor ligands on self-administration of ethanol in an operant procedure in rats. *Pharmacol Biochem Behav* **66**: 129–36.

Tomkins D M, Sellers E M, Fletcher P J (1994b). Median and dorsal raphe injections of the 5-HT1A agonist, 8-OH-DPAT, and the GABAA agonist, muscimol, increase voluntary ethanol intake in Wistar rats. *Neuropharmacology* **33**: 349–58.

Trigo J M, Renoir T, Lanfumey L, *et al.* (2007). 3,4-Methylenedioxymethamphetamine self-administration is abolished in serotonin transporter knockout mice. *Biol Psychiatry* **62**: 669–79.

Uhl G R, Hall F S, Sora I (2002). Cocaine, reward, movement and monoamine transporters. *Mol Psychiatry* **7**: 21–6.

Wellman C L, Izquierdo A, Garrett J E, *et al.* (2007). Impaired stress-coping and fear extinction and abnormal corticolimbic morphology in serotonin transporter knock-out mice. *J Neurosci* **27**: 684–91.

Wilson A W, Neill J C, Costall B (1998). An investigation into the effects of 5-HT agonists and receptor antagonists on ethanol self-administration in the rat. *Alcohol* **16**: 249–70.

Wise R A, Bozarth M A (1987). A psychomotor stimulant theory of addiction. *Psychol Rev* **94**: 469–92.

Wozniak K M, Pert A, Linnoila M (1990). Antagonism of 5-HT3 receptors attenuates the effects of ethanol on extracellular dopamine. *Eur J Pharmacol* **187**: 287–9.

Xu F, Gainetdinov R R, Wetsel W C, *et al.* (2000). Mice lacking the norepinephrine transporter are supersensitive to psychostimulants. *Nat Neurosci* **3**: 465–71.

Yan Q, Reith M E, Yan S (2000). Enhanced accumbal dopamine release following 5-HT(2A) receptor stimulation in rats pretreated with intermittent cocaine. *Brain Res* **863**: 254–8.

Yan Q S (2000). Activation of 5-HT2A/2C receptors within the nucleus accumbens increases local dopaminergic transmission. *Brain Res Bull* **51**: 75–81.

Yan Q S, Yan S E (2001). Activation of 5-HT(1B/1D) receptors in the mesolimbic dopamine system increases dopamine release from the nucleus accumbens: a microdialysis study. *Eur J Pharmacol* **418**: 55–64.

Yan Q S, Zheng S Z, Yan S E (2004). Involvement of 5-HT1B receptors within the ventral tegmental area in regulation of mesolimbic dopaminergic neuronal activity via GABA mechanisms: a study with dual-probe microdialysis. *Brain Res* **1021**: 82–91.

Yoshimoto K, McBride W J, Lumeng L, Li T K (1992). Alcohol stimulates the release of dopamine and serotonin in the nucleus accumbens. *Alcohol* **9**: 17–22.

Zhao S, Edwards J, Carroll J, *et al.* (2006). Insertion mutation at the C-terminus of the serotonin transporter disrupts brain serotonin function and emotion-related behaviors in mice. *Neuroscience* **140**: 321–34.

Zhou F C, Lesch K P, Murphy D L (2002). Serotonin uptake into dopamine neurons via dopamine transporters: a compensatory alternative. *Brain Res* **942**: 109–19.

Zhou F M, Liang Y, Salas R, Zhang L, De Biasi M, Dani J A (2005). Corelease of dopamine and serotonin from striatal dopamine terminals. *Neuron* **46**: 65–74.

Zhou Q Y, Palmiter R D (1995). Dopamine-deficient mice are severely hypoactive, adipsic, and aphagic. *Cell* **83**: 1197–209.

JUSTIN L. LAPORTE, RENEE F. REN-PATTERSON, DENNIS L. MURPHY AND ALLAN V. KALUEFF

9

Modeling SERT × BDNF interactions in brain disorders: single BDNF gene allele exacerbates brain monoamine deficiencies and increases stress abnormalities in serotonin transporter knock-out mice

ABSTRACT

There is growing clinical evidence that many psychiatric illnesses have overlapping genetic mechanisms. Understanding these mechanisms is important to the improvement of psychiatric treatment and preventions of the disorders, and animal genetic models continue to be a critical avenue of research towards these ends. As serotonin is a key neurotransmitter with important roles in normal behavioral processes and has been implicated in the pathogenesis of psychopathological conditions such as depression, anxiety, and addiction, it is a prime target for investigation in behavioral neurogenetics. The serotonin transporter (SERT) is a key brain protein that regulates the amount of serotonin that can activate the receptor. It is becoming evident that SERT interacts with brain-derived neurotrophic factor (BDNF), an important modulator of dopaminergic, cholinergic, and serotonergic neurons, which has been linked to memory function, activity, eating behavior, depression, and anxiety. The pivotal roles played by these two brain molecules have resulted in the development of numerous mutant animal models that have reduced function of SERT, BDNF, or both. Interestingly, SERT × BDNF mutant mice show numerous different behavioral phenotypes that are distinct from either SERT mutants or

Experimental Models in Serotonin Transporter Research, eds. A. V. Kalueff and J. L. LaPorte.
Published by Cambridge University Press.

BDNF mutants alone, displaying phenotypes that are highly relevant to human clinical scenarios and bringing them added validity. This chapter will provide data from numerous experiments utilizing these rodent models and will explain their relevance and validity for research into the genetics of neuropsychiatric disorders.

INTRODUCTION

Various genetic animal models are used in neuroscience research for screening psychotropic drugs, testing neurobiological hypotheses, and finding candidate genes for stress-related brain disorders (Crawley, 1999; Kaiser *et al.*, 2001; Kalueff and Tuohimaa, 2004; Van Meer and Raber, 2005; Vetter *et al.*, 2002). Mounting data indicate that many brain disorders represent overlapping pathogenetic pathways with common genetic determinants and clinical manifestations (Kalueff and Nutt, 1996; Kalueff and Tuohimaa, 2004; Kalueff *et al.*, 2007b), raising the possibility that several distinct but interacting domains may contribute to clinical and experimental phenotypes. This also implies that a closer in-depth analysis of different domains may stimulate new, clinically relevant genetic experimental modeling of neuropsychiatric disorders. This chapter will focus on two key brain molecules – serotonin transporter (SERT) and brain-derived neurotrophic factor (BDNF) – that have been implicated in multiple neuropsychiatric disorders, and discusses how their genetic animal models may optimize further experimental research in this field.

Serotonin (5-HT) is a key brain neurotransmitter (Adayev *et al.*, 2005; Aghajanian, 1990; Aghajanian and Marek, 1997, 1999; Lauder, 1990; Turlejski, 1996; Whitaker-Azmitia, 1991, 2001). Clusters of serotonergic cell bodies are located along the midline of the brain stem known as the raphe nuclei, and their axonal projections are distributed throughout the central nervous system (CNS). The dorsal and median raphe nuclei send their projections to diverse regions including the cortex, hippocampus, limbic structure, striatum, thalamus, midbrain, and hypothalamus. Although found in only a small percentage (about 1–2%) of neurons in the brain, 5-HT is an important morphogenetic contributor to the developing brain (Ansorge *et al.*, 2004; Bonnin *et al.*, 2006, 2007; Vitalis *et al.*, 2007; Vitalis and Parnavelas, 2003; Whitaker-Azmitia, 1999, 2001; Whitaker-Azmitia *et al.*, 1996). Disrupted signaling of this neurotransmitter during early development produces enduring changes in the morphology and function of the CNS (Gross and Hen, 2004a, 2004b; Gross *et al.*, 2002).

Altered developmental and postnatal 5-HT affects numerous facets of cognition and emotional regulation (Graeff *et al.*, 1996; Gross and Hen, 2004a, 2004b; Gross *et al.*, 2000, 2002; Lucki, 1998; Owens and Nemeroff, 1994), as evidenced by its implication in the pathogenesis of many brain disorders such as anxiety, depression, mania, addiction, schizophrenia, autism, and obsessive compulsive disorder (OCD) (Firk and Markus, 2007; Kennedy *et al.*, 2003; Lesch, 2005a, 2005b; Lesch and Mossner, 2006; Lesch *et al.*, 2003; Meyer, 2007; Senkowski *et al.*, 2003; Shiah and Yatham, 2000; Yatham *et al.*, 2000).

The uptake of synaptic 5-HT into nerve terminals – the most important mechanism of serotonergic regulation – is mediated by SERT, a high-affinity plasma membrane serotonin transporter (Lesch, 2005b; Murphy *et al.*, 2001, 2003, 2004; Rudnick, 2006a, 2006b; Zhou *et al.*, 2002). In humans, a common SERT polymorphism in the promoter region, a variable-number tandem repeat in intron 2, and a coding region mutation have been reported to be associated with a variety of neuropsychiatric diseases, including anxiety, autism, OCD, and depression (Firk and Markus, 2007; Glatt *et al.*, 2001; Glatt and Reus, 2003; Hariri and Holmes, 2006; Holmes and Hariri, 2003; Kalueff *et al.*, 2007a; Murphy *et al.*, 2003; Ozaki *et al.*, 2003).

Previous studies have demonstrated that BDNF is the most abundant brain neurotrophic factor and that reduced expression of BDNF in mice can affect brain synaptic vesicle function, synaptic plasticity, and can lead to specific alterations in hippocampus-based spatial learning as well as hypothalamus-regulated eating behavior and motor activity (Angelucci *et al.*, 2000, 2005; Berton *et al.*, 2006; Bonhoeffer, 1996; Kernie *et al.*, 2000; Ren-Patterson *et al.*, 2006). In addition, loss of the BDNF receptor, TrkB, leads to more severe changes through neuronal loss and cortical degenerative abnormalities (Vitalis *et al.*, 2002; Xu *et al.*, 2000).

Similarly, decreased serum levels of BDNF have been found in patients under stress and in patients with mood disorders (Karege *et al.*, 2002; Licinio and Wong, 2002; Martinowich and Lu, 2008; Martinowich *et al.*, 2007; Nestler *et al.*, 2002). A recent study found that only the BDNF gene was identified as a potential risk gene out of 76 candidate genes studied in a bipolar disorder sample (Sklar *et al.*, 2002), supporting the hypothesis that BDNF plays a primary role in mood disorders. In addition, a val66met BDNF human gene variant has been shown to be associated with changes in memory and abnormal hippocampal activation assessed by fMRI (Egan *et al.*, 2003). This variant of the BDNF gene is also associated with several neuropsychiatric disorders

(Hall *et al.*, 2003; Kim *et al.*, 2007; Lohoff *et al.*, 2005; Neves-Pereira *et al.*, 2005). BDNF has also been found to directly affect the brain serotonergic system. For example, intracortically administered BDNF produces localized increases in serotonin axon density (Mamounas *et al.*, 1995). Several cultured cell models indicate that BDNF enhances the differentiation of a serotonergic phenotype (Eaton and Whittemore, 1996; Galter and Unsicker, 2000a, 2000b; Rumajogee *et al.*, 2002, 2004, 2005, 2006). BDNF also modulates serotonin transporter (SERT) function in cultured cell lines (Mossner *et al.*, 2000; Ren-Patterson *et al.*, 2005b). Pre-administration of BDNF prevents the formation of serotonergic axonal lesions produced by the serotonin neurotoxin parachloramphetamine (Mamounas *et al.*, 1995, 2000). Moreover, abnormal thalamocortical axon overgrowth, which is a consequence of excess serotonin availability during certain stages of brain development in mice with a targeted deletion of the MAO-A gene, is exacerbated by inter-breeding these MAO-A gene-deleted mice with mice lacking the BDNF receptor, TrkB (Vitalis *et al.*, 2002).

To extend these studies of brain plasticity and of specific interactions between BDNF and the serotonergic and dopaminergic systems (Berton *et al.*, 2006; Lyons *et al.*, 1999; Ren-Patterson *et al.*, 2005a), we investigated whether an endogenous BDNF gene difference might play a role in the consequences of a serotonin transporter deficit found in SERT knock-out mice.

Notably, BDNF is an important modulator of dopaminergic, cholinergic, and serotonergic neurons, implicated in synaptic vesicle function and synaptic plasticity. Leading to specific alterations in behaviors, including memory, activity, eating behavior, depression, and anxiety (Aloe *et al.*, 2000; Angelucci *et al.*, 2000, 2004, 2005; Bartoletti *et al.*, 2002; Berton *et al.*, 2006; Bonhoeffer, 1996; Chourbaji *et al.*, 2004; Kernie *et al.*, 2000; Kuipers and Bramham, 2006; McAllister, 1999; Minichiello *et al.*, 1999; Murphy *et al.*, 2004; Pozzo-Miller *et al.*, 1999; Yamada *et al.*, 2002). Prominent physiological changes have been observed in a double SERT−/− BDNF+/− knock-out mouse model (Ren-Patterson *et al.*, 2005a, 2005b, 2006), strongly supporting the importance of SERT–BDNF interactions.

LOSS OF BDNF SINGLE GENE EXACERBATES 5-HT DEFICIENCIES IN MALE SERT × BDNF (SB) DOUBLE-MUTANT MICE, BUT NOT IN FEMALE MICE

Serotonin (5-HT) concentrations in the four brain regions for both genders and four genotypes (SB = SERT+/+ BDNF+/+; Sb = SERT+/+

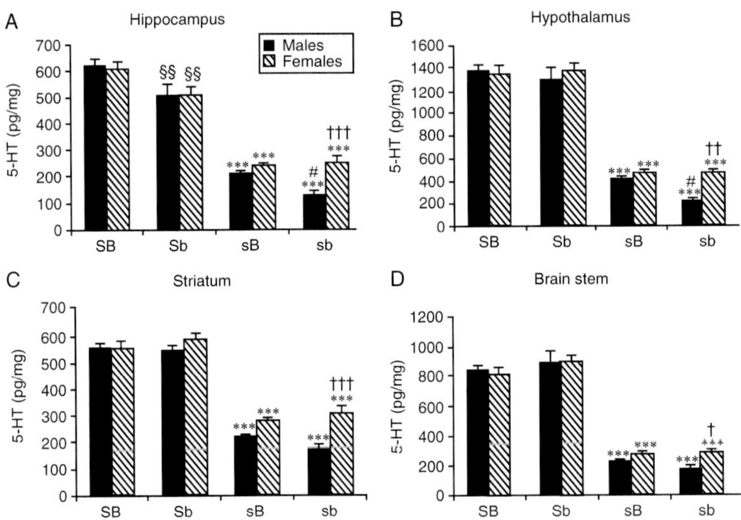

Figure 9.1 5-HT concentrations in different brain regions were significantly reduced (pg/mg protein, mean ± SEM, n = 5–6) in sb double-mutant mice compared to SB and Sb mice (SB = SERT+/+ BDNF+/+; Sb = SERT+/+ BDNF+/−; sB = SERT−/− BDNF+/+; and sb = SERT−/− BDNF+/− mice). Hippocampus −79%, hypothalamus −80%, brain stem −79%, striatum −69%. A significant further serotonin reduction of 37% in hippocampus and 43% in hypothalamus was observed in sb mice compared to sB mice. In addition, male compared to female sb mice had a significant reduction of 5-HT concentrations in hippocampus and striatum, †††$p<0.001$, in hypothalamus, ††$p<0.01$, in brain stem, †$p<0.04$. Furthermore, both genders of sB mice had significant reductions in all four brain regions (***$p<0.001$) relative to SB mice. Sb mice compared to SB controls had significant reductions of 5-HT in only the hippocampus (§§$p<0.008$), but not in other brain regions.

BDNF+/−; sB = SERT−/− BDNF+/+; and sb = SERT−/− BDNF+/−) are presented in Figure 9.1A–D. Significant gender × genotype interactions were found in hippocampus ($F_{3,46}=4.2$, $p<0.01$) and striatum ($F_{3,46}=4.6$, $p<0.006$). Significant genotype-related 5-HT reductions were found in sB and sb mice relative to the SB controls in multiple brain regions: hippocampus ($F_{3,46}=189.9$, $p<0.001$), striatum ($F_{3,46}=177.3$, $p<0.001$), hypothalamus ($F_{3,46}=224.5$, $p<0.001$), and brain stem ($F_{3,46}=200.5$, $p<0.001$). Post-hoc analyses revealed that significant serotonin reductions of 37% in hippocampus ($p<0.01$) and 43% in hypothalamus ($p<0.02$) were observed in male sb double-mutant mice compared to male sB SERT knock-out mice (Ren-Patterson *et al.*, 2005a). In contrast, female sb mice had no further significant reductions in serotonin concentrations compared to female sB mice. Serotonin concentrations in these female sb mice differed significantly from male sb mice in all four brain regions studied (Figure 9.1).

DOPAMINE AND METABOLITES SHOW GENDER-BASED DIFFERENCES IN SERT × BDNF (SB) DOUBLE-MUTANT MICE IN STRIATUM

A significant gender × genotype interaction for dopamine concentrations was found in striatum ($F_{3,46}=5.07$, $p<0.004$). Significant genotype-related reductions in dopamine were observed ($F_{3,46}=3.0$, $p<0.04$). While male mice had significant reductions of dopamine of 32% (Figure 9.2) relative to SB mice ($p<0.001$) and Sb mice ($p<0.001$), and of 25% relative to sB mice ($p<0.004$), female sb mice had no reductions of dopamine in striatum. Thus, male sb mice compared to sb female mice had significantly reduced striatal dopamine ($p<0.001$). Dopamine concentrations were unaltered in other brain regions.

Furthermore, both DOPAC (a primary dopamine metabolite) and HVA (a major catecholamine metabolite) concentrations in striatum were altered, with significant gender × genotype interactions: DOPAC ($F_{3,46}=4.2$, $p<0.01$); HVA ($F_{3,46}=4.1$, $p<0.01$). For both DOPAC ($F_{3,46}=8.2$, $p<0.001$) and HVA ($F_{3,46}=12.7$, $p<0.001$), significant reductions were observed only in male sb relative to male SB mice, but not in female mice. Significant genotype-related DOPAC and HVA reductions were found in sB ($p<0.004$) and sb ($p<0.001$) mice relative to the Sb controls. However, significant gender differences were only found in double-mutant mice: both DOPAC and HVA ($p<0.001$) were significantly different in post-hoc comparisons of sb male with sb female mice.

ANXIETY-LIKE BEHAVIORS ARE GENDER-DEPENDENT IN SERT × BDNF-DEFICIENT MALE, BUT NOT FEMALE, MICE

Behavioral changes observed in a double sb (SERT−/− BDNF+/−) knock-out mouse model further strongly support the importance of SERT–BDNF interactions. Several results based on this model reflect SERT–BDNF interplay and illustrate the utility of dissecting individual domains and studying them as a system of interacting endophenotypes. For example, the elevated plus-maze (EPM) data (Figure 9.3 A–C) show a significant gender × genotype interaction for the percentage of time the animal spent in the open arm areas ($F_{3,91}=2.67$, $p<0.05$). While male

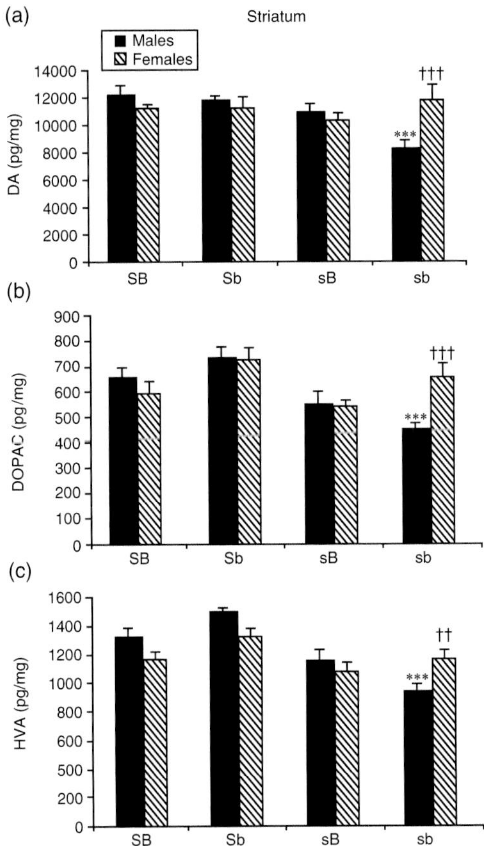

Figure 9.2 Dopamine (DA) concentrations were significantly reduced by 32% (***$p<0.0001$) only in male sb double-mutant mice compared to SB, Sb, and sB mice. DA concentrations in female sb mice were significantly different compared to sb male mice (†††$p<0.0004$). DOPAC and HVA concentrations were also significantly reduced by 32% (***$p<0.001$) and 30% (***$p<0.001$) only in male sb mice compared to SB, Sb, and sB mice. In contrast, DOPAC (†††$p<0.001$) and HVA (††$p<0.01$) concentrations in female sb mice were significantly different compared to male sb mice.

sb mice spent less time on the open arms than male SB mice ($p<0.006$; Figure 9.3A) and also made fewer open entries compared to SB mice ($F_{3,91}=5.35$, $p<0.001$; Figure 9.3B), female sb double-mutant mice showed no differences from their littermate controls on either open arm time or open arm entries percentages. Thus, there were significant differences between the male and female sb mice on percent open arm time ($p<0.001$), but not on open arm entries.

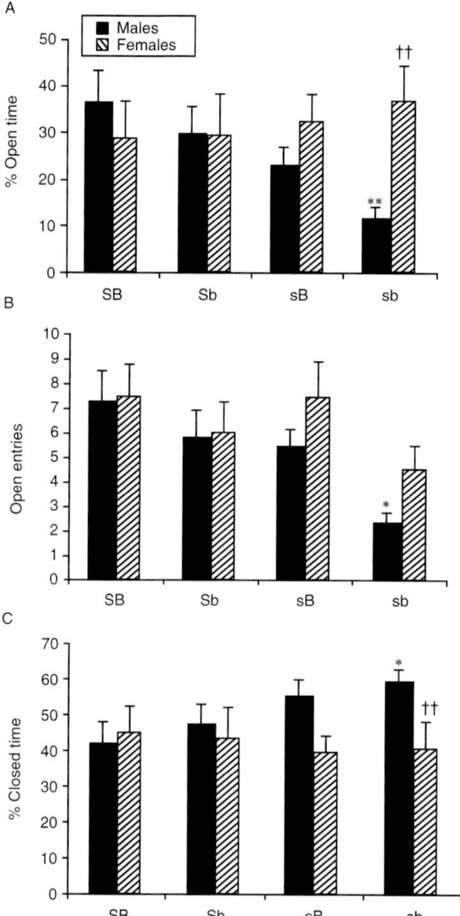

Figure 9.3 Male sb double-mutant mice showed heightened anxiety-like behavior in the elevated plus-maze test relative to SB controls. sb double-mutant male mice spent less time on the open arms ($^{**}p<0.006$) and made fewer open arm entries ($^{*}p<0.003$) compared to SB or Sb controls. Female sb double-mutant mice were not different from their littermate controls, but female sb double mutant mice were significantly different from male sb mice in percent open time ($^{\dagger\dagger}p<0.001$). Male sb double-mutant mice spent more time on the closed arm than male SB mice ($p<0.05$). In addition, sb male mice were significantly different from female sb mice ($p<0.02$). Data (also in Figures 9.4–9.5) are means ± SEM, $n = 12$–15 males and $n = 10$–12 females per genotype.

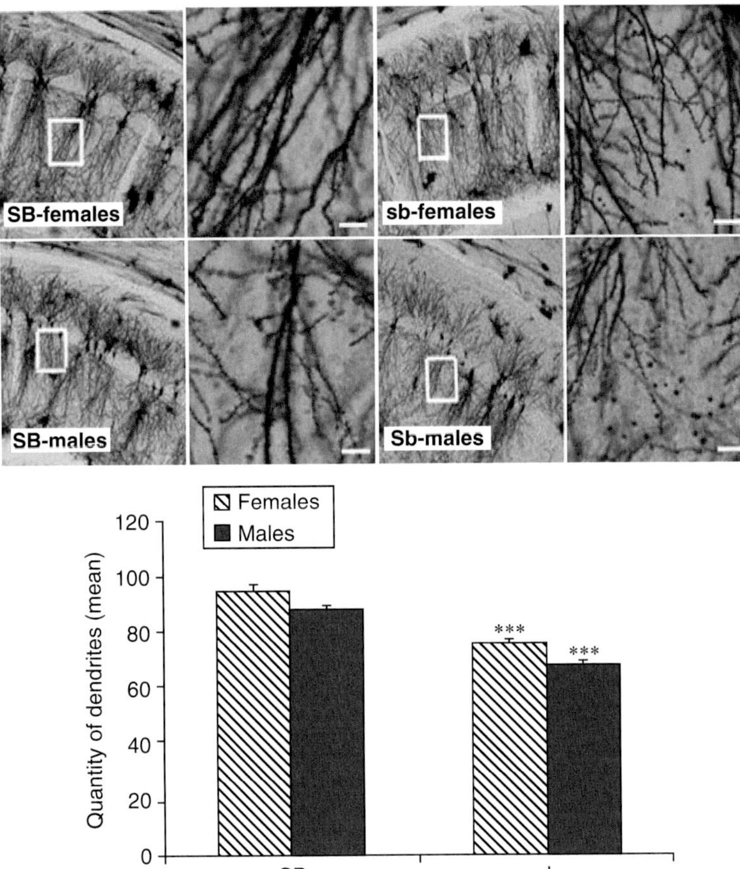

Figure 9.4 Reductions of 5-HT and BDNF affect development of neuronal dendritic branches in sb mice. The morphology of brain neuronal hippocampal near dentate gyrus dendrites and spines was evaluated in 20 fields. (Scale bars = 10 μm). The quantity of dendrites in brain sections with Golgi impregnation. Both genders had significant reductions in sb mice (***$p<0.0001$) compared to SB mice using two-way ANOVA test (see legend for Figure 9.3 for details).

On the other hand, as can be seen in Figure 9.3C, a significant gender difference was found for percentage of time spent in the closed arm ($F_{1,91}=4.5$, $p<0.04$), but no genotype or gender × genotype interaction was found. Thus, male sb mice spent more time on the closed arm than female sb mice ($p<0.01$). For the closed arm entries endpoint,

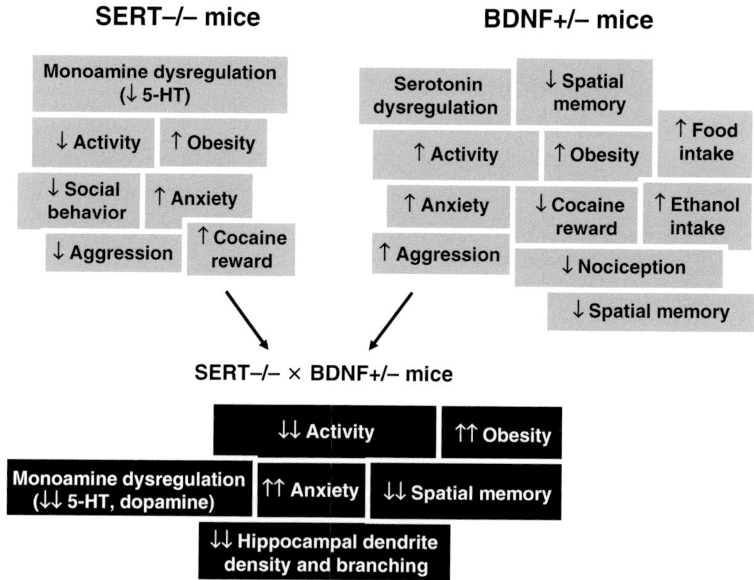

Figure 9.5 Domain architectonics in 5-HT transporter knock-out (SERT−/−), brain-derived neurotrophic factor heterozygous knock-out (BDNF +/−), and double mutant (SERT−/− BDNF+/−) mice. Note that only selected disordered domains are presented (gray) for each genetic model (↑, increased, ↓, decreased profile). Exacerbation of the respective known domains in the double knock-out (SERT−/− BDNF+/−) model, as a result of genetic interactions, is marked with black color and double arrows (see legend for Figure 9.3 for details).

a significant genotype difference was found ($F_{3,91}$=7.71, p<0.001), but no gender or gender × genotype interaction. Thus sb mice of both genders made significantly fewer closed arm entries than SB mice (p<0.01). In contrast, female sb double-mutant mice showed no differences from their littermate controls on either closed arm time or closed arm entries percentages.

TARGETING SERT- AND BDNF-MEDIATED BRAIN DISORDERS

Figure 9.4 shows marked morphological alterations in neurons of mice with combined SERT and BDNF knock-out (see further). Figure 9.5 compares several altered domains in SERT−/− and BDNF+/− gene-targeted mice, outlining their possible interplay in SERT−/− BDNF+/− double-mutant mice. For example, SERT−/− BDNF+/− mutant mouse data show that reduced BDNF availability during development exaggerates the consequences of absent SERT function, leading to increased anxiety and obesity (Murphy *et al.*, 2003; Ren-Patterson *et al.*, 2005a). Interestingly, using neonatal models, Garoflos *et al.* (2005) examined the effects of early developmental experience on spatial learning and memory, food intake, hippocampal glucocorticoid, mineralocorticoid and 5-HT1A receptors, and BDNF. They found that neonatal handling has a beneficial effect in male mice, improving their cognitive ability, accompanied by increased hippocampal gluco/mineralocorticoid receptors ratio and BDNF. Another pathway causing the anti-stress effects of handling may involve upregulated 5-HT1A receptors that prevent stress-induced hyperphagia, obesity, and resistance to leptin (Garoflos *et al.*, 2005; Panagiotaropoulos *et al.*, 2004).

These findings are consistent with our observations that SERT × BDNF double-mutant mice have larger stress-induced increases in plasma adrenocorticotropic hormone (than any single-knock-out mice) (Murphy *et al.*, 2003), confirming that the multiple gene interactions affect many systems (including the neuroendocrine system) co-modulating the animal behavioral and physiological phenotypes. Importantly, BDNF, SERT, and 5-HT are present not only in the brain, but also in peripheral tissues involved in metabolic functions and responses to stress (Tjurmina *et al.*, 2002; Tonra *et al.*, 1999). Thus, both central and peripheral 5-HT/BDNF-mediated mechanisms are affected in the double-mutant SERT × BDNF mice. One of the mechanisms for this may be mediated by corticotropin-releasing hormone that originates from hypothalamus paraventricular nucleus, which in turn results in the release of adrenocorticotropic hormone from the pituitary into general circulation. Furthermore, stress-induced obesity (Bjorntorp, 2001; Bjorntorp and Rosmond, 2000; Rosmond *et al.*, 1998) is believed to be associated with glucocorticoid-induced resistance to leptin (Solano and Jacobson, 1999), although other important neuroendocrine mechanisms (Dutton *et al.*, 2006; Kuo *et al.*, 2007a, 2007b), potentially associated with 5-HT, SERT, and BDNF, have recently been reported.

As BDNF plays a central role in the development and plasticity of neuronal circuits in the central nervous system, analysis of neuronal morphology showed that hypothalamus and hippocampus neurons exhibited 25–30% reductions in dendrites (especially in multiple, highly ordered dendrites branches) in double-mutant mice compared with BDNF+/− mice (Figure 9.4). These morphological changes imply that the deletion of BDNF × SERT genes significantly affects the development and growth of dendrites – the structural elements that are crucial for synaptogenesis. Furthermore, a more focused examination of the dendrites and spines in the hippocampus near the dentate gyrus in female and male sb mice compared to SB mice (Figure 9.4) revealed a significant 20–23% genotype-related reduction in spines relative to SB wildtype. Also, these double-mutant mice showed poorer performance in the radial arm maze (compared with any single-mutant mice; R. Ren-Patterson *et al.*, unpublished data). This may indicate aberrant hippocampal memory caused by irregular hippocampal morphology (but also does not exclude other hippocampal abnormalities, such as impaired navigation and exploration). Clearly, a further dissection of diverse domains may be possible in this model, elucidating the role of the two genes in their regulation and co-modulation.

CONCLUDING REMARKS

In addition to the fundamental roles that SERT and BDNF play independently of each other, it is clear that SERT and BDNF interact at numerous levels and play an integral part in the regulation of physiological and behavioral functions as seen in both clinical and experimental studies (Berton *et al.*, 2006; Kaufman *et al.*, 2006; Ren-Patterson *et al.*, 2005a, 2005b, 2006). This evidence, as summarized in this chapter, effectively demonstrates that this related involvement allows for the effective co-modulation of a range of neural mechanisms. However, genetic interactions also play an active part in this regulatory process, adding another interesting dimension to the interplay between SERT and BDNF. The elucidation of such mechanisms offers encouraging potential for novel avenues of investigation into the pathogenesis of common and devastating brain maladies. With the possibilities for inventive exploration, there arises the obligation for developing relevant animal models that foster treatment-oriented research. Given the importance that genetic interactions have on the development and perpetuation of many disorders, genetic models based on mutant or transgenic mice are ideal candidates for this task. As clearly summarized in this chapter, SERT, BDNF, and SERT × BDNF mutant mice emerge as particularly promising models pertinent to many prevalent human disorders.

ACKNOWLEDGMENTS

This study is supported by the Intramural Research Program of the National Institute of Mental Health (NIMH/NIH, USA) and NARSAD YI Award (to AVK).

REFERENCES

Adayev T, Ranasinghe B, Banerjee P (2005). Transmembrane signaling in the brain by serotonin, a key regulator of physiology and emotion. *Bioscience Reports* **25**: 363–85.

Aghajanian G K (1990). Serotonin-induced inward current in rat facial motoneurons: evidence for mediation by G proteins but not protein kinase C. *Brain Res* **524**: 171–4.

Aghajanian G K, Marek G J (1997). Serotonin induces excitatory postsynaptic potentials in apical dendrites of neocortical pyramidal cells. *Neuropharmacology* **36**: 589–99.

Aghajanian G K, Marek G J (1999). Serotonin, via 5-HT2A receptors, increases EPSCs in layer V pyramidal cells of prefrontal cortex by an asynchronous mode of glutamate release. *Brain Res* **825**: 161–71.

Aloe L, Iannitelli A, Angelucci F, Bersani G, Fiore M (2000). Studies in animal models and humans suggesting a role of nerve growth factor in schizophrenia-like disorders. *Behav Pharmacol* **11**: 235–42.

Angelucci F, Aloe L, Vasquez P J, Mathe A A (2000). Mapping the differences in the brain concentration of brain-derived neurotrophic factor (BDNF) and nerve growth factor (NGF) in an animal model of depression. *Neuroreport* **11**: 1369–73.

Angelucci F, Brene S, Mathe A A (2005). BDNF in schizophrenia, depression and corresponding animal models. *Mol Psychiatry* **10**: 345–52.

Angelucci F, Mathe A A, Aloe L (2004). Neurotrophic factors and CNS disorders: findings in rodent models of depression and schizophrenia. *Progr Brain Res* **146**: 151–65.

Ansorge M S, Zhou M, Lira A, Hen R, Gingrich J A (2004). Early-life blockade of the 5-HT transporter alters emotional behavior in adult mice. *Science* **306**: 879–81.

Bartoletti A, Cancedda L, Reid S W, *et al.* (2002). Heterozygous knock-out mice for brain-derived neurotrophic factor show a pathway-specific impairment of long-term potentiation but normal critical period for monocular deprivation. *J Neurosci* **22**: 10 072–7.

Berton O, McClung C A, Dileone R J, *et al.* (2006). Essential role of BDNF in the mesolimbic dopamine pathway in social defeat stress. *Science* **311**: 864–8.

Bjorntorp P (2001). Do stress reactions cause abdominal obesity and comorbidities? *Obes Rev* **2**: 73–86.

Bjorntorp P, Rosmond R (2000). Obesity and cortisol. *Nutrition Burbank, Los Angeles County, Calif* **16**: 924–36.

Bonhoeffer T (1996). Neurotrophins and activity-dependent development of the neocortex. *Curr Opin Neurobiol* **6**: 119–26.

Bonnin A, Peng W, Hewlett W, Levitt P (2006). Expression mapping of 5-HT1 serotonin receptor subtypes during fetal and early postnatal mouse forebrain development. *Neuroscience* **141**: 781–94.

Bonnin A, Torii M, Wang L, Rakic P, Levitt P (2007). Serotonin modulates the response of embryonic thalamocortical axons to netrin-1. *Nat Neurosci* **10**: 588–97.

Chourbaji S, Hellweg R, Brandis D, *et al.* (2004). Mice with reduced brain-derived neurotrophic factor expression show decreased choline acetyltransferase activity, but regular brain monoamine levels and unaltered emotional behavior. *Brain Res Mol Brain Res* **121**: 28–36.

Crawley J N (1999). Behavioral phenotyping of transgenic and knockout mice: experimental design and evaluation of general health, sensory functions, motor abilities, and specific behavioral tests. *Brain Res* **835**: 18–26.

Dutton M A, Lee E W, Zukowska Z (2006). NPY and extreme stress: lessons learned from posttraumatic stress disorder. *Exs*: 213–22.

Eaton M J, Whittemore S R (1996). Autocrine BDNF secretion enhances the survival and serotonergic differentiation of raphe neuronal precursor cells grafted into the adult rat CNS. *Exp Neurol* **140**: 105–14.

Egan M F, Kojima M, Callicott J H, *et al.* (2003). The BDNF val66met polymorphism affects activity-dependent secretion of BDNF and human memory and hippocampal function. *Cell* **112**: 257–69.

Firk C, Markus C R (2007). Review: Serotonin by stress interaction: a susceptibility factor for the development of depression? *J Psychopharmacol* **21**: 538–44.

Galter D, Unsicker K (2000a). Brain-derived neurotrophic factor and TrkB are essential for cAMP-mediated induction of the serotonergic neuronal phenotype. *J Neurosci Res* **61**: 295–301.

Galter D, Unsicker K (2000b). Sequential activation of the 5-HT1(A) serotonin receptor and TrkB induces the serotonergic neuronal phenotype. *Mol Cell Neurosci* **15**: 446–55.

Garoflos E, Panagiotaropoulos T, Pondiki S, Stamatakis A, Philippidis E, Stylianopoulou F (2005). Cellular mechanisms underlying the effects of an early experience on cognitive abilities and affective states. *Ann Gen Psychiatry* **4**: 8.

Glatt C E, DeYoung J A, Delgado S, *et al.* (2001). Screening a large reference sample to identify very low frequency sequence variants: comparisons between two genes. *Nat Genet* **27**: 435–8.

Glatt C E, Reus V I (2003). Pharmacogenetics of monoamine transporters. *Pharmacogenomics* **4**: 583–96.

Graeff F G, Guimaraes F S, De Andrade T G, Deakin J F (1996). Role of 5-HT in stress, anxiety, and depression. *Pharmacol Biochem Behav* **54**: 129–41.

Gross C, Hen R (2004a). The developmental origins of anxiety. *Nature Rev* **5**: 545–52.

Gross C, Hen R (2004b). Genetic and environmental factors interact to influence anxiety. *Neurotox Res* **6**: 493–501.

Gross C, Santarelli L, Brunner D, Zhuang X, Hen R (2000). Altered fear circuits in 5-HT(1A) receptor KO mice. *Biol Psychiatry* **48**: 1157–63.

Gross C, Zhuang X, Stark K, *et al.* (2002). Serotonin1A receptor acts during development to establish normal anxiety-like behavior in the adult. *Nature* **416**: 396–400.

Hall D, Dhilla A, Charalambous A, Gogos J A, Karayiorgou M (2003). Sequence variants of the brain-derived neurotrophic factor (BDNF) gene are strongly associated with obsessive-compulsive disorder. *Am J Human Genet* **73**: 370–6.

Hariri A R, Holmes A (2006). Genetics of emotional regulation: the role of the serotonin transporter in neural function. *Trends Cogn Sci* **10**: 182–91.

Holmes A, Hariri A R (2003). The serotonin transporter gene-linked polymorphism and negative emotionality: placing single gene effects in the context of genetic background and environment. *Genes Brain Behav* **2**: 332–5.

Kaiser A, Fedrowitz M, Ebert U, *et al.* (2001). Auditory and vestibular defects in the circling (ci2) rat mutant. *Eur J Neurosci* **14**: 1129–42.

Kalueff A, Nutt D J (1996). Role of GABA in memory and anxiety. *Depress Anxiety* **4**: 100–10.

Kalueff A V, Ren-Patterson R F, Murphy D L (2007a). The developing use of heterozygous mutant mouse models in brain monoamine transporter research. *Trends Pharmacol Sci* **28**: 122–7.

Kalueff A V, Tuohimaa P (2004). Experimental modeling of anxiety and depression. *Acta Neurobiol Exp (Wars)* **64**: 439–48.

Kalueff A V, Wheaton M, Murphy D L (2007b). What's wrong with my mouse model? Advances and strategies in animal modeling of anxiety and depression. *Behav Brain Res* **179**: 1–18.

Karege F, Perret G, Bondolfi G, Schwald M, Bertschy G, Aubry J M (2002). Decreased serum brain-derived neurotrophic factor levels in major depressed patients. *Psychiatry Res* **109**: 143–8.

Kaufman J, Yang B Z, Douglas-Palumberi H, *et al.* (2006). Brain-derived neurotrophic factor-5-HTTLPR gene interactions and environmental modifiers of depression in children. *Biol Psychiatry* **59**: 673–80.

Kennedy J L, Farrer L A, Andreasen N C, Mayeux R, St George-Hyslop P (2003). The genetics of adult-onset neuropsychiatric disease: complexities and conundra? *Science* **302**: 822–6.

Kernie S G, Liebl D J, Parada L F (2000). BDNF regulates eating behavior and locomotor activity in mice. *EMBO J* **19**: 1290–300.

Kim J M, Stewart R, Kim S W, *et al.* (2007). Interactions between life stressors and susceptibility genes (5-HTTLPR and BDNF) on depression in Korean elders. *Biol Psychiatry* **62**: 423–8.

Kuipers S D, Bramham C R (2006). Brain-derived neurotrophic factor mechanisms and function in adult synaptic plasticity: new insights and implications for therapy. *Current Opini Drug Discov Dev* **9**: 580–6.

Kuo L E, Abe K, Zukowska Z (2007a). Stress, NPY and vascular remodeling: implications for stress-related diseases. *Peptides* **28**: 435–40.

Kuo L E, Kitlinska J B, Tilan J U, *et al.* (2007b). Neuropeptide Y acts directly in the periphery on fat tissue and mediates stress-induced obesity and metabolic syndrome. *Nature Med* **13**: 803–11.

Lauder J M (1990). Ontogeny of the serotonergic system in the rat: serotonin as a developmental signal. *Ann NY Acad Sci* **600**: 297–313; discussion 314.

Lesch K P (2005a). Genetic alterations of the murine serotonergic gene pathway: the neurodevelopmental basis of anxiety. *Handb Exp Pharmacol* **169**: 71–112.

Lesch K P (2005b). Serotonergic gene inactivation in mice: models for anxiety and aggression? *Novartis Found Symp* **268**: 111–40; discussion 140–6, 167–70.

Lesch K P, Mossner R (2006). Inactivation of 5HT transport in mice: modeling altered 5HT homeostasis implicated in emotional dysfunction, affective disorders, and somatic syndromes. *Handb Exp Pharmacol* **175**: 417–56.

Lesch K P, Zeng Y, Reif A, Gutknecht L (2003). Anxiety-related traits in mice with modified genes of the serotonergic pathway. *Eur J Pharmacol* **480**: 185–204.

Licinio J, Wong M L (2002). Brain-derived neurotrophic factor (BDNF) in stress and affective disorders. *Mol Psychiatry* **7**: 519.

Lohoff F W, Sander T, Ferraro T N, Dahl J P, Gallinat J, Berrettini W H (2005). Confirmation of association between the Val66Met polymorphism in the brain-derived neurotrophic factor (BDNF) gene and bipolar I disorder. *Am J Med Genet B Neuropsychiatr Genet* **139**: 51–3.

Lucki I (1998). The spectrum of behaviors influenced by serotonin. *Biol Psychiatry* **44**: 151–62.

Lyons W E, Mamounas L A, Ricaurte G A, *et al.* (1999). Brain-derived neurotrophic factor-deficient mice develop aggressiveness and hyperphagia in conjunction with brain serotonergic abnormalities. *Proc Natl Acad Sci USA* **96**: 15 239–44.

Mamounas L A, Altar C A, Blue M E, Kaplan D R, Tessarollo L, Lyons W E (2000). BDNF promotes the regenerative sprouting, but not survival, of injured serotonergic axons in the adult rat brain. *J Neurosci* **20**: 771–82.

Mamounas L A, Blue M E, Siuciak J A, Altar C A (1995). Brain-derived neurotrophic factor promotes the survival and sprouting of serotonergic axons in rat brain. *J Neurosci* **15**: 7929–39.

Martinowich K, Lu B (2008). Interaction between BDNF and serotonin: role in mood disorders. *Neuropsychopharmacology* **33**: 73–83.

Martinowich K, Manji H, Lu B (2007). New insights into BDNF function in depression and anxiety. *Nat Neurosci* **10**: 1089–93.

McAllister A K (1999). Subplate neurons: a missing link among neurotrophins, activity, and ocular dominance plasticity? *Proc Natl Acad Sci USA* **96**: 13 600–02.

Meyer J H (2007). Imaging the serotonin transporter during major depressive disorder and antidepressant treatment. *J Psychiatry Neurosci* **32**: 86–102.

Minichiello L, Korte M, Wolfer D, *et al.* (1999). Essential role for TrkB receptors in hippocampus-mediated learning. *Neuron* **24**: 401–14.

Mossner R, Daniel S, Albert D, *et al.* (2000). Serotonin transporter function is modulated by brain-derived neurotrophic factor (BDNF) but not nerve growth factor (NGF). *Neurochem Int* **36**: 197–202.

Murphy D L, Lerner A, Rudnick G, Lesch K P (2004). Serotonin transporter: gene, genetic disorders, and pharmacogenetics. *Mol Interv* **4**: 109–23.

Murphy D L, Li Q, Engel S, *et al.* (2001). Genetic perspectives on the serotonin transporter. *Brain Res Bull* **56**: 487–94.

Murphy D L, Uhl G R, Holmes A, *et al.* (2003). Experimental gene interaction studies with SERT mutant mice as models for human polygenic and epistatic traits and disorders. *Genes Brain Behav* **2**: 350–64.

Nestler E J, Barrot M, DiLeone R J, Eisch A J, Gold S J, Monteggia L M (2002). Neurobiology of depression. *Neuron* **34**: 13–25.

Neves-Pereira M, Cheung J K, Pasdar A, *et al.* (2005). BDNF gene is a risk factor for schizophrenia in a Scottish population. *Mol Psychiatry* **10**: 208–12.

Owens M J, Nemeroff C B (1994). Role of serotonin in the pathophysiology of depression: focus on the serotonin transporter. *Clin Chem* **40**: 288–95.

Ozaki N, Goldman D, Kaye W H, *et al.* (2003). Serotonin transporter missense mutation associated with a complex neuropsychiatric phenotype. *Mol Psychiatry* **8**: 933–6.

Panagiotaropoulos T, Papaioannou A, Pondiki S, Prokopiou A, Stylianopoulou F, Gerozissis K (2004). Effect of neonatal handling and sex on basal and chronic stress-induced corticosterone and leptin secretion. *Neuroendocrinology* **79**: 109–18.

Pozzo-Miller L D, Gottschalk W, Zhang L, *et al.* (1999). Impairments in high-frequency transmission, synaptic vesicle docking, and synaptic protein distribution in the hippocampus of BDNF knockout mice. *J Neurosci* **19**: 4972–83.

Ren-Patterson R F, Cochran L W, Holmes A, Lesch K P, Lu B, Murphy D L (2006). Gender-dependent modulation of brain monoamines and anxiety-like behaviors in mice with genetic serotonin transporter and BDNF deficiencies. *Cell Mol Neurobiol* **26**: 755–80.

Ren-Patterson R F, Cochran L W, Holmes A, *et al.* (2005a). Loss of brain-derived neurotrophic factor gene allele exacerbates brain monoamine deficiencies and increases stress abnormalities of serotonin transporter knockout mice. *J Neurosci Res* **79**: 756–71.

Ren-Patterson R F, Kim D K, Zheng X, *et al.* (2005b). Serotonergic-like progenitor cells propagated from neural stem cells in vitro: survival with SERT protein expression following implantation into brains of mice lacking SERT. *Faseb J* **19**: 1537–9.

Rosmond R, Dallman M F, Bjorntorp P (1998). Stress-related cortisol secretion in men: relationships with abdominal obesity and endocrine, metabolic and hemodynamic abnormalities. *J Clin Endocrinol Metab* **83**: 1853–9.

Rudnick G (2006a). Serotonin transporters – structure and function. *J Membr Biol* **213**: 101–10.

Rudnick G (2006b). Structure/function relationships in serotonin transporter: new insights from the structure of a bacterial transporter. *Handb Exp Pharmacol* **175**: 59–73.

Rumajogee P, Madeira A, Verge D, Hamon M, Miquel M C (2002). Up-regulation of the neuronal serotoninergic phenotype in vitro: BDNF and cAMP share TrkB-dependent mechanisms. *J Neurochem* **83**: 1525–8.

Rumajogee P, Verge D, Darmon M, Brisorgueil M J, Hamon M, Miquel M C (2005). Rapid up-regulation of the neuronal serotoninergic phenotype by brain-derived neurotrophic factor and cyclic adenosine monophosphate: relations with raphe astrocytes. *J Neurosci Res* **81**: 481–7.

Rumajogee P, Verge D, Hamon M, Miquel M C (2006). Somato-dendritic distribution of 5-HT(1A) and 5-HT(1B) autoreceptors in the BDNF- and cAMP-differentiated RN46A serotoninergic raphe cell line. *Brain Res* **1085**: 121–6.

Rumajogee P, Verge D, Hanoun N, *et al.* (2004). Adaption of the serotoninergic neuronal phenotype in the absence of 5-HT autoreceptors or the 5-HT transporter: involvement of BDNF and cAMP. *Eur J Neurosci* **19**: 937–44.

Senkowski D, Linden M, Zubragel D, Bar T, Gallinat J (2003). Evidence for disturbed cortical signal processing and altered serotonergic neurotransmission in generalized anxiety disorder. *Biol Psychiatry* **53**: 304–14.

Shiah I S, Yatham L N (2000). Serotonin in mania and in the mechanism of action of mood stabilizers: a review of clinical studies. *Bipolar Disord* **2**: 77–92.

Sklar P, Gabriel S B, McInnis M G, *et al.* (2002). Family-based association study of 76 candidate genes in bipolar disorder: BDNF is a potential risk locus. Brain-derived neutrophic factor. *Mol Psychiatry* **7**: 579–93.

Solano J M, Jacobson L (1999). Glucocorticoids reverse leptin effects on food intake and body fat in mice without increasing NPY mRNA. *Am J Physiol* **277**: E708–16.

Tjurmina O A, Armando I, Saavedra J M, Goldstein D S, Murphy D L (2002). Exaggerated adrenomedullary response to immobilization in mice with targeted disruption of the serotonin transporter gene. *Endocrinology* **143**: 4520–6.

Tonra J R, Ono M, Liu X, *et al.* (1999). Brain-derived neurotrophic factor improves blood glucose control and alleviates fasting hyperglycemia in C57BLKS-Lepr (db)/lepr(db) mice. *Diabetes* **48**: 588–94.

Turlejski K (1996). Evolutionary ancient roles of serotonin: long-lasting regulation of activity and development. *Acta Neurobiol Exp (Wars)* **56**: 619–36.

Van Meer P, Raber J (2005). Mouse behavioral analysis in systems biology. *Biochem J* **389**: 593–610.

Vetter D E, Li C, Zhao L, *et al.* (2002). Urocortin-deficient mice show hearing impairment and increased anxiety-like behavior. *Nat Genet* **31**: 363–9.

Vitalis T, Cases O, Gillies K, *et al.* (2002). Interactions between TrkB signaling and serotonin excess in the developing murine somatosensory cortex: a role in tangential and radial organization of thalamocortical axons. *J Neurosci* **22**: 4987–5000.

Vitalis T, Cases O, Passemard S, Callebert J, Parnavelas J G (2007). Embryonic depletion of serotonin affects cortical development. *Eur J Neurosci* **26**: 331–44.

Vitalis T, Parnavelas J G (2003). The role of serotonin in early cortical development. *Dev Neurosci* **25**: 245–56.

Whitaker-Azmitia P M (1991). Role of serotonin and other neurotransmitter receptors in brain development: basis for developmental pharmacology. *Pharmacol Rev* **43**: 553–61.

Whitaker-Azmitia P M (1999). The discovery of serotonin and its role in neuroscience. *Neuropsychopharmacology* **21**: 2S–8S.

Whitaker-Azmitia P M (2001). Serotonin and brain development: role in human developmental diseases. *Brain Res Bull* **56**: 479–85.

Whitaker-Azmitia P M, Druse M, Walker P, Lauder J M (1996). Serotonin as a developmental signal. *Behav Brain Res* **73**: 19–29.

Xu B, Zang K, Ruff N L, *et al.* (2000). Cortical degeneration in the absence of neurotrophin signaling: dendritic retraction and neuronal loss after removal of the receptor TrkB. *Neuron* **26**: 233–45.

Yamada K, Mizuno M, Nabeshima T (2002). Role for brain-derived neurotrophic factor in learning and memory. *Life Sci* **70**: 735–44.

Yatham L N, Liddle P F, Shiah I S, *et al.* (2000). Brain serotonin2 receptors in major depression: a positron emission tomography study. *Arch Gen Psychiatry* **57**: 850–8.

Zhou F C, Lesch K P, Murphy D L (2002). Serotonin uptake into dopamine neurons via dopamine transporters: a compensatory alternative. *Brain Res* **942**: 109–19.

KHALISA N. HERMAN, JAMES T. WINSLOW AND STEPHEN J. SUOMI

10

Primate models in serotonin transporter research

ABSTRACT

Numerous studies provide persuasive evidence that a polymorphism in the serotonin promoter, 5-HTTLPR, interacts with environmental risk factors to produce heightened rates of depression, anxiety, antisocial and borderline personality disorders, and substance abuse in adults and adolescents. Investigations with the rhesus monkey have demonstrated similar gene–environment (G×E) interactions on both behavioral and biological outcomes. In this chapter, we review the history of primate models in serotonin transporter (5-HTT) research. Work with non-human primates has noted associations between behavioral differences and variation in serotonin metabolism (5-hydroxyindole acetic acid, 5-HIAA). Investigations in several non-human primate species have also indicated that manipulation of early experience results in changes in behavior along with alterations in serotonergic functioning. These lines of research have contributed to the discovery of short (*s*) and long (*l*) forms within the serotonin promoter (rh5-HTTLPR) in the rhesus monkey. Researchers have since documented associations between the *l*/*s* or *s*/*s* genotypes and reduced cognitive flexibility, greater impulsivity, and anxious-like behavior, as well as higher rates of alcohol consumption. Furthermore, multiple G×E interactions have been documented for levels of 5-HIAA, hypothalamic–pituitary–adrenocortical (HPA) axis activity, alcohol consumption, rates of behavioral pathology, social play, aggression, and infant temperament. In most cases, these interactions were due to worse outcomes in *l*/*s* subjects that had been subjected to early maternal deprivation. This program

Experimental Models in Serotonin Transporter Research, eds. A. V. Kalueff and J. L. LaPorte. Published by Cambridge University Press.

of research demonstrates that *l/s* monkeys are more vulnerable to the effects of early-life stress, whereas *l/l* monkeys are more resilient.

INTRODUCTION

Durable primate societies adhere to complex rules and relationships (Maestripieri *et al.*, 2007). Using these rules, individuals respond to the behavior of others and choose courses of action fitting current circumstances. Collectively, our actions have the power to influence the direction of our lives, as well as the quality of our experiences. One way that quality of life can be seriously impaired is by the emergence of psychopathology (USDHHS, 2000). Many mental disorders are thought to emerge from a dynamic interaction between our genetic predispositions and our cumulative history of adverse and positive life experiences (O'Hara *et al.*, 2007). Exposure to adversity during infancy and childhood appears to have a powerful influence on the emergence of disorders throughout the life span, an influence which is believed to grow in proportion with the duration and significance of the adverse circumstances (Heim *et al.*, 2001; Rutter *et al.*, 2006a). For these reasons, it is important to study how experiential factors, especially those encountered early in the lifespan, interact with genetic predispositions for disease.

A number of disorders, including depression, anxiety, disruptive behavior, and suicide attempts, have been linked to altered functioning of the neurotransmitter serotonin (Kruesi *et al.*, 1990; Malison *et al.*, 1998; Roy *et al.*, 1986). More recently, investigators have examined variations in genes that give rise to altered serotonergic function and potentially influence the progress of psychopathologies (Roy *et al.*, 2007). Together, these efforts suggest that – as in much physical pathology – individuals may be more or less vulnerable to mental illness depending on genetic factors, including those regulating serotonergic systems and interacting with unique developmental histories (Rutter *et al.*, 2006b; Shanahan and Hofer, 2005).

One important regulator of serotonin activity is the serotonin transporter protein (5-HTT) (Heils *et al.*, 1996; Murphy *et al.*, 2004). The serotonin transporter protein regulates the amount of serotonin that is available in the synaptic space by binding excess transmitter and transporting it back into the cell body for processing (reuptake). Recently, researchers determined that the promoter region of the human serotonin transporter protein gene (SLC6A4) contains a polymorphism with a variable number of repeats in one element (Heils *et al.*,

1996). The variant with the greatest number of repeats (the long allele) is associated with a higher transcription rate of serotonin transporter gene (5-HTTLPR) than the variant with fewer repeats (the short allele) (Heils *et al.*, 1996). Subsequent studies suggest that incidence of this particular species of polymorphism is unique and highly conserved in human and some simian primates (Lesch *et al.*, 1997).

The presence of the short allele of the serotonin transporter polymorphism in humans was originally found to be moderately correlated with anxiety symptoms in adults (Lesch *et al.*, 1996). Subsequent studies have revealed that the relationship between the short-allele genotype and anxious phenotypes is considerably more complex (Ebstein, 2006; Hariri *et al.*, 2002, 2005). Furthermore, the presence of the short allele has also been linked to conduct disorders in adolescents (Sakai *et al.*, 2006) and childhood aggression (Beitchman *et al.*, 2003; Haberstick *et al.*, 2006), which suggests that the association between 5HTTLPR polymorphisms and emotionality do not conform to a "one gene, one disorder" model of psychopathology.

One emerging strategy adopted to simplify complex interactions between genetic, neural, and behavioral processes in mental illness has been to identify neural and behavioral elemental "units" contributing to disorders, or endophenotypes (Gottesman and Shields, 1973; Iarocci *et al.*, 2007). The validity of an endophenotype clearly depends on its capacity to predict the emergence of psychopathology and, for our purposes, to explain the interaction between genetic risk and developmental experiences.

Researchers have identified a number of potential neural and behavioral endophenotypes that are associated with variation in the serotonin transporter polymorphism as well as psychopathology. For example, carriers of the short allele exhibit a heightened startle response to unexpected sounds (Brocke *et al.*, 2006), increased amygdala activity to fearful, threatening faces and novel neutral stimuli (Hariri *et al.*, 2002, 2005; Heinz *et al.*, 2007), and a greater coupling between the amygdala and ventromedial prefrontal cortex when viewing both aversive and pleasant images compared to individuals homozygous for the long allele (Heinz *et al.*, 2005; Pezawas *et al.*, 2005). Intriguingly, elevated startle response has also been associated with post-traumatic stress disorder (MacTurk and Morgan, 1995; Morgan *et al.*, 1996) and with elevated risk for mood disorders (Grillon *et al.*, 2005). Together, these findings suggest that the short allele may be associated with heightened sensitivity to emotionally provocative stimuli and adverse experience.

Another approach to simplify complex interactions in the emergence of mental illness has been to examine how adversity differentially affects individuals with the short variant of the serotonin transporter polymorphism. Numerous studies have reported that this serotonin transporter polymorphism interacts with environmental risk factors to produce heightened rates of depression, anxiety, antisocial and borderline personality disorders, and substance abuse in adults and adolescents (Caspi *et al.*, 2003; Kaufman *et al.*, 2004; Kendler *et al.*, 2005; Lyons-Ruth *et al.*, 2007; Sjoberg *et al.*, 2006; Wilhelm *et al.*, 2006), as well as reticent behavior around peers (Fox *et al.*, 2005). Some epidemiological studies employing large samples have reported that this interaction may be further influenced by gender (Eley *et al.*, 2004; Grabe *et al.*, 2005), while others have failed to replicate the interaction (Gillespie *et al.*, 2005; Surtees *et al.*, 2006).

There are many potential explanations for a complexity in the interaction between experience and genotype, such as the presence of additional unidentified, epistatic gene variants that confer heightened resilience against or sensitivities to disease, differences in sensitivity to the severity or length of exposure to adversity, and/or the action of protective cultural or environmental constraints buffering the effect of adverse environmental experience. Investigations employing human subjects have generated compelling correlational data, but are often limited by the inability to examine the contribution of experience or genetic risk using controlled experimental methodologies.

In contrast, researchers using non-human models are not restricted by the same methodological limitations as those who study human subjects. For example, infant monkeys possessing risk-conferring alleles can be randomly assigned to tightly controlled rearing conditions and can then be studied prospectively throughout development. In addition, biological indicators of serotonergic activity can be sampled, and functional differences in serotonergic neural circuitry can be examined using techniques not yet available to clinical researchers.

While rodent models are critically important to understanding fundamental brain–behavior relationships, it is difficult to generalize from rodent behavior to the complex social and cognitive activities of humans. For this reason, it is important to extend these studies to non-human primates. Two further unique features of primate biology argue for the appropriateness of examining the interaction of early developmental experience and 5HTTLPR gene polymorphisms in the non-human primate: (1) the spontaneous polymorphism described in humans is closely related to a homologous polymorphism in some old-world monkeys evidently stemming from a common ancestral genetic event (Lesch *et al.*, 1997); and (2) many of the behavioral alterations associated with the polymorphism in humans appear to involve inhibitory processes typically associated with cortical structures not extensively developed in rodents (Fuster, 2002; Izquierdo *et al.*, 2007).

In this chapter, we will summarize some of what is known about the role of serotonergic activity in social and emotional behavior from studies that have employed non-human primate models. Research with several new- and old-world non-human primate species strongly suggests that serotonin is involved in the expression of emotional behavior by non-human primates. This work is consistent with studies of rodent brain serotonin and behavioral studies using sophisticated molecular technologies (Ferrari *et al.*, 2005; Gingrich and Hen, 2001; Lucki, 1998).

ASSOCIATIONS BETWEEN MEASURES OF SEROTONERGIC ACTIVITY AND BEHAVIORAL TRAITS OF MONKEYS

Over the years, primate investigators have examined the relationship between serotonin and social or emotional behavior by examining correlations between behavior and serotonergic measures in plasma and/or cerebrospinal fluid (CSF). Serotonin production and metabolism in the periphery and brain are independent (Udenfriend and Weissbach, 1958). Nevertheless, investigators have determined that plasma measures, particularly of the serotonin metabolite 5-hydroxyindolaceatic acid (5-HIAA), can be highly correlated with 5-HIAA measures detected in brain homogenates of mice (Pietraszek *et al.*, 1992) and CSF in primates (Yan *et al.*, 1993) when collected concurrently. Consequently, plasma 5-HIAA can serve as an adequate model of central serotonergic activity for some purposes (Anderson, 2004). In non-human primates, for example, CSF and plasma 5-HIAA levels within individual monkeys appear to be highly correlated and remarkably stable across development and contexts, suggesting that central serotonergic activity may be trait-like and contribute to individual differences in behavioral temperament (Higley *et al.*, 1997; Kaplan *et al.*, 2000). That said, neither plasma nor CSF serotonergic measures can serve as more than crude proxies for complex activity at the synaptic level or even the level of brain regions. Recently, advancements in in vivo imaging have put access to analysis of alterations in regional brain serotonergic activity within reach (Ichise *et al.*, 2006).

A number of associations have been reported between central and peripheral serotonergic functioning and specific behavioral traits among non-human primates living in a number of contexts. Rhesus macaques living in the wild are more likely to risk injury by engaging in long leaps between trees if they have chronically low CSF 5-HIAA (Mehlman *et al.*, 1995). They are also more likely to emigrate from their natal troops earlier in development, and to die before reaching maturity as a result of wounds from aggressive encounters, if they have low levels of CSF 5-HIAA (Higley *et al.*, 1996a; Howell *et al.*, 2007). Adolescent macaques with low levels of CSF 5-HIAA also exhibit high rates of impulsivity and rapidly escalated aggressive behavior in social groups compared to monkeys with high levels (Higley *et al.*, 1996b). Low 5-HIAA monkeys also engage in fewer social interactions, which may be both a cause and a consequence of greater aggressive behavior (Higley *et al.*, 1996a), as well as higher rates of alcohol consumption (Higley *et al.*, 1996d). Similarly, vervet macaques living in large social groups with low CSF 5-HIAA levels are also characterized by high levels of impulsivity, particularly in the presence of a novel adult male vervet (Fairbanks *et al.*, 2001).

Captive male rhesus macaques with low CSF 5-HIAA levels reach more quickly into a novel box than subjects with higher 5-HIAA levels (Bennett *et al.*, 1998b). Similarly, captive female adult cynomolgus monkeys with elevated aggressive and defensive behavior display reduced serotonergic responsivity as measured by a fenfluramine challenge test (Shively *et al.*, 1995). In contrast, new-world marmoset monkeys with high rather than low levels of platelet 5-HIAA and platelet 5-HT displayed high levels of behavioral inhibition to a novel conspecific (Kinnally *et al.*, 2006).

Primate social and emotional behavior is comparably affected when serotonergic levels are modulated chronically through diet or pharmacological treatment. For example, marmoset monkeys fed a tryptophan-free diet leading to reduced serotonin production display a higher rate of perseverative errors (i.e. disrupted behavioral inhibition) on a reversal learning task (Clarke *et al.*, 2004). Marmosets treated with fluoxetine for 2 weeks display reduced whole blood 5-HIAA and 5-HT levels as well as altered social behavioral inhibition (Kinnally *et al.*, 2006). Similarly, vervet monkeys are also less likely to approach a novel adult male intruder if they have a history of receiving daily fluoxetine treatment for 8 weeks, suggesting that increased serotonergic activity may reduce social impulsivity (Fairbanks *et al.*, 2001).

HOW MANIPULATIONS OF ENVIRONMENTAL EXPERIENCE CAN LEAD TO ALTERED SEROTONERGIC EXPRESSION

Early experiences, especially of an adverse nature, are linked to alterations in a variety of rodent brain systems (McEwen, 2007) including, and perhaps particularly, serotonin pathways (Konno *et al.*, 2007). Similarly, studies of differential rearing experiences in non-human primates have revealed robust and reliable alterations in indices of neural activity (Sanchez, 2006; Sanchez, *et al.* 1998). One of the more prominent differential rearing models involves raising infant rhesus macaques in a nursery setting with continuous exposure to conspecific peers in lieu of maternal care for 6–7 months after birth (Chamove *et al.*, 1973). Infants that are prevented from having access to a primary attachment figure are thought to lack homeostatic mechanisms when interacting with peers or provocations (Hofer, 1994). As a result, the limbic hypothalamic–pituitary–adrenocortical axis (LHPA) may be chronically aroused, which in turn may result in permanent changes in the way that stressors impact the brain ("allostatic load") (McEwen, 2006). Peer-reared subjects are found to exhibit greater LHPA activation to a brief separation from their peer-partners compared to a mother–infant separation (Higley *et al.*, 1991) and have also been characterized by consistently lower CSF 5-HIAA levels (Higley *et al.*, 1996d; Kraemer and Clarke, 1996; Shannon *et al.*, 2005). Recently, nursery rearing was also associated with reduced 5-HTT (SERT) binding across selected regions of the brain including the raphe nuclei – structures within the corpus striatum – and other limbic subcortical areas as measured by positron emission tomography (Ichise *et al.*, 2006).

Behaviorally, macaques with a history of peer-rearing tend to exhibit higher levels of impulsive and aggressive behavior, low social dominance, greater social isolation, and less social play (Higley *et al.*, 1996c, 1996d; Suomi, 1979), but this is not always found (Barr *et al.*, 2003b), relative to mother-reared subjects. Additionally, peer-reared subjects consume more alcohol than mother-reared subjects, and those that display high rates of drinking tend to be less socially competent (Higley *et al.*, 1996d). Similarly, a provocative and elegant "neglect" model developed by Rosenblum and Paully (1984) and Rosenblum and Andrews (1994) used varying foraging demands on bonnet macaque mothers to make it difficult for mothers to provide continuous care to infants even when present in the same environment. Relatively modest levels of neglect and unpredictability were associated with altered 5-HIAA (although elevated) levels in adulthood for affected infants

(Coplan *et al.*, 1998). Additional studies using this model suggest that the developmental timing of the "neglect" experience may be a critical determinant of both the amount and direction of change measured in CSF indices of neural activity (Mathew *et al.*, 2002).

Finally, supportive findings have emerged in naturalistic populations where mothers with poor or abusive maternal skills produce offspring with low 5-HIAA levels and a high incidence of solitary play, even when the offspring are cross-fostered to these moms (Maestripieri *et al.*, 2006b). These latter findings confirm that early adverse experience alone may be sufficient to imbue persistent altered brain and social/emotional development.

ASSOCIATIONS BETWEEN RH5-HTTLPR AND BEHAVIORAL TRAITS IN THE RHESUS MACAQUE

The rhesus macaque 5-HTTLPR gene (rh5-HTTLPR) is located on chromosome 16, is orthologous to the human (Rogers *et al.*, 2006), and also contains a polymorphism consisting of a 21 base-pair insertion/deletion event expressed as short (*s*) and long (*l*) forms that function similarly to the human variants (Lesch *et al.*, 1997). Bennett *et al.* (2002) have reported that the *s* variant expresses approximately half the number of serotonin transporters as the *l* variant, and is associated with lower levels of 5-HIAA (Bennett *et al.*, 2002).

Similar to findings in humans, the presence of two copies of the *s* allele has also been associated with impulsivity and anxious-like behavior. For example, infant monkeys with the *s/s* genotype were found to exhibit significantly greater behavioral inhibition compared to subjects with heterozygous or homozygous dominant genotypes (Bethea *et al.*, 2004). In a series of tests designed to assess variation in anxious behavior, *s/s* subjects were found to engage in significantly less play during an individual free-play period involving novel toys, and they also exhibited significantly greater levels of fear displays and lipsmacking behavior during a remote control car test. No associations were found between the *s* allele and fear responses to a human intruder, or in the latency to touch novel fruit or to reach over a rubber snake or spider to obtain familiar fruit. Two other studies have also found no effect of the *s* allele on anxiety-like behavior (Izquierdo *et al.*, 2007; Rogers *et al.*, 2008), but did detect evidence of elevated aggressive behavior (Izquierdo *et al.*, 2007).

Researchers have also compared associations between polymorphisms in the serotonin transporter protein and global measures of aggression in seven species of macaque (Thierry *et al.*, 2000; Wendland *et al.*, 2006). The rhesus macaque was the only species found to possess both the *s* variant of rh5-HTTLPR and to have high levels of variation in rates of aggression. Since the *s* allele is associated with lower 5-HIAA, it is surprising that they did not find higher overall rates of aggression in rhesus compared to the six other macaque species. Instead, they found greater variability in aggression, which suggests a role for additional genetic variation besides the serotonin transporter or perhaps environmental modification of genetic differences.

The presence of the *s*/*s* genotype has recently been associated with impaired cognitive performance in adult rhesus macaques on several cognitive tasks involving the Wisconsin General Testing Apparatus (Izquierdo *et al.*, 2007). More specifically, *s*/*s* monkeys made more errors on a task called the Object Discrimination Reversal Learning (ODRL), which tests the monkeys' ability to adapt to changes in reward contingencies. Subjects with the *s*/*s* genotype also took longer to stop looking for a food reward on an extinction task which tests how many trials it takes for a subject to stop looking under a testing well for a reward. No effect of genotype was found on a reinforcer devaluation task, which tests the ability of subjects to associate two different positive foods with particular objects. These deficits are consistent with impulse control deficits previously measured as escalated aggression or other high-risk behaviors in monkeys with low CSF 5-HIAA (Higley *et al.*, 1996b, 1997). Taken together, these studies implicate serotonin in the expression of social behavior and cognition.

GENE–ENVIRONMENT INTERACTIONS INVOLVING RH5-HTTLPR

A number of studies in rhesus monkeys have demonstrated that the influence of the serotonin transporter polymorphism on behavior is modified by early experience. For example, gene–environment interactions involving the serotonin transporter polymorphism have been reported for rates of behavioral pathologies and propensity for alcoholism (Spinelli *et al.*, 2007). A variety of developmental milestones are also impacted by this interaction, including indices of infant temperament and social competence with peers (Barr *et al.*, 2003a, 2003b, 2004a; Champoux *et al.*, 2002). These early developmental changes suggest that *l*/*s* and *s*/*s* subjects may be at heightened risk of developing negative social relationships (Higley *et al.*, 1996d).

Before reviewing the effects of early stress on genotype–behavior associations, we will first describe several studies that have investigated biological measures of interactions between rearing and rh5-HTTLPR.

An initial study using the radioligand [(I)123] beta-CIT ([(I)123] methyl 3beta-(4-iodophenyl) tropane-2-carboxylate) for PET imaging of the availability of serotonin transporters in the brain stem found no effect of rh5-HTTLPR variation on the availability in the brainstem raphe areas of adult macaques reared without their mothers (Heinz *et al.*, 1998). Interestingly, decreased CSF 5-HIAA concentrations were also detected. The study was somewhat weakened by the absence of a mother-reared control group, which makes interpretation of these findings relative to normal monkeys unclear.

Subsequent studies suggest that alteration in serotonergic systems are associated with nursery rearing and are further linked to the presence or absence of the *s* allele on rh5-HTTLPR (Bennett *et al.*, 2002). Subjects with the *l/s* genotype were found to have the lowest 5-HIAA levels, but only if they also experienced peer-rearing in lieu of maternal care. Remarkably, no main effect for rearing on 5-HIAA levels was found, suggesting that only those subjects with the *s* allele that already transcribe less 5-HTT protein are influenced by early social stress.

More recently, Kinnally and her colleagues (2008) used quantitative reverse transcription PCR techniques to examine levels of 5-HTT expression in lymphocyte samples collected at 2.5 and 8 h after the onset of a social separation of differentially reared monkeys. A significant overall rearing effect was found, such that only mother-reared subjects upregulated lymphocyte 5-HTT during the social separation. However, no main genotype effect or interaction effect between rearing and genotype was detected.

The effects of a short-term social separation on HPA measures of stress vary based on an interaction between genotype and rearing experience (Barr *et al.*, 2003a). In this study, when monkeys were 6 months of age, all subjects underwent four 4-day long separations punctuated by 3-day reunion periods. Mothers were removed from the social groups so that the infants were left with other group members, while members of the peer-only condition were separated physically into four separate quadrants that still permitted sensory contact between subjects. Adrenocorticotropic hormone (ACTH) and cortisol were measured from blood samples collected at baseline, after the first hour and then again 4 days into the separation. Monkeys with the *l/s* genotype that were subjected to peer-rearing appeared to be most strongly affected by the separation measured as the highest ACTH levels during the separation, although these subjects also had higher ACTH levels at baseline.

Subsequently, Barr and colleagues (2004b) found that female macaques appear to be more vulnerable than males to the stressful effects of the social separation. Males with the *l/s* genotype were found to have higher ACTH responses to separation than *l/l* males, regardless of rearing background. By contrast, *l/s* females only displayed a heightened ACTH response relative to *l/l* subjects if they were subjected to peer-rearing. The authors concluded that females with the *l/s* genotype may be more vulnerable to the affects of adversity than males. An additional implication of these findings is that females with the *l/s* genotype are less affected by a short-term stressor than males if they are not subjected to adverse rearing. In other words, males with the *l/s* genotype experience separations more stressfully than *l/l* subjects, while females only do if they also have a history of adverse rearing.

A separate analysis of behavioral data from this study confirms that social separations are stressful experiences for differentially reared young rhesus macaques (Spinelli *et al.*, 2007). Peer-reared *l/s* monkeys were found to exhibit higher levels of pathological behaviors such as self-directed behaviors and pacing during both the acute and chronic phases of the separation paradigm. Interestingly, peer-reared infants displayed greater despair-like behaviors during both phases of the separation if they had the *l/l* genotype. The authors mentioned that these high levels of despair-like behaviors may promote coping by helping the subjects reduce their levels of anxiety. Alternatively, high levels of infant despair during a social separation may indicate a more adaptive response, as it may decrease the likelihood of being detected by predators.

Champoux *et al.* (2002) reported that nursery-reared infants with the *s* variant of rh5-HTTLPR have less-developed orientation skills when investigating a novel toy. Across rearing conditions, *l/s* infants also have been found to engage in higher rates of vocalizations than *l/l* infants. This study demonstrated that maternal deprivation has greater costs on visual processing for infants with the *l/s* genotype, which suggests that these infants may pay less attention to their peer playmates later in development and consequently develop less social competence.

There are also data demonstrating an interaction between rearing and rh5-HTTLPR on the development of social competence in juvenile rhesus macaques (Barr *et al.*, 2003b). Barr *et al.* observed captive rhesus macaques living with their mothers in social groups or in groups of four to five same-age and gender peers. They rated the subjects on social play and aggressive behaviors and they also genotyped subjects for rh5-HTTLPR. Peer-reared infants were found to engage in higher rates of social play than mother-reared infants, which the authors attributed to greater peer experience (Suomi, 1979). Additionally, *l/s* infants were found to engage in less social play, but only if they were peer-reared. The authors interpreted this result as an indicator of greater reticence in *l/s* infants. They also reported a significantly greater incidence of aggression in peer-reared *l/s* infants than infants in all other groups. This study demonstrates that adversity negatively impacts the serotonergic system and thereby the development of social competence. Incidentally, the adverse effects may also place these subjects at greater risk of developing a dependence to alcohol (Higley *et al.*, 1996d).

Researchers investigating risk factors for alcoholism have discovered that rh5-HTTLPR interacts with peer-only rearing to produce altered drinking patterns in adolescent macaques (Barr *et al.*, 2003a). A large number of subjects were rated for their intoxication levels after receiving intravenous injections of alcohol. The investigators found greater sensitivity to alcohol in *l/s* compared to *l/l* subjects. Additionally, a comparison involving only the peer-reared animals revealed that *l/s* subjects had higher intoxication scores than *l/l* subjects. Researchers have also noted that mother-reared *l/s* monkeys may drink less alcohol than *l/s* peer-reared subjects, suggesting a protective effect of nurturing maternal care (Barr *et al.*, 2003a; Bennett *et al.*, 1998a). However, in a follow up study, the same group of researchers found the interaction between rearing and rh5-HTTLPR on alcohol consumption only held up for female macaques (Barr *et al.*, 2004a). These studies demonstrate that individuals with the *l/s* genotype are more susceptible to the addictive properties of alcohol, but only if they are exposed to early-life stress.

Several studies demonstrate that adversity, including fetal alcohol exposure, can influence serotonergic activity and thereby developmental outcomes both prenatally and during early infancy. Fetal alcohol exposure differentially affects developmental milestones of infants with different rh5-HTTLPR genotypes. During four weekly social separations, both mother- and nursery-reared infants were tested on the Primate Neonatal Neurobehavioral Assessment (Kraemer *et al.*, 2008). This work is important because most women of childbearing age drink alcoholic beverages, and many do not learn of their pregnancies until they are well past the first month of gestation (Ebrahim *et al.*, 1999; Forrest, 1994). The study randomly assigned female rhesus macaques to either alcohol exposure during pregnancy or to a control condition, as well as to either a social separation when their infants were 6 months of age or to a control condition. During the first month after birth, the researchers conducted temperament tests on the infants using the Primate Neonatal Neurobehavioral Assessment (Schneider *et al.*, 1991), an adaptation of the human Neonatal Behavioral Assessment Scale (Brazelton and Nugent, 1995). Kramer *et al.* (2007) reported that *l/s* infants that were exposed prenatally to alcohol had significantly higher irritability scores on their Brazelton tests than *l/l* infants, but there were no genotype differences for infants from the control condition. Additionally, they reported that *l/s* infants exposed to alcohol in utero also displayed higher ACTH and cortisol responses to the social separation relative to all other groups of infants. Thus variations in early experience can help modulate associations between 5-HTT and biological and behavioral outcomes.

CONCLUDING REMARKS

Taken together, the findings from the studies described above demonstrate that non-human primates, and in particular rhesus macaques, are excellent models for studying genetic and experiential contributions to traits associated with atypical serotonergic activity. Much progress has been made over the past decade in understanding how individual variation in serotonergic activity is associated with a variety of biological and behavioral measures. Even so, more studies are needed to replicate the findings that have been reported for rhesus macaques, and to investigate how intermediate developmental milestones are linked to later reproductive fitness.

We see a need for more studies that will further examine the interaction of the serotonin transporter polymorphism and environmental experience, in particular the long-term sequelae of early adverse experience, genotype, and subsequent risk for mental illness and addiction. It is critically important to identify neural and behavioral endophenotypes capable of predicting the emergence of behavioral pathologies. In vivo imaging is likely to be a particularly informative group of technologies in this regard.

Future research on interactions involving rh5-HTTLPR and early experience should examine the effects of additional genes such as monoamine oxidase A (MAOA) as well as additional environmental factors such as quality of peer relationships (e.g. G×G×E or E×E×G) (Kinnally, 2007). For example, a positive peer relationship may remedy some initial deficits stemming from maternal deprivation (Suomi and Harlow, 1972). Finally, in an effort to improve the generalizability of these data to humans, studies are needed to examine gene–environment interaction effects for macaques that have been subjected to adversity that is within the realm of normative experience. For instance, researchers could examine whether infants subjected to high levels of rejection by their mothers are at greater risk of developing adverse outcomes if they possess the *l/s* genotype (Maestripieri *et al.*, 2006a).

The mere presence of a maternal figure having a protective effect against alcoholism for *l/s* macaques suggests that infants with the *s* variant of rh5-HTTLPR may also benefit from nurturing maternal care or enrichment (Belsky, 2005; Bennett *et al.*, 1998a). One study from our laboratory (which unfortunately lacks genetic data) found that offspring of highly reactive and punitive mothers are more likely to be behaviorally precocious and enterprising when cross-fostered to mothers high in affiliative grooming toward previous infants (Suomi, 1987). Perhaps the *s* variant of rh5-HTTLPR continues to exist in populations of rhesus macaques precisely because it allows developmental outcomes to be partly determined by the quality of the environmental circumstances under which infants are developing?

In sum, there is good experimental evidence of gene–environment interactions involving the serotonin transporter polymorphism in macaques for both biological and behavioral measures. This suggests that when interactions are not found in human populations, the lack of evidence may be due to buffering effects, such as unmeasured positive life experiences. Research with non-human primates is therefore improving (markedly) our knowledge of human disorders involving the serotonin system.

REFERENCES

Anderson G M (2004). Peripheral and central neurochemical effects of the selective serotonin reuptake inhibitors (SSRIs) in humans and nonhuman primates: assessing bioeffect and mechanisms of action. *Int J Dev Neurosci* **22**: 397–404.

Barr C S, Newman T K, Becker M L, *et al.* (2003a). Serotonin transporter gene variation is associated with alcohol sensitivity in rhesus macaques exposed to early-life stress. *Alcohol Clin Exp Res* **27**: 812–7.

Barr C S, Newman T K, Becker M L, *et al.* (2003b). The utility of the non-human primate model for studying gene by environment interactions in behavioral research. *Genes Brain Behav* **2**: 336–40.

Barr C S, Newman T K, Lindell S, *et al.* (2004a). Interaction between serotonin transporter gene variation and rearing condition in alcohol preference and consumption in female primates. *Arch Gen Psychiatry* **61**: 1146–52.

Barr C S, Newman T K, Schwandt M, *et al.* (2004b). Sexual dichotomy of an interaction between early adversity and the serotonin transporter gene promoter variant in rhesus macaques. *Proc Natl Acad Sci USA* **101**: 12 358–63.

Beitchman J H, Davidge K M, Kennedy J L, *et al.* (2003). The serotonin transporter gene in aggressive children with and without ADHD and nonaggressive matched controls. *Ann NY Acad Sci* **1008**: 248–51.

Belsky J (2005). Differential susceptibility to rearing influence: an evolutionary hypothesis and some evidence. In Ellis B, Bjorklund D, editors. *Origins of the social mind: evolutionary psychology and child development.* New York: Guilford Press, pp. 139–63.

Bennett A J, Lesch K P, Heils A, Linnoila M V (1998a). Serotonin transporter gene variation, CSF 5-HIAA concentrations, and alcohol-related aggression in rhesus monkeys (*Macaca mulatta*). *Am J Primatol* **45**: 168–9.

Bennett A J, Lesch K P, Heils A, *et al.* (2002). Early experience and serotonin transporter gene variation interact to influence primate CNS function. *Mol Psychiatry* **7**: 118–22.

Bennett A J, Tsai T, Pierre P J, Suomi S J, Shoaf S E, Linnoila M V (1998b). Behavioral response to novel objects varies with CSF monoamine concentrations in rhesus monkeys. *Soc Neurosci Abstr* **24**: 954.

Bethea C L, Streicher J M, Coleman K, Pau F K, Moessner R, Cameron J L (2004). Anxious behavior and fenfluramine-induced prolactin secretion in young rhesus macaques with different alleles of the serotonin reuptake transporter polymorphism (5HTTLPR). *Behav Genet* **34**: 295–307.

Brazelton T B, Nugent J K (1995). *Neonatal behavioral assessment scale.* Cambridge: Cambridge University Press.

Brocke B, Armbruster D, Muller J, *et al.* (2006). Serotonin transporter gene variation impacts innate fear processing: acoustic startle response and emotional startle. *Mol Psychiatry* **11**: 1106–12.

Caspi A, Sugden K, Moffitt T E, *et al.* (2003). Influence of life stress on depression: moderation by a polymorphism in the 5-HTT gene. *Science* **301**: 386–9.

Chamove A S, Rosenblum L A, Harlow H F (1973). Monkeys (*Macaca mulatta*) raised only with peers: a pilot study. *Anim Behav* **21**: 316–25.

Champoux M, Bennett A, Shannon C, Higley J D, Lesch K P, Suomi S J (2002). Serotonin transporter gene polymorphism, differential early rearing, and behavior in rhesus monkey neonates. *Mol Psychiatry* **2002**: 1058–63.

Clarke H F, Dalley J W, Crofts H S, Robbins T W, Roberts A C (2004). Cognitive inflexibility after prefrontal serotonin depletion. *Science* **304**: 878–80.

Coplan J D, Trost R C, Owens M J, *et al.* (1998). Cerebrospinal fluid concentrations of somatostatin and biogenic amines in grown primates reared by mothers exposed to manipulated foraging conditions. *Arch Gen Psychiatry* **55**: 473–7.

Ebrahim S H, Diekman S T, Floyd R L, Decoufle P (1999). Comparison of binge drinking among pregnant and nonpregnant women, United States, 1991–1995. *Am J Obstet Gynecol* **180**: 1–7.

Ebstein R P (2006). The molecular genetic architecture of human personality: beyond self-report questionnaires. *Mol Psychiatry* **11**: 427–45.

Eley T C, Sugden K, Corsico A, *et al.* (2004). Gene–environment interaction analysis of serotonin system markers with adolescent depression. *Mol Psychiatry* **9**: 908–15.

Fairbanks L A, Melega W P, Jorgensen M J, Kaplan J R, McGuire M T (2001). Social impulsivity inversely associated with CSF 5-HIAA and fluoxetine exposure in vervet monkeys. *Neuropsychopharmacology* **24**: 370–8.

Ferrari P F, Palanza P, Parmigiani S, de Almeida R M, Miczek K A (2005). Serotonin and aggressive behavior in rodents and nonhuman primates: predispositions and plasticity. *Eur J Pharmacol* **526**: 259–73.

Forrest J D (1994). The role of hormonal contraceptives: epidemiology of unintended pregnancy and contraceptive use. *Am J Obstet Gynecol* **170**: 1485–9.

Fox N A, Nichols K E, Henderson H A, *et al.* (2005). Evidence for a gene–environment interaction in predicting behavioral inhibition in middle childhood. *Psychol Sci* **16**: 921–6.

Fuster J M (2002). Frontal lobe and cognitive development. *J Neurocytol* **31**: 373–85.

Gillespie N A, Whitfield J B, Williams B, Heath A C, Martin N G (2005). The relationship between stressful life events, the serotonin transporter (5-HTTLPR) genotype and major depression. *Psychol Med* **35**: 101–11.

Gingrich J A, Hen R (2001). Dissecting the role of the serotonin system in neuropsychiatric disorders using knockout mice. *Psychopharmacology (Berl.)* **155**: 1–10.

Gottesman I I, Shields J (1973). Genetic theorizing and schizophrenia. *Br J Psychiatry* **122**: 15–30.

Grabe H J, Lange M, Wolff B, *et al.* (2005). Mental and physical distress is modulated by a polymorphism in the 5-HT transporter gene interacting with social stressors and chronic disease burden. *Mol Psychiatry* **10**: 220–4.

Grillon C, Warner V, Hille J, *et al.* (2005). Families at high and low risk for depression: a three-generation startle study. *Biol Psychiatry* **57**: 953–60.

Haberstick B C, Smolen A, Hewitt J K (2006). Family-based association test of the 5HTTLPR and aggressive behavior in a general population sample of children. *Biol Psychiatry* **59**: 836–43.

Hariri A R, Drabant E M, Munoz K E, *et al.* (2005). A susceptibility gene for affective disorders and the response of the human amygdala. *Arch Gen Psychiatry* **62**: 146–52.

Hariri A R, Mattay V S, Tessitore A, *et al.* (2002). Serotonin transporter genetic variation and the response of the human amygdala. *Science* **297**: 400–3.

Heils A, Teufel A, Petri S, *et al.* (1996). Allelic variation of human serotonin transporter gene expression. *J Neurochem* **66**: 2621–4.

Heim C, Newport D J, Bonsall R, Miller A H, Nemeroff C B (2001). Altered pituitary–adrenal axis responses to provocative challenge tests in adult survivors of childhood abuse. *Am J Psychiatry* **158**: 575–81.

Heinz A, Braus D F, Smolka M N, *et al.* (2005). Amygdala–prefrontal coupling depends on a genetic variation in the serotonin transporter. *Nat Neurosci* **8**: 20–1.

Heinz A, Higley J D, Gorey J G, *et al.* (1998). In vivo association between alcohol intoxication, aggression, and serotonin transporter availability in nonhuman primates. *Am J Psychiatry* **155**: 1023–8.

Heinz A, Smolka M N, Braus D F, *et al.* (2007). Serotonin transporter genotype (5-HTTLPR): effects of neutral and undefined conditions on amygdala activation. *Biol Psychiatry* **61**: 1011–4.

Higley J D, Linnoila M, Stoff D M, Mann J J (1997). Low central nervous system serotonergic activity is traitlike and correlates with impulsive behavior: a nonhuman primate model investigating genetic and environmental influences on neurotransmission. In Stoff D M, Mann J J, editors. *Neurobiology of suicide: from the bench to the clinic. Ann NY Acad Sci* **836**: 39–56.

Higley J D, Mehlman P T, Higley S B, *et al.* (1996a). Excessive mortality in young free-ranging male nonhuman primates with low cerebrospinal fluid 5-hydroxyindoleacetic acid concentrations. *Arch Gen Psychiatry* **53**: 537–43.

Higley J D, Mehlman P T, Poland R E, *et al.* (1996b). CSF testosterone and 5-HIAA correlate with different types of aggressive behaviors. *Biol Psychiatry* **40**: 1067–82.

Higley J D, Suomi S J, Linnoila M (1996c). A nonhuman primate model of type II alcoholism? Part 2. Diminished social competence and excessive aggression correlates with low cerebrospinal fluid 5-hydroxyindoleacetic acid concentrations. *Alcohol Clin Exp Res* **20**: 643–50.

Higley J D, Suomi S J, Linnoila M (1996d). A nonhuman primate model of type II excessive alcohol consumption? Part 1. Low cerebrospinal fluid 5-hydroxyindoleacetic acid concentrations and diminished social competence correlate with excessive alcohol consumption. *Alcohol Clin Exp Res* **20**: 629–42.

Higley J D, Suomi S J, Linnoila M (1991). CSF monoamine metabolite concentrations vary according to age, rearing, and sex, and are influenced by the stressor of social separation in rhesus monkeys. *Psychopharmacology (Berl.)* **103**: 551–6.

Hofer M A (1994). Early relationships as regulators of infant physiology and behavior. *Acta Paediatr (Suppl)* **397**: 9–18.

Howell S, Westergaard G, Hoos B, *et al.* (2007). Serotonergic influences on life-history outcomes in free-ranging male rhesus macaques. *Am J Primatol* **69**: 851–65.

Iarocci G, Yager J, Elfers T (2007). What gene–environment interactions can tell us about social competence in typical and atypical populations. *Brain Cogn* **65**: 112–27.

Ichise M, Vines D C, Gura T, *et al.* (2006). Effects of early life stress on [11C]DASB positron emission tomography imaging of serotonin transporters in adolescent peer- and mother-reared rhesus monkeys. *J Neurosci* **26**: 4638–43.

Izquierdo A, Newman T K, Higley J D, Murray E A (2007). Genetic modulation of cognitive flexibility and socioemotional behavior in rhesus monkeys. *Proc Natl Acad Sci USA* **104**: 14 128–33.

Kaplan J R, Martin L J, Comuzzie A G, Manuck S B, Mann J J, Rogers J (2000). Heritability of monoaminergic metabolites measured in the cerebrospinal fluid of baboons. *Social Neurosci Abstr* **26**: 1439.

Kaufman J, Yang B-z, Douglas-Palumberi H, *et al.* (2004). Social supports and serotonin transporter gene moderate depression in maltreated children. *Proc Nat Acad Sci* **101**: 17 316–21.

Kendler K S, Kuhn J W, Vittum J, Prescott C A, Riley B (2005). The interaction of stressful life events and a serotonin transporter polymorphism in the prediction of episodes of major depression: a replication. *Arch Gen Psychiatry* **62**: 529–35.

Kinnally E L (2007). *Genetic and environmental factors that impact infant temperamental features and parameters of the serotonergic system associated with adult impulsivity in rhesus macaques* (Macaca mulatta). Davis, CA: Department of Psychology, University of California at Davis. 100 pp.

Kinnally E L, Jensen H A, Ewing J H, French J A (2006). Serotonin function is associated with behavioral response to a novel conspecific in marmosets. *Am J Primatol* **68**: 812–24.

Kinnally E L, Lyons L A, Abel K, Mendoza S, Capitanio J P (2008). Effects of early experience and genotype on serotonin transporter regulation in infant rhesus macaques. *Genes Brain Behav* **7**: 481–6.

Konno K, Matsumoto M, Togashi H, *et al.* (2007). Early postnatal stress affects the serotonergic function in the median raphe nuclei of adult rats. *Brain Res* **1172**: 60–6.

Kraemer G W, Clarke A S (1996). Social attachment, brain function, and aggression. *Ann NY Acad Sci* **794**: 121–35.

Kraemer G W, Moore C F, Newman T K, Barr C S, Schneider M L (2008). Moderate level fetal alcohol exposure and serotonin transporter gene promoter polymorphism affect neonatal temperament and limbic–hypothalamic–pituitary–adrenal axis regulation in monkeys. *Biol Psychiatry* **63**: 317–24.

Kruesi M J, Rapoport J L, Hamburger S, *et al.* (1990). Cerebrospinal fluid monoamine metabolites, aggression, and impulsivity in disruptive behavior disorders of children and adolescents. *Arch Gen Psychiatry* **47**: 419–26.

Lesch K P, Bengel D, Heils A, *et al.* (1996). Association of anxiety-related traits with a polymorphism in the serotonin transporter gene regulatory region. *Science* **274**: 1527–31.

Lesch K P, Meyer J, Glatz K, *et al.* (1997). The 5-HT transporter gene-linked polymorphic region (5-HTTLPR) in evolutionary perspective: alternative biallelic variation in rhesus monkeys. Rapid communication. *J Neural Transm* **104**: 1259–66.

Lucki I (1998). The spectrum of behaviors influenced by serotonin. *Biol Psychiatry* **44**: 151–62.

Lyons-Ruth K, Holmes B M, Sasvari-Szekely M, Ronai Z, Nemoda Z, Pauls D (2007). Serotonin transporter polymorphism and borderline or antisocial traits among low-income young adults. *Psychiatr Genet* **17**: 339–43.

MacTurk R H, Morgan G A (1995). *Mastery motivation: origins, conceptualizations, and applications*. Norwood, NJ: Ablex, pp. xiii, 376 pp.

Maestripieri D, Higley J D, Lindell S G, Newman T K, McCormack K M, Sanchez M M (2006a). Early maternal rejection affects the development of monoaminergic systems and adult abusive parenting in rhesus macaques (*Macaca mulatta*). *Behav Neurosci* **120**: 1017–24.

Maestripieri D, Lindell S G, Higley J D (2007). Intergenerational transmission of maternal behavior in rhesus macaques and its underlying mechanisms. *Dev Psychobiol* **49**: 165–71.

Maestripieri D, McCormack K, Lindell S G, Higley J D, Sanchez M M (2006b). Influence of parenting style on the offspring's behavior and CSF monoamine metabolite levels in crossfostered and noncrossfostered female rhesus macaques. *Behav Brain Res* **175**: 90–5.

Malison R T, Price L H, Berman R, *et al.* (1998). Reduced brain serotonin transporter availability in major depression as measured by [123I]-2 beta-carbomethoxy-3 beta-(4-iodophenyl)tropane and single photon emission computed tomography. *Biol Psychiatry* **44**: 1090–8.

Mathew S J, Coplan J D, Smith E L, *et al.* (2002). Cerebrospinal fluid concentrations of biogenic amines and corticotropin-releasing factor in adolescent non-human primates as a function of the timing of adverse early rearing. *Stress* **5**: 185–93.

McEwen B S (2006). Protective and damaging effects of stress mediators: central role of the brain. *Dialog Clin Neurosci* **8**: 367–81.

McEwen B S (2007). Physiology and neurobiology of stress and adaptation: central role of the brain. *Physiol Rev* **87**: 873–904.

Mehlman P T, Higley J D, Faucher I, *et al.* (1995). Correlation of CSF 5-HIAA concentration with sociality and the timing of emigration in free-ranging primates. *Am J Psychiatry* **152**: 907–13.

Morgan C A, 3rd, Grillon C, Southwick S M, Davis M, Charney D S (1996). Exaggerated acoustic startle reflex in Gulf War veterans with posttraumatic stress disorder. *Am J Psychiatry* **153**: 64–8.

Murphy D L, Lerner A, Rudnick G, Lesch K P (2004). Serotonin transporter: gene, genetic disorders, and pharmacogenetics. *Mol Interv* **4**: 109–23.

O'Hara R, Schroder C M, Mahadevan R, *et al.* (2007). Serotonin transporter polymorphism, memory and hippocampal volume in the elderly: association and interaction with cortisol. *Mol Psychiatry* **12**: 544–55.

Pezawas L, Meyer-Lindenberg A, Drabant E M, *et al.* (2005). 5-HTTLPR polymorphism impacts human cingulate–amygdala interactions: a genetic susceptibility mechanism for depression. *Nat Neurosci* **8**: 828–34.

Pietraszek M H, Takada Y, Yan D, Urano T, Serizawa K, Takada A (1992). Relationship between serotonergic measures in periphery and the brain of mouse. *Life Sci* **51**: 75–82.

Rogers J, Kaplan J, Garcia R, Shelledy W, Nair S, Cameron J (2006). Mapping of the serotonin transporter locus (SLC6A4) to rhesus chromosome 16 using genetic linkage. *Cytogenet Genome Res* **112**: 341A.

Rogers J, Shelton S E, Shelledy W, Garcia R, Kalin N H (2008). Genetic influences on behavioral inhibition and anxiety in juvenile rhesus macaques. *Genes Brain Behav* **7**: 463–9.

Rosenblum L A, Andrews M (1994). Influences of environmental demand on maternal behavior and infant development. *Acta Paediatr* **397**: 57–63.

Rosenblum L A, Paully G S (1984). The effects of varying environmental demands on maternal and infant behavior. *Child Dev* **55**: 305–14.

Roy A, Hu X Z, Janal M N, Goldman D (2007). Interaction between childhood trauma and serotonin transporter gene variation in suicide. *Neuropsychopharmacology* **32**: 2046–52.

Roy A, Virkkunen M, Guthrie S, Linnoila M (1986). Indices of serotonin and glucose metabolism in violent offenders, arsonists, and alcoholics. *Ann NY Acad Sci* **487**: 202–20.

Rutter M, Marshall P J, Fox N A (2006a). *The psychological effects of early institutional rearing. The development of social engagement: neurobiological perspectives.* New York: Oxford University Press, pp. 355–91.

Rutter M, Moffitt T E, Caspi A (2006b). Gene–environment interplay and psychopathology: multiple varieties but real effects. *J Child Psychol Psychiatry* **47**: 226–61.

Sakai J T, Young S E, Stallings M C, *et al.* (2006). Case-control and within-family tests for an association between conduct disorder and 5HTTLPR. *Am J Med Genet B Neuropsychiatr Genet* **141**: 825–32.

Sanchez M M (2006). The impact of early adverse care on HPA axis development: nonhuman primate models. *Horm Behav* **50**: 623–31.

Sanchez M M, Hearn E F, Do D, Rilling J K, Herndon J G (1998). Differential rearing affects corpus callosum size and cognitive function of rhesus monkeys. *Brain Res* **812**: 38–49.

Schneider M L, Moore C F, Suomi S J, Champoux M (1991). Laboratory assessment of temperament and environmental enrichment in rhesus monkey infants (*Macaca mulatta*). *Am J Primatol* **25**: 137–55.

Shanahan M J, Hofer S M (2005). Social context in gene–environment interactions: retrospect and prospect. *J Gerontol B Psychol Sci Soc Sci* **60** Spec No **1**: 65–76.

Shannon C, Schwandt M L, Champoux M, *et al.* (2005). Maternal absence and stability of individual differences in CSF 5-HIAA concentrations in rhesus monkey infants. *Am J Psychiatry* **162**: 1658–64.

Shively C A, Fontenot M B, Kaplan J R (1995). Social status, behavior, and central serotonergic responsivity in female cynomolgus monkeys. *Am J Primatol* **37**: 333–9.

Sjoberg R L, Nilsson K W, Nordquist N, *et al.* (2006). Development of depression: sex and the interaction between environment and a promoter polymorphism of the serotonin transporter gene. *Int J Neuropsychopharmacol* **9**: 443–9.

Spinelli S, Schwandt M L, Lindell S G, *et al.* (2007). Association between the recombinant human serotonin transporter linked promoter region polymorphism and behavior in rhesus macaques during a separation paradigm. *Dev Psychopathol* **19**: 977–87.

Suomi S J (1979). Peers, play, and primary prevention in primates. In Kent M, Rolf J, editors. *Primary prevention of psychopathology: Social competence in children*. Hanover, NH: Press of New England, pp. 127–49.

Suomi S J (1987). Genetic and maternal contributions to individual differences in rhesus monkey biobehavioral development. In Krasnegor N A, Blass E M, Hofer M A, editors. *Perinatal development: a psychobiological perspective*. San Diego, CA: Academic Press, pp. 397–419.

Suomi S J, Harlow H F (1972). Social rehabilitation of isolate-reared monkeys. *Dev Psychol* **6**: 487–96.

Surtees P G, Wainwright N W, Willis-Owen S A, Luben R, Day N E, Flint J (2006). Social adversity, the serotonin transporter (5-HTTLPR) polymorphism and major depressive disorder. *Biol Psychiatry* **59**: 224–9.

Thierry B, Iwaniuk A N, Pellis S M (2000). The influence of phylogeny on the social behavior of macaques (Primates: Cercopithecidae, genus *Macaca*). *Ethology* **106**: 713–28.

Udenfriend S, Weissbach H (1958). Turnover of 5-hydroxytryptamine (serotonin) in tissues. *Proc Soc Exp Biol Med* **97**: 748–51.

USDHHS (2000) Mental health: a report of the Surgeon General. In USDoHaH, editor. U.S. Department of Health and Human Services, Substance Abuse and Mental Health Services Administration, Center for Mental Health Services, National Institutes of Health, National Institute of Mental Health.

Wendland J R, Lesch K P, Newman T K, *et al.* (2006). Differential functional variability of serotonin transporter and monoamine oxidase a genes in macaque species displaying contrasting levels of aggression-related behavior. *Behav Genet* **36**: 163–72.

Wilhelm K, Mitchell P B, Niven H, *et al.* (2006). Life events, first depression onset and the serotonin transporter gene. *Br J Psychiatry* **188**: 210–5.

Yan D, Urano T, Pietraszek M H, *et al.* (1993). Correlation between serotonergic measures in cerebrospinal fluid and blood of subhuman primate. *Life Sci* **52**: 745–9.

KLAUS-PETER LESCH

11

The role of serotonin transporter in modeling psychiatric disorders: focus on depression, emotion regulation, and the social brain

ABSTRACT

Depression is an etiologically and clinically heterogeneous syndrome frequently co-occurring in a wide spectrum of psychiatric disorders. Characterized by a wide range of symptoms that reflect alterations in cognitive, emotional, and psychomotor processes, this syndrome is moderately to highly heritable, and caused by interaction of genes and adverse life events. Differentiation of risk-related psychobiological and neuropsychological markers is essential for the dissection of the complex genetic susceptibility to depression and comorbid disorders. A brain serotonin (5-HT) system dysfunction is thought to be involved in the pathogenesis of depression by modulating cognitive dysfunction, stress response, neuroadaptive processes, and resulting pervasive emotional disturbance. A regulatory variation in the gene encoding the 5-HT transporter (5-HTT), the master controller in the fine-tuning of 5-HT signaling, is not only associated with anxiety-related traits, but also modifies the risk of developing disorders of emotion regulation. Yet the neural and molecular mechanisms underlying gene × environment interaction are poorly understood. This paper investigates innate variability of brain 5-HTT function from an interdisciplinary perspective blending behavioral genetics and cognitive neuroscience. Following an appraisal of imaging neural correlates of genomic variation and epigenetic mechanisms as a strategy for psychiatric disorder risk assessment, future challenges for biosocial sciences in the perspective

Experimental Models in Serotonin Transporter Research, eds. A. V. Kalueff and J. L. LaPorte.

of the complex genetic architecture of emotional behavior and social interaction in non-human primates and humans are defined.

INTRODUCTION

Research on the role of the serotonin (5-HT) transporter (5-HTT, SERT, SLC6A4) in the pathophysiology of depression, a prototypical stress-linked disorder of emotion regulation with far-reaching consequences for social cognitive processes, has come a long way (Figure 11.1). In the wake of the ground-breaking discovery of presynaptic neurotransmitter uptake by Hertting and Axelrod (1961) and shortly after its identification as the initial target of antidepressant drug action (Raisman *et al.*, 1979), 5-HTT was first linked to the etiology and pathophysiology of depression by Langer, Briley, and associates (Langer *et al.*, 1981). Following characterization of the rat 5-HTT gene (*Slc6a4*) (Blakely *et al.*, 1991), the era of molecular genetic studies of emotion regulation began with three high-impact papers in 1996 that reported associations between *5-HTT* variation and anxiety-related traits (Lesch *et al.*, 1996) as well as depression (Collier *et al.*, 1996; Ogilvie *et al.*, 1996).

In the years following the first report linking *5-HTT* variation to anxiety-related traits, numerous clinical cohorts have been studied for association with disorders of emotion regulation (including depression, bipolar affective disorder, alcohol dependence, suicide, eating disorders, and autism) or disorders related to morphogenetic actions of 5-HT in other organ systems apart from the brain, such as heart, blood vessels, bowel, and bone. Modest effect sizes typical of non-Mendelian traits, polygenic patterns of inheritance, epistatic and epigenetic interactions, and heterogeneity between studies lead to inconsistent success in replication and considerably confounded attempts to reach agreement regarding the role of 5-HTT in the pathophysiology of these diseases. Nevertheless, 5-HTT has become a model *par excellence* in cognitive, biosocial, and psychiatric neuroscience, and the current status of *5-HTT* genetics is by no means discouraging. The demonstration that early life stress and other modes of gene × environmental interaction uniquely reinforce or even uncover links between *5-HTT* variation, behavior, and psychopathology in both humans and non-human primates is particularly outstanding, and heralds a new era of behavioral genetics. Several recent studies suggest that 5-HTT variation interacts with deleterious early rearing experience in rhesus macaques to influence attentional and emotional resources, sensitivity to ethanol, and stress response.

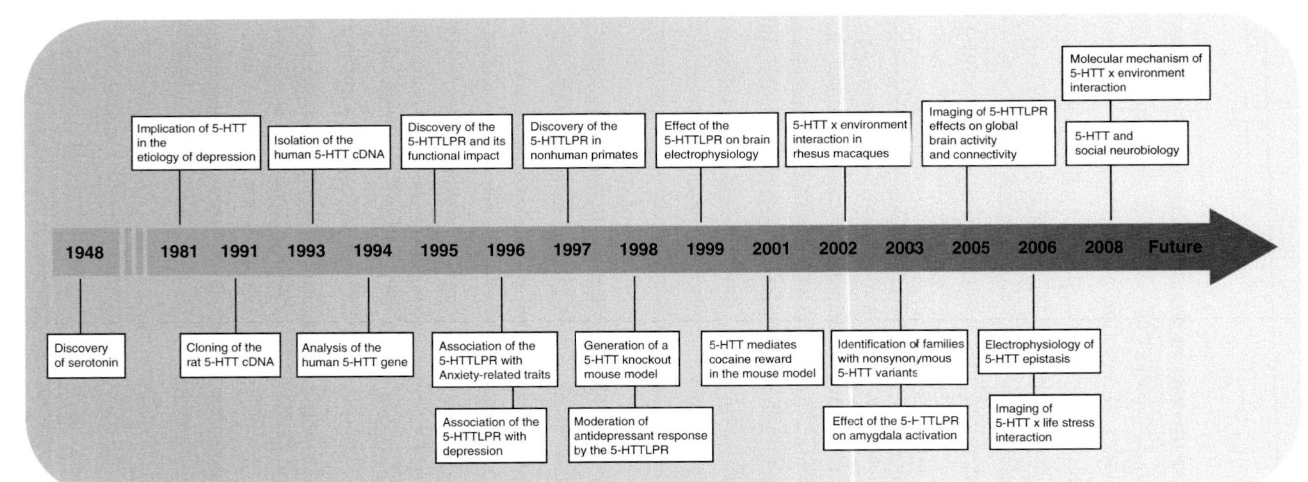

Figure 11.1 Timeline: 60 years after the discovery of serotonin and nearly 30 years of serotonin transporter research in depression.

The identification of *5-HTT* as a susceptibility gene for depression is a first step en route to an explanation of the molecular dimension of personality and behavior at risk, outlines strategies to identify physiologic pathways and mechanisms that lead to other disorders of cognitive function and emotion regulation, provides tools to dissect the interactive effects of genes and environment in the development of affective spectrum disorders, and holds the potential to predict response to antidepressant therapy and other treatments.

Early small steps of behavioral genetics are contrasted by giant leaps in a postgenomic era still in its infancy. The application of paradigms novel to neurogenetic approaches including neurophysiology, neuropsychology, and functional neuroimaging, as well as inclusion of a more extensive phenotypic spectrum (e.g. higher cognitive functions, communication skills, social competence, longevity, etc.) have strengthened the connection between *5-HTT*, social cognition and emotionality, and continue to enable a more profound understanding of how common genetic variation modulates human behavior. Finally, studies in genetically modified mice have begun to underscore the central role of 5-HT and its fine-tuning by 5-HTT function in embryonic patterning events, brain development, and synaptic plasticity, particularly in neurocircuitries related to social cognitive and emotional processes. Potential relevance of *5-HTT* variation in social cognition, the construct comprising processes employed to conform with essential norms and procedures of the social world, is currently transcending the borders of behavioral genetics to embrace biosocial science. As analyses of the genomes of humans, non-human primates, and other species has contributed fundamentally to understanding how humans have evolved. The next level of complexity concerns the nature of genetic variation among humans and its influence on inter-individual differences, as well as the relative impact of genetic and environmental determinants on social competence and behavior.

This paper focuses – from a *neurodevelopmental perspective* – on the nature of an inborn variability in brain 5-HTT function that predisposes to emotional dysregulation, depression, and a wide spectrum of psychiatric disorders with comorbid depression. The various psychobiological facets of *5-HTT* variation and resulting clinical phenomes will be reviewed critically with emphasis on meta-analyses. The relevance of *gene × environment interaction* in the etiology of depression is also highlighted. and an appraisal of *functional imaging* of emotionality and its potential for depression risk assessment is provided. Evidence for neural modularity of social cognitive processes and emotion regulation is also taken into consideration. Finally, pertinent views of *biosocial sciences* will be discussed in the perspective of the complex genetic architecture of emotional behavior and social interaction in non-human primates and humans.

DEPRESSION HERITABILITY

Among affective spectrum disorders, depression is the most prevalent and clinically relevant condition. Depression is an etiologically heterogeneous group of brain disorders that are characterized by a wide range of symptoms that reflect alterations in cognitive, psychomotor, and emotional processes. Affected individuals differ remarkably in the profile of clinical features, severity, and course of illness, as well as response to drug treatment and reintegration efforts. Genetic epidemiology has assembled convincing evidence that affective spectrum disorders, including depression, are influenced substantially by genetic factors. Population prevalence is 2–19% and an age-adjusted risk for first-degree relatives is estimated at 5–25%. The heritability of unipolar recurrent depression is remarkable, with estimates between 40% and 70%.

Twin and family-based studies have accrued considerable evidence that a complex genetic mechanism is involved, and that specific environmental factors are critical in the susceptibility to depression and comorbid disorders (for review see Kendler, (1998); Lyons *et al.*, (1998); Malhi *et al.*, 2000; McGuffin *et al.*, 1996; Silberg *et al.*, 1999) (Figure 11.2). In a meta-analysis of five large and rigorously selected family studies of major depression, familiality was demonstrated by a relative risk of 2.8 for affected subject versus first-degree relative status (Sullivan *et al.*, 2000). Early age of onset and multiple episodes of depression increase the familial aggregation, and different affective spectrum disorders are often present in the same family (Kovacs *et al.*, 1997). Depression-associated genetic factors are largely shared with generalized anxiety disorder, while environmental determinants seem to be distinct (Kendler, 1996; Kendler *et al.*, 1999). This concept is consistent with recent models of emotion regulation, which view depression and anxiety as sharing common vulnerabilities, but differing on dimensions including focus on attentional and cognitive processes or psychosocial liability. Because the mode of inheritance of depression is complex, it has been concluded that multiple genes of modest effect, in interaction with each other and in conjunction with environmental factors, produce vulnerability to the disorder. Although adverse life events may precipitate depression, examination of familial risk along with social adversity revealed

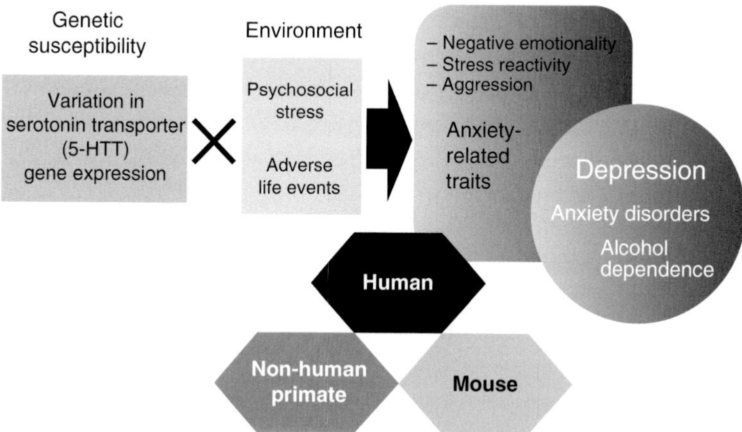

Figure 11.2 Neither genes nor environment act alone: interaction between serotonin transporter gene variation and environmental factors (G × E) in the susceptibility of depression and related comorbid disorders. *5-HTT* × E has been demonstrated in humans as well as in the non-human primate and mouse model.

that environmental effects tend to be contaminated by genetic influences: predisposition to suffer life events is likely influenced by shared family environment, and some events may be associated with genetic factors.

State-of-the-art genome-wide linkage scans have identified several chromosomal loci of interest, including 1p36, 12q22–q24.11, 13q31.1–q31.3, and 15q25.3–26.2 (Abkevich *et al.*, 2003; Holmans *et al.*, 2004; McGuffin *et al.*, 2005; Zubenko *et al.*, 2003). Although some of these chromosomal regions meet criteria for suggestive evidence of linkage, narrowing the regions and identifying candidate genes have proven difficult, and no genes have yet been demonstrated to influence risk for depression conclusively. The inconsistencies appear to result from still widely underestimated genetic heterogeneity and insufficient statistical power to detect genes with modest effects. On the other hand, the clinical (categorical) diagnosis of depression, no matter how carefully assessed, does not reflect neurobiological (dimensional) processes and may therefore not be the appropriate phenotype for genetic analysis. To alleviate these limitations, the definition of more homogeneous clinical subtypes, or intermediate (endo)phenotypes derived from neuropsychological and neuroimaging paradigms with less genetic complexity, preferably biologically measurable, but not necessarily exclusive for the disease, is required.

While molecular genetic research has typically focused on severe clinical phenotypes, such as early-onset recurrent depression or depression-related traits, with few investigations evaluating the genetic and environmental relationship between the two, it is crucial to answer the question whether a certain quantitative trait etiopathogenetically influences the disorder, or whether the trait is a syndromal dimension of the disorder. This concept also supports the hypothesis that a genetic predisposition, coupled with early life stress, in critical stages of development may result in a phenotype that is neurobiologically vulnerable to stress and may lower an individual's threshold for developing depression on additional stress exposure.

PERSONALITY AND DEPRESSION-RELATED TRAITS

Individual differences in behavioral predispositions, referred to as personality traits, are relatively enduring, continuously distributed, and substantially heritable, and are therefore likely to result from the interplay of genetic variations with environmental influences. This perspective has increasingly encouraged the pursuit of dimensional approaches to behavioral genetics, in addition to the traditional strategy of studying individuals with categorically defined psychiatric disorders. The relative influence of genetic and environmental factors on human personality and resulting behavioral differences is among the most prolonged and contentious controversies in intellectual debate. Although current views emphasize the joint influence of genes and environmental stressors, the complexities of gene × gene and gene × environment interactions (genotypes may *respond* differentially to different environments) as well as gene–environment correlations (genotypes may be *exposed* differentially to environments) represent emergent research areas (Bouchard, 1994; Loehlin, 1992; McGue and Bouchard, 1998; Plomin *et al.*, 1994).

A growing body of evidence implicates personality traits of the anxiety-related cluster (neuroticism) in the comorbidity of affective spectrum disorders (Figure 11.2) (Kendler *et al.*, 1995; Thapar and McGuffin, 1997). The dimensional structure of neuroticism comprising fearfulness, depression, negative emotionality, and stress reactivity has been delineated by systematic research (Costa and McCrae, 1992). As indexed by the personality scale of neuroticism, general vulnerability is likely to overlap genetically with both anxiety and depression. Categorical separation of depression from anxiety- and depression-related personality disorders in current consensual diagnostic systems therefore enhanced interest in the link between temperament, personality, and affective spectrum disorders as well as the impact of this inter-relationship on the heterogeneity within diagnostic entities, prediction of long-term course, and treatment response. This concept may predict that when a quantitative trait locus (QTL) is found for neuroticism, the same QTL should be associated with symptoms of anxiety and depression (Plomin *et al.*, 1994). Anxiety and mood disorders are therefore likely to represent the extreme end of variation in negative emotionality. The genetic factor contributing to the extreme ends of dimensions of variation commonly recognized as a disorder may be quantitatively, not qualitatively, different from the rest of the distribution. This vista has important implications for identifying genes for complex traits related to a distinct disorder.

Because the power of linkage analysis to detect small gene effects is considered to be quite limited – at least with realistic cohort sizes – molecular genetic research in depression has relied simultaneously on association analysis using genetic variation in or near candidate genes with etiological or pathophysiological relevance. Gene variants with a significant impact on the functionality of components of brain monoamine neurotransmission, such as the serotonin system, have been a rational starting point for this effort.

SEROTONIN SYSTEM IN EMOTION REGULATION

A neural circuit composed of several regions of the ventromedial prefrontal cortex, anterior cingulate cortex, amygdala, hippocampus, ventral striatum, hypothalamus, and several other interconnected structures involving multiple neurotransmitter systems have been implicated in emotion regulation. While a complex developmental program controls the formation and function of this circuitry, the amygdala is central to processes of cognition, emotion, and learning to associate stimuli with events that are either punishing or rewarding (Phelps, 2006).

Representing a phylogenetically ancient signaling molecule, serotonin (5-hydroxtryptamine, 5-HT) is the most widely distributed neurotransmitter in the brain. Serotonergic neurons of cells of the raphe complex project diffusely to a variety of brain regions, particularly comprising neurocircuits implicated in emotion regulation (Lowry *et al.*, 2005). Moreover, substantial evidence has been accumulated in humans, non-human primates, and other mammals that the serotonergic signaling pathway integrates not only basic physiological functions including circadian rhythms of food intake, sleep, and reproductive activity, but also elementary brain tasks of sensory processing, cognition, emotion regulation, and motor activity. 5-HT is an important regulator of morphogenetic activities during early brain development as well as during adult neurogenesis and plasticity, including cell proliferation, migration, differentiation, and synaptogenesis (Azmitia and Whitaker-Azmitia, 1997; Gaspar *et al.*, 2003; Gould, 1999; Lauder, 1990). As 5-HT shapes various brain systems during develoment, it thus sets the stage for function – above all, the emotion-regulating limbic system circuitry. With its unsurpassed complexity, 5-HT neurotransmission is a major modulator of emotional behavior including anxiety and stress response, as well as impulsivity and aggression, and considerable evidence links serotonergic dysfunction to depression and comorbid conditions such as alcohol dependence, from the very beginning of development and throughout the life cycle.

The diversity of these functions is due to the capacity of 5-HT to orchestrate the activity and its interaction with several other neurotransmitter systems, particularly activity-, cognition-, and reward-related dopaminergic pathways. While 5-HT may be viewed as a "team player" within this highly complex system of neural communication mediated by 14 pre- and postsynaptic receptor subtypes with a multitude of isoforms and subunits, its action as a chemical messenger is terminated primarily by the "bottleneck" of reuptake via the 5-HT transporter (5-HTT).

SEROTONIN TRANSPORTER – BOTTLENECK OR MASTER CONTROLLER?

The level of 5-HT in the synaptic cleft (and extrasynaptic space) is restricted by the synchronized action of at least three components. Firing of raphe 5-HT neurons is controlled by 5-HT$_{1A}$ autoreceptors located in the somatodendritic section of neurons. Release of 5-HT at the terminal fields is regulated by the 5-HT$_{1B}$ receptor. Once released, 5-HT is taken up by the 5-HTT located at the terminals (as well as the somatodendritic fraction) of 5-HT neurons, where it is eventually metabolized by monoamine oxidase A (MAOA). The action of 5-HT as a messenger is tightly regulated by its synthesizing and metabolizing enzymes, and, more directly, by the 5-HTT. It is therefore likely that genetically driven variation in 5-HTT function affects extracellular levels of 5-HT and its role as a moderator of cognition and emotionality dramatically. Consistent with this view, the brain 5-HTT is the initial site of action of widely used 5-HT reuptake inhibiting antidepressant and anti-anxiety drugs, as well as a target of psychomotor stimulants, such as amphetamines and cocaine.

The 5-HTT (solute carrier family 6 member 4, SLC6A4) belongs to the sodium:neurotransmitter symporter family (SNF). The human SLC6A4 is encoded by a single gene (*5-HTT, SERT, SLC6A4*) located on chromosome 17q11.2 (25,549,033–25,586,831), which is composed of 14 exons spanning at least 38 kb, and encodes an integral membrane protein of 630 amino acids with 12 transmembrane domains (TMDs) (Lesch *et al.*, 1993, 1994). Alternative promoters in combination with differential splicing involving exons 1A, B, and C in brain versus gut, and alternate polyadenylation site usage resulting in multiple mRNA species are likely to participate in the regulation of gene expression in humans (Heils *et al.*, 1995; Ozsarac *et al.*, 2002).

In addition to several regulatory domains controlling selective expression in 5-HT neurons, transcriptional activity of the human *5-HTT* is modulated by a length variation of a repetitive sequence, the *5-HTT*-linked polymorphic region (5-HTTLPR), located ~1.4 kb upstream of the transcription start site, which is comprised of a predominantly short (s) and long (l) variant resulting in differential *5-HTT* expression (Figure 11.3). The GC-rich sequence and unique structure of the 5-HTTLPR may give rise to the formation of a DNA secondary structure (e.g. cation-dependent tetrastrands aggregation) that has the potential to regulate the transcriptional activity of the downstream *5-HTT* promoter. Additional potentially functional variations have been described in the 5-HTTLPR (single nucleotide polymorphism, SNP rs25531), in intron 2 (variable number of a 16/17 base pair tandem repeat, VNTR-17) (Lesch *et al.*, 1994; Wendland *et al.*, 2006b), and several rare non-synonymous single nucleotide polymorphisms (SNPs) throughout the coding region (Di Bella *et al.*, 1996; Glatt *et al.*, 2001; Sutcliffe *et al.*, 2005). A predominantly Caucasian population displayed allele frequencies of 57% for the long (l) allele and 43% for the short (s) allele with a 5-HTTLPR genotype distribution of 32% ll, 49% ls, and 19% ss (Lesch *et al.*, 1996); different allele and genotype distributions are found in other populations (Gelernter *et al.*, 1997; Ishiguro *et al.*, 1997; Kunugi *et al.*, 1997).

Comparison of different mammalian species confirmed the presence of the 5-HTTLPR in platyrrhini and catarrhini (hominoids, cercopithecoids), but not in prosimian primates and other mammals (Figure 11.4) (Lesch *et al.*, 1997). The 5-HTTLPR is unique to humans and simian primates. The majority of alleles are composed of either 14 or 16 repeat elements in humans (s and l variants, respectively), while alleles with 15, 18, 19, 20 or 22 repeat elements are rare. The great apes, including the orangutan, gorilla, and chimpanzee, display a high prevalence of 18 and 20 repeat alleles. In hominoids, all alleles originate

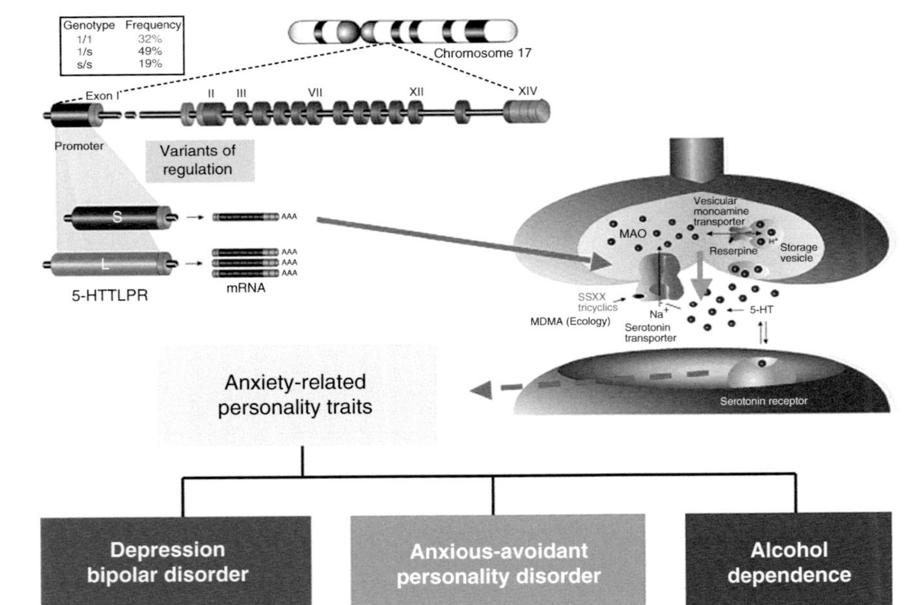

Figure 11.3 Allelic variation of serotonin transporter function in anxiety-related personality, depression, and other disorders of emotion regulation.

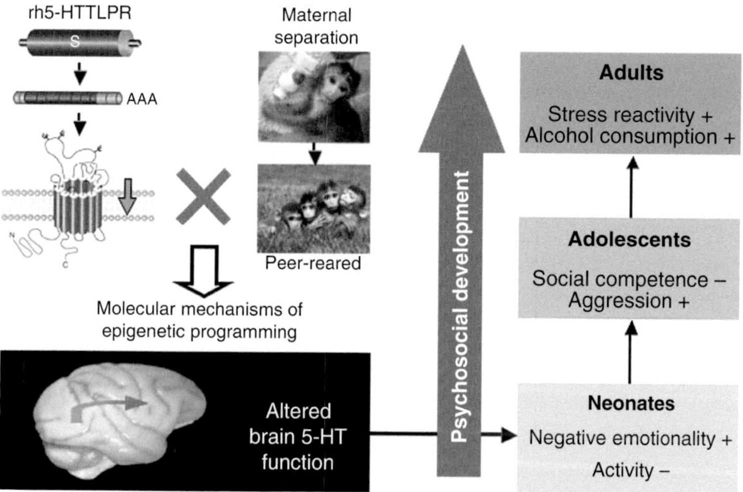

Figure 11.4 Effect of interaction between maternal separation and rh5-HTTLPR genotype on psychosocial development, including brain 5-HT function, emotion regulation, social competence, stress reactivity, behavior, and psychopathology, across the lifespan of rhesus macaques.

from variation at a single site (polymorphic locus 1, PL1), whereas an alternative location for a 21-bp length variation (PL2) within the 5-HTTLPR was found in the *5-HTT* of rhesus macaques located on chromosome 16 (Lesch *et al.*, 1997; Rogers *et al.*, 2006). Somewhat surprising, and yet meaningfully paralleling the human condition (but likely based on an independent molecular event), the length variation of the rh5-HTTLPR is once more basically biallelic with the majority of alleles composed of either 22 or 23 repeats (likewise, s and l variants). The presence of the rh5-HTTTLPR and resulting allelic variation of 5-HTT activity in rhesus monkeys provides a unique model to dissect the relative contribution of genes and environmental stressors to central 5-HT function and related behavioral outcomes.

When fused to a luciferase reporter gene and transfected into human 5-HTT-expressing cell lines, the s and l 5-HTTLPR variants differentially modulate transcriptional activity of the 5-HTT gene promoter (Lesch *et al.*, 1996). The effect of 5-HTTLPR length variability on 5-HTT function was determined by studying the relationship between the 5-HTTLPR genotype, 5-HTT gene transcription, and 5-HT uptake activity in human lymphoblastoid cell lines. Cells homozygous for the l variant of the 5-HTTLPR produced higher concentrations of 5-HTT mRNA than cells containing one or two copies of the s form. Membrane preparations from ll lymphoblasts showed higher inhibitor binding than did ss cells. Furthermore, the rate of specific 5-HT uptake was more than twofold higher in cells homozygous for the l form of the 5-HTTLPR than in cells carrying one or two copies of the s variant of the promoter. Further evidence from studies of 5-HTT promoter activity in other cell lines (Mortensen *et al.*, 1999), mRNA concentrations in the raphe complex of human postmortem brain (Little *et al.*, 1998), platelet 5-HT uptake and content (Greenberg *et al.*, 1999; Hanna *et al.*, 1998; Nobile *et al.*, 1999), and in vivo SPECT imaging of human brain 5-HTT (Heinz *et al.*, 1999) confirmed that the s form is associated with lower 5-HTT expression and function. Also associated with allelic variation of 5-HTT function are adaptive changes of human brain 5-HT_{1A} receptor revealed by pharmacological challenge tests and PET imaging (David *et al.*, 2005; Lesch and Gutknecht, 2004).

The orthologous murine *5-HTT* (*Slc6a4*) located in a syntenic region on chromosome 11qB5 (76,814,792–76,848,536) is composed of 14 exons extending more than 34 kb. A TATA-like motif within 26–31 bp with respect to the transcription initiation site and several potential binding sites for transcription factors as well as cAMP-responsive element- (CRE-) and glucocortized-responsive- (GRE)-like motifs are present in the GC-rich 5′-flanking region (Bengel *et al.*, 1997). Functional mapping of the transcriptional control region indicated constitutive promoter activity and several cell-specific enhancer/repressor elements within ~2 kb of *5-HTT*'s 5′-flanking sequence (Heils *et al.*, 1998). While comparison of the human and murine *SLC6A4* genes revealed a striking conservation of both the exon/intron organization and the 5′-flanking transcriptional control region, a 5-HTTLPR-like sequence similar to the one in humans (or non-human primates) is absent.

SEROTONIN TRANSPORTER IN PERSONALITY AND DISORDERS OF EMOTION REGULATION

Based on converging lines of evidence that the 5-HTT fine-tunes serotonergic signaling and is involved in a myriad of processes during brain development as well as synaptic plasticity throughout the life cycle, emotional behavior and depression-related predispositions are likely to be influenced by genetically driven variability of 5-HTT function. Consequently, the impact of genetic variation of the 5-HTT to inter-individual differences in personality dimensions and to the risk of psychiatric and other disorders has been investigated extensively over the past decade (Figure 11.3).

The contribution of the 5-HTTLPR to individual phenotypic differences in personality traits was explored initially in two independent population and family-based genetic studies. Anxiety-related and other personality traits were assessed by the NEO personality inventory – revised (NEO-PI-R), a self-report inventory based on the five-factor model of personality ("Big Five") (Costa and McCrae, 1992). The five factors assessed by the NEO are: Neuroticism (emotional instability), Extraversion, Agreeableness (cooperation, reciprocal alliance formation), Openness (intellect, problem-solving), and Conscientiousness (will to achieve). In 1996, population and within-family associations between the low-expressing 5-HTTLPR s variant and Neuroticism, the trait related to anxiety, hostility, and depression, on the NEO-PI-R were first reported in a primarily male population ($n = 505$) (Lesch *et al.*, 1996). Individuals with either one or two copies of the 5-HTTLPR s variant (group S) had significantly greater levels of Neuroticism, defined as proneness to negative emotionality, including anxiety, hostility, and depression, than those homozygous for the 5-HTTLPR l genotype (group L) in the sample as a whole and also within sibships. Individuals with group S genotypes also had significantly decreased NEO Agreeableness.

In a subsequent investigation this association was also found in an independent family-based sample ($n = 397$, 84% female, primarily sib-pairs) (Greenberg *et al.*, 2000). The findings replicated the association between the 5-HTTLPR and NEO Neuroticism. Combined data from the two studies ($n = 902$), which were corrected for ethnicity and age, gave a highly significant association between the s allele and anxiety-related traits both across individuals and within families, reflecting a genuine genetic influence rather than an artifact of ethnic admixture. Another association encountered in the original study between the s allele and lower scores of NEO Agreeableness was also replicated and was even more robust in the primarily female replication sample. Gender-related differences in 5-HTTLPR-personality trait associations are possible since several lines of evidence demonstrate sexual dichotomy in central 5-HT system function in humans and rodents.

The effect sizes for the 5-HTTLPR–personality associations, which were comparable in the two samples, indicate that this gene variation has only a modest influence on the behavioral predispositions of approximately 0.30 standard deviation units. This corresponds to 3–4% of the total variance and 7–9% of the genetic variance, based on estimates from twin studies using these and related measures which have consistently demonstrated that genetic factors contribute 40–60% of the variance in neuroticism and other related personality traits.

Although the genetic effect suggests that the 5-HTTLPR represents an above-average sized QTL, the associations represent only a small portion of the genetic contribution to anxiety-related persoality traits. If additional genes were hypothesized to contribute similar gene–dose effects to anxiety, at least 10–15 genes are predicted to be involved, but assuming a 0.1–1% QTL threshold, up to 100 genes are more likely. Thus, the results are consistent with the view that the influence of a single, common polymorphism on continuously distributed traits is likely to be modest, if not minimal (Plomin *et al.*, 1994; Reif and Lesch, 2003).

At first sight, association between the high-activity 5-HTTLPR l variant with lower Neuroticism and related traits seems to be counter-intuitive with regard to the known antidepressant and anxiolytic effects of 5-HTT inhibitors (SRIs). Likewise, Knutson *et al.* (1998) reported that long-term inhibition of the 5-HTT by the selective SRI paroxetine reduced indices of hostility through a more general decrease in negative affect, a personality dimension related to neuroticism. The same individuals also demonstrated an increase in directly measured social cooperation after paroxetine treatment, an interesting finding in view of the association between the 5-HTTLPR genotype and agreeableness. The fact that a drug inhibiting 5-HTT lessens negative emotionality and increases social cooperation appears to conflict with findings that the 5-HTTLPR long allele, which confers higher 5-HTT expression, is associated with lower NEO Neuroticism and higher NEO Agreeableness. However, this apparent contradiction may be due to the fact that both 5-HT and 5-HTT play critical roles in brain development that differ from their functions in regulating neurotransmission in the adult.

In subsequent studies, attempts to replicate the original findings have been reported, although only a few studies used large populations with sufficient statistical power (Jorm *et al.*, 1998; Mazzanti *et al.*, 1998). Three out of the four adequately powered studies found evidence congruent with an influence of the 5-HTTLPR on Neuroticism and related traits (Greenberg *et al.*, 2000; Lesch *et al.*, 1996; Mazzanti *et al.*, 1998), whereas a large population study not employing a within-family design (Jorm *et al.*, 1998) did not. Smaller population-based studies have had variable, but generally negative, results. Interpretation of these studies is complicated by their use of relatively small or unusual samples, and the lack of within-family designs that may minimize population stratification artifacts. Other efforts to detect associations between the 5-HTTLPR and personality traits have been complicated by the use of small sample sizes, heterogeneous subject populations, and differing methods of personality assessment. Furthermore, the subject selection in two studies (Ball *et al.*, 1997; Dreary *et al.*, 1999) was unusual in that subjects at the high or low ends of the distribution for Neuroticism were selected on the assumption that the 5-HTTLPR affects the trait uniformly across its distribution. However, re-analysis of the data from the initial study revealed that the contribution of the 5-HTTLPR to NEO Neuroticism is greatest in the central range of the distribution and actually decreases at the extremes (Sirota *et al.*, 1999). This illustrates the need to obtain genotypes from individuals across the distribution of a trait, and suggests caution in the use of extreme populations in attempting to establish genetic influences on traits that are continuously distributed across the population. A role of 5-HTTLPR-dependent 5-HTT function in personality traits of negative emotionality was finally confirmed by meta-analyses of the published data (Schinka *et al.*, 2004; Sen *et al.*, 2004).

Difficulties in interpretation of population-based association studies due to ethnic differences in 5-HTTLPR allele frequencies, which are most prominent in the Japanese population with ll genotype frequencies arround 5%, have also been expressed (Katsuragi *et al.*, 1999). From an evolutionary psychological perspective, anxiety is a pervasive and innately driven form of distress that arises in response to actual or threatened exclusion from social groups (Baumeister and Tice, 1990; Buss, 1991). Notably, Nakamura and associates (1997) have discussed the higher prevalence of the anxiety- and depression-associated 5-HTTLPR ls and ss genotypes in the context of extraordinary emotional restraint and interpersonal sensitivity in the Japanese population as a possible population-typical adaptation to prevent social exclusion (Ono *et al.*, 1996).

An association of the 5-HTTLPR and affective illnesses including depression and bipolar disorder was first reported by Collier and coworkers in 1996 and subsequently confirmed in a considerable number of, but not all, studies (for review see Levinson, 2006). An impact of allelic variation of 5-HTT function on disease risk was further underscored by several meta-analyses of the published data (Cho *et al.*, 2005; Lotrich and Pollock, 2004). Likewise, a small but pathophysiologically relevant impact of regulatory and structural *5-HTT* variation has been suggested in a variety of diseases such as anxiety disorders, eating disorders, substance abuse including alcohol dependence, autism, schizophrenia, and neurodegenerative disorders (Lesch and Mossner, 1998; Murphy *et al.*, 2004). The most promising findings to date, however, indicate an association between the 5-HTTLPR and the response to 5-HT reuptake inhibitors (SRIs) and possibly other antidepressant treatment strategies in patients with depression and comorbid disorders (Lesch and Gutknecht, 2005; Serretti *et al.*, 2005).

Variations that alter the structure of 5-HTT protein are rare; nevertheless, several non-synonymous SNPs changing the coding sequence were found to segregate with a complex 5-HT dysfunction-associated phenotype including obsessive compulsive disorder (OCD), autism, depression, and other "5-HT spectrum disorders" (Di Bella *et al.*, 1996; Ozaki *et al.*, 2003; Sutcliffe *et al.*, 2005). OCD is characterized by either obsessions or compulsions that cause marked distress and are time-consuming or significantly interfere with an individual's normal routine or functioning. Obsessions are recurrent and persistent ideas, thoughts, impulses, or images that an individual attempts to ignore or suppress; whereas compulsions are repetitive, purposeful, and intentional behaviors performed in response to an obsession to neutralize or prevent discomfort, worry and anxiety, or some dreaded event. OCD often co-occurs with other disorders such as depression. Autism is a spectrum of disorders exhibiting deficits in development of language and social cognition as well as patterns of repetitive, restricted behaviors or interests and resistance to change similar to OCD.

A missense mutation resulting in a conserved Ile425Val substitution in 5-HTT was detected in two affected individuals and their family members with OCD and related disorders including autism, social phobia, anorexia nervosa, tic disorder, depression, and alcohol dependence (Ozaki *et al.*, 2003). The evolutionary conserved Ile425Val substitution is located in transmembrane domain 8 (TMD8) and modifies the α-helical secondary structure of the 5-HTT protein and consequently transport function. These findings indicate that gain-of-function mutations of the 5-HTT protein may contribute to the expression of psychopathology related to 5-HT dysfunction in some families. Interestingly, two brothers from one of the families suffering from OCD and autism and carrying the Ile425Val variant were also homozygous for the 5-HTTLPR l genotype, which was previously found to be associated with or preferentially transmitted in both OCD (Bengel *et al.*, 1999; Bloch *et al.*, 2008; McDougle *et al.*, 1998) and autism (Klauck *et al.*, 1997). Moreover, a Leu255Met substitution located in TMD4 was detected in a patient with delusional depression, who was also found to be a homozygous carrier of the 5-HTTLPR s genotype (Di Bella *et al.*, 1996). Low 5-HTT gene expression in interaction with the Leu255Met variant, which is highly conserved among various species, could additively perturb 5-HTT function. These examples of co-occurence and possible cooperativity of allelic variation in gene expression and protein structure might represent a "double hit", with functional consequences in the same gain- and loss-of-function direction for both of these 5-HTT variations.

SEROTONIN TRANSPORTER, EPIGENETIC INTERACTION, AND DEVELOPMENT: SETTING THE STAGE FOR EMOTION REGULATION

While the impact of biology on social sciences has been ever-increasing, the transition from complicated correlations to useful prediction is now the basic challenge. Biosocial concepts (Wilson, 1975, 1978) paved the way for an increasing interest in human personality, particularly the "Big Five" personality dimensions, from an evolutionary perspective (Buss, 1991). These five dimensions define the framework for adapting to other people in a given social context, a crucial task in long-term reproductive success. Extraversion and agreeableness are important to the formation of social structures ranging from pair bonds to coalitions of groups; emotional stability and conscientiousness are critical to the endurance of these structures; openness may reflect the capacity for innovation. Since the genetic basis of present-day personality and behavioral traits is already laid out in all mammalian species ranging phylogenetically from rodents to non-human primates, and therefore may reflect selective forces among our remote ancestors, recently, research efforts have been focused on non-human primates, especially rhesus macaques (*Macaca mulatta*). In this primate model, environmental influences are probably less complex, can be more easily controlled for, and are thus less likely to confound associations between genes and behavior. All forms of emotionality in rhesus monkeys – the major categories are anxiety and aggression – appear to be modulated by environmental factors, and marked disruption of the mother–infant relationship likely confers increased risk.

In rhesus monkeys, maternal separation and replacement of the mother by an inanimate surrogate during the first months of life results in long-term consequences for brain 5-HT system function. This early life trauma causes anxiety- and depression-related behavior, resulting in deficient social adaptation and peer interaction (Higley *et al.*, 1991). As a parameter of the impact of severe stress on the function of brain 5-HT system, cisterna cerebrospinal fluid (CSF) concentrations of 5-hydroxyindoleacetic acid (5-HIAA), the major metabolite of 5-HT, was studied in rhesus macaques suffering from maternal separation. Previous work had revealed that CSF 5-HIAA shows a strong heritable component and is trait-like, with demonstrated stability over an individual's lifespan (Higley *et al.*, 1992; Kraemer *et al.*, 1989). As indicated by low CSF 5-HIAA levels, the stressful experience of maternal separation is associated with robust and long-term consequences for central 5-HT function.

Given the presence of the orthologous repeat length variation in the transcriptional control region of the rhesus *5-HTT* gene (rh5-HTTLPR, Figure 11.4) (Lesch *et al.*, 1997) and the potential of the maternal separation model to study gene × environment interaction, several rhesus monkey cohorts were tested for associations between early life stress, 5-HT function, and rh5-HTTLPR genotype. Initial findings suggested that the low-activity s variant of the rh5-HTTLPR is predictive of CSF 5-HIAA concentrations, but that early experiences make unique contributions to variation in later 5-HT system function and thus provided evidence of an environment-dependent association between the *5-HTT* and a direct measure of brain 5-HT function (Bennett *et al.*, 2002). The consequences of the deleterious early experiences of maternal separation seem consistent with the notion that the 5-HTTLPR influences the risk for disorders of social cognition and emotion regulation.

For exploration of the contribution of genetics and early rearing environment to the shaping of behavioral traits, studies were extended to the neonatal period of rhesus macaques, a time in early development when environmental influences are modest and least likely to confound gene–behavior associations. Between postnatal days 7–30, mother-reared and maternally separated neonates were assessed on a standardized neurobehavioral test designed to measure orienting, motor maturity, reflex functioning, and temperament in primates. The main effects of genotype and, in some cases, interactions between rearing condition and genotype were demonstrated for items indicative of orienting, attention, and temperament. In general, infants with the s form of the rh-HTTLPR displayed higher behavioral stress-reactivity compared to l variant homozygotes, reflected by diminished orientation, lower attentional capabilities, and increased affective responding (Champoux *et al.*, 2002). However, the genotype effects were more pronounced for animals raised in the neonatal nursery than for animals reared by their mothers. These results demonstrate the contributions of rearing environment and genetic background, and their interaction, in a non-human primate model of behavioral development.

Beyond the neonatal period, particularly during the adolescence of rhesus monkeys, evidence for a complex interplay between inter-individual differences in 5-HT system function and social success has been accumulated. Impaired 5-HT signaling, as indicated by low CSF 5-HIAA levels, is associated with lower rank within a social group, less competent social behavior, and greater impulsive aggression. While subjects with low 5-HIAA are no more likely to engage in competitive aggression than other monkeys, aggressive behavior frequently escalates to violent and hazardous intensity. The interactive effect of rh5-HTTLPR genotype and early rearing environment on social play and competition-elicited aggression was also explored (Figure 11.4) (Barr *et al.*, 2003). Infant rhesus monkeys homozygous for the l variant were more likely to engage in rough play than were s variant carriers with significant interaction between rh5-HTTLPR genotype and rearing condition. Peer-reared s variant carriers were less likely to play with peers than those homozygous for the l allele, whereas the rh5-HTTLPR genotype had no effect on the incidence of social play among mother-reared monkeys. Socially dominant mother-reared monkeys were more likely than their peer-reared counterparts to engage in aggression. In contrast, peer-reared but not mother-reared monkeys carrying the s variant exhibited more aggressive behaviors than their l homozygote counterparts. This rh5-HTTLPR genotype × rearing interaction for aggressive behavior indicates that peer-reared subjects with the s variant, while unlikely to win in a competitive encounter, are more inclined to persist in aggression once it begins.

Since allelic variation of 5-HTT function is associated with anxiety-related traits as well as an increased risk for developing depression in the face of adversity, the impact of rh5-HTTLPR × rearing condition interaction on stress-elicited endocrine responses was determined in infant rhesus macaques. ACTH and cortisol levels in monkeys reared with their mothers or in peer-only groups were determined at baseline and during separation stress at 6 months of age. Cortisol levels increased during separation, and there was a main effect of rearing conditions, with decreased cortisol levels among peer-reared macaques. Monkeys carrying the rh5-HTTLPR s variant had higher ACTH levels. ACTH levels increased during separation, and there was a maternal deprivation × rh5-HTTLPR interaction, such that peer-reared s carriers had higher ACTH levels during separation than l homozygotes. A confirmatory study further revealed that this interaction is sexually dichotomous and the interactive effect may underlie the increased incidence of certain stress-related disorders of emotion regulation in women (Barr *et al.*, 2004b). These findings confirm the data from studies in human populations that allelic variation of 5-HTT function affects hypothalamic–pituitary–adrenal (HPA) axis activity and that the influence of rh5-HTTLPR on hormonal responses during stress is modulated by early experience and displays gender specificity.

Previous research has also revealed that peer-reared primates consume more alcohol as young adults and maternally deprived female rhesus macaques have exaggerated HPA axis responses to alcohol (Higley and Linnoila, 1997). Because their environments can be controlled, use of the macaque model permits investigation of independent influences as well as potential interactions between 5-HT system-related genes, maternal deprivation, and stress in the etiology of alcohol dependence. Given that 5-HT signaling and HPA axis hormones are involved in the reinforcement of alcohol intake and contribute to the risk for symptoms of withdrawal and relapse in alcohol dependence in a gender-specific manner, the interactive effect of rh5-HTTLPR genotype and early rearing environment on the patterns of preference and consumption across a 6-week alcohol consumption paradigm was examined (Barr *et al.*, 2004a). Female rhesus macaques were reared with their mothers in social groups or in peer-only groups and as young adults, they were given the choice of an alcohol solution or vehicle. Interactions between rearing condition and rh5-HTTLPR genotype with dramatically higher levels of ethanol preference were demonstrated in s variant carriers. An effect of rearing condition on alcohol consumption during the 6 weeks as well as a phase × rearing interaction, such that peer-reared animals progressively increased their levels of consumption was also found. This was especially evident for peer-reared females carrying the rh5-HTTLPR s variant. These data confirm an interaction between 5-HT system activity and early experience in the vulnerability to alcohol dependence.

Taken together, these findings provide evidence of an environment-dependent association between allelic variation of 5-HTT expression and central 5-HT function, and illustrate how this specific genetic variation moderates 5-HT-mediated behavior and psychosocial development in rhesus macaques (Figure 11.4). Because rhesus monkeys exhibit personality and behavioral traits that parallel anxiety, depression, and aggression-related personality dimensions associated in humans with the low-actitvity s variant of the 5-HTTLPR, it may be possible to search for evolutionary continuity in this genetic mechanism for individual differences. Non-human primate studies are therefore useful to help identify environmental factors that either compound the vulnerability conferred by a particular genetic makeup or, conversely, may act to improve the behavioral outcome associated with a distinct genetic makeup.

Consequently, the impact of genetic variation on social cognition and emotionality (including anxiety and depression) depends on interactions between genes and the environment, and such interactions lead to the expression of environmental effects only in the presence of a permissive genetic background. Not unexpectedly, a recent study by Caspi and coworkers (2003) robustly confirmed that individuals with one or two short versions of the 5-HTTLPR are up to twofold more likely to become depressed after stressful events such as bereavement, romantic disasters, illnesses, or losing their job. Moreover, childhood maltreatment significantly increased the probability of developing depressive syndromes in later life in individuals with the low-activity short allele of the 5-HTTLPR. These results further support the notion of how a combination of genetic disposition and specific life events may interact to facilitate the development of mental illness. What went largely unnoticed, though, was its implications for the relevance of studying the genetics of personality. Depression is strongly associated with anxiety- and depression-related traits, the factual personality dimensions that have been linked to allelic variation of the 5-HTT. Given the high comorbidity between anxiety and depression and the evidence for their modulation by common genetic factors (Kendler, 1996), it is likely that predisposition to mood disorders will also be determined by environmental influences whose impact on the brain is under genetic control.

Particularly interesting is that early trauma inflicted by childhood maltreatment is interacting with allelic variation of 5-HTT function to increase vulnerability to develop mood disorders (Caspi *et al.*, 2003; for review, also see Uher and McGuffin, 2008). A remarkable body of evidence suggests that emotionality and stress response can be influenced by experiences early in life, and it has long been supposed that severe early-life trauma may increase the risk for anxiety and affective disorders (Brown and Harris, 2008). For example, adults experiencing 4 out of a list of 7 severe early traumatic events showed a more than 4-fold increased risk for depressive symptoms and about a 12-fold increased risk for attempted suicide (Felitti *et al.*, 1998). No direct correlation between any specific childhood trauma and a specific adult anxiety or affective disorder could be made, however, suggesting that other, possibly genetic, factors determine the precise pathology that is precipitated by the traumatic event. The observation that during early developmental stages individuals are particularly susceptible to adverse environmental influences is confirmed by rodent studies that have demonstrated influential effects of the quality of maternal care on lifelong brain function, emotional behavior, and disease risk.

Of related relevance, functional variation in another gene of the 5-HT signaling pathway, encoding the 5-HT-metabolizing enzyme MAOA, has been implicated in aggression-related cluster B personality disorders (Jacob *et al.*, 2005), as well as in antisocial and aggressive behavior of alcohol dependence (Samochowiec *et al.*, 1999; Schmidt *et al.*, 2000), particularly when associated with early adverse experiences (Caspi *et al.*, 2002; Meyer-Lindenberg *et al.*, 2006; Reif *et al.*, 2007). Interestingly, an interaction between this *MAOA* variation and the 5-HTTLPR influencing alcohol binge drinking risk in young women was reported recently (Herman *et al.*, 2005). Transcription of *MAOA* in rhesus monkeys is modulated by an orthologous polymorphism (rhMAOALPR) in its upstream regulatory region. In a recent study, male rhesus monkeys raised with or without their mothers were tested for competitive and social group aggression. High- and low-activity variants of the rhMAOALPR showed a genotype × environment interaction effect on aggressive behavior, such that mother-reared male monkeys with the low-activity variant had higher aggression scores (Newman *et al.*, 2005). Similar to the findings with the *5-HTT*, these results suggest that the behavioral expression of allelic variation in MAOA activity is sensitive to social experiences early in development, and that its functional outcome might depend on social context.

VARIATION OF SEROTONIN SIGNALING AND SOCIAL ORGANIZATION IN MACAQUE SPECIES

Macaques exhibit exceptional inter-species variation in aggression-related behavior, as illustrated by recent studies showing overlapping patterns of aggression-based social organization grades and macaque phylogeny. For macaques, like humans, survival depends on effective social functioning. Social skills facilitate access to sustenance, protection, and mates. Socially adept individuals tend to be healthier and live longer. Geographically, one of the most widely distributed species of non-human primates, rhesus macaques exhibit a degree of variation in aggression-related behavior that is unequaled in other primate species (de Waal and Luttrell, 1989; Thierry, 1990). Thierry (2000) proposed a 4-grade classification scheme for describing social organization across 16 species of the genus *Macaca*. This classification is based on the extent and asymmetry of aggression-related behavior within specific macaque species. Grade 1 species exhibit highly hierarchical and nepotistic societies as well as low levels of conciliatory behaviors, while grade 4 species can be considered to be more tolerant, displaying relaxed dominance, open relationships, and high levels of conciliatory behaviors. For example, the risk of a retaliatory attack from a subordinate is much higher in grade 4 species than in grade 1 after an initial attack by a dominant, but the retaliatory attack will likely be much less severe, and the probability of reconciliation much higher, in grade 4 than grade 1 macaques. By mapping this distribution of social style grades onto phylogenetic trees (Morales and Melnick, 1998), a significant association with phylogeny was shown for 7 out of 16 traits used for the classification, including patterns of female rank acquisition and male–female dominance relationships (Thierry *et al.*, 2000).

Moreover, it was shown for this genus that social organization and behavior have changed little during several hundred thousand years (Thierry *et al.*, 2000). Ecological and climatic conditions are likely to have varied considerably during such a long period of time, and if one assumed that macaque behavior and social organization were solely influenced by environment, one should also expect changes in behavior as an expression of adjustment to changing peristasis. Instead, the influence of phylogeny was proposed by several studies (Matsumura, 1999; Thierry *et al.*, 2000). In line with this hypothesis, Thierry and coworkers (2000) demonstrated a significant association of his classification of social aggression in macaques based on two independently derived phylogenies. This led to the conclusion that the structure of macaque social organization is influenced more by phylogeny than environment, and that polymorphisms in genes of the 5-HT signaling pathway are likely to contribute to the variability in species-characteristic social behavior. To search for the molecular basis for this hypothesis, variation at the 5-HTTLPR and MAOALPR was determined in seven macaque species representing the entire spectrum of different social organization grades (Figure 11.5) (Wendland *et al.*, 2006a). Macaque species displaying tolerant societies, with relaxed dominance and high levels of conciliatory tendency, were monomorphic for the 5-HTTLPR (and the MAOALPR). In contrast, those species known to exhibit intolerant, hierarchical, and nepotistic societies were polymorphic at one or more of these loci. Rhesus monkeys, the most intolerant and hierarchical species of macaques, showed the greatest degree of allelic variation in both genes. These findings suggest that genetic variation of 5-HT neurotransmission affects key elements of macaque social behavior, in particular the exceptional level of inter-species variation in aggression-related behavior. In a similar approach investigating rodents of the genus *Microtus* (prairie vole) known to display strong species differences in social structure, an effect of a polymorphic repeat upstream of the

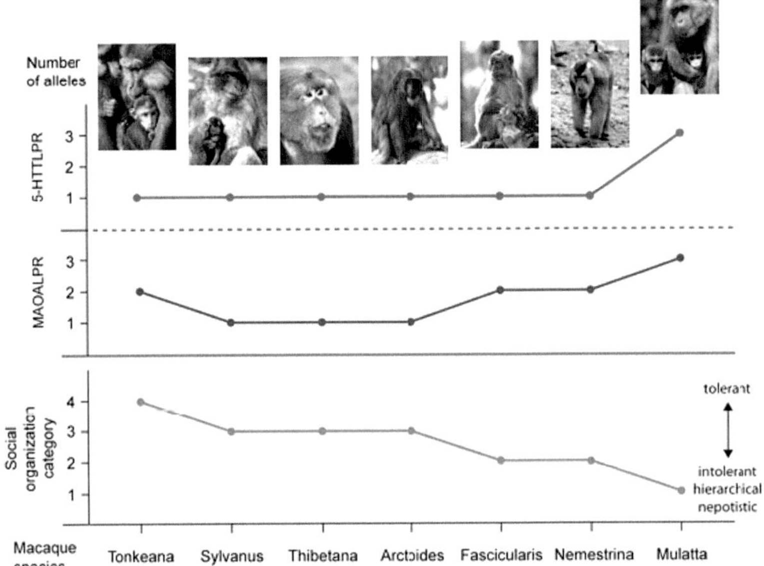

Figure 11.5 Degree of variation in two genes of the 5-HT signaling pathway (5-HT transporter and monoamine oxidase A), aggression and social organization in seven macaque species.

gene encoding the vasopressin 1a receptor (Avpr1a), social engagement and bonding behavior were recently demonstrated (Hammock and Young, 2005). A role of 5-HTT function (in interaction with *AVPR1a* variation) in the evolution of social skills was recently confirmed in one of humankind's most ancient and universal behavioral traits – the propensity and need for dancing – which comprises a complex phenotype of social communication, courtship, spirituality, and sensorimotor integration (Bachner-Melman *et al.*, 2005).

IMAGING OF EMOTIONALITY: A RISK ASSESSMENT STRATEGY FOR DEPRESSION?

Imaging techniques become increasingly elaborate in displaying the genomic influence on brain system activation in response to environmental cues, thus representing tools to bridge the gap between multiple alleles with small effects and complex behavior, as well as psychopathological dimensions. Evidence for a modulatory effect of the 5-HTTLPR on prefrontal cortex activity suggests that genotype–phenotype correlations may be accessible to structural and functional imaging of the brain. In two subsequent studies, Fallgatter and coworkers (1999, 2004) were the first to report an association between 5-HTTLPR genotype and prefrontal cortex–limbic excitability detected by event-related potentials (ERPs) with two different tasks of cognitive response control (Go–NoGo and error-processing task). Individuals with one or two s alleles of the 5-HTTPLR showed higher prefrontal brain activity as compared to subjects homozygous for the l variant, thus indicating that the low-activity s variant is associated with enhanced responsiveness of the prefrontal cortex, particularly the anterior cingulate cortex (ACC). These findings strongly suggest a relationship between cognitive processing and allelic variation of 5-HTT function.

Using functional magnetic resonance imaging (fMRI), Hariri and associates (2002) likewise observed that individuals with one or two copies of the low-activity s variant of the 5-HTTLPR exhibit greater neuronal activity of the human amygdala, a brain system central to emotionality and social behavior, in response to fearful stimuli compared with individuals homozygous for the l variant. These 5-HTTLPR-related effects on the response bias of amygdala reactivity to environmental threat were subsequently confirmed in a large cohort of both healthy men and women, indicating that the allelic variation of 5-HTT function may represent a classic susceptibility factor for affective spectrum disorders by biasing the functional reactivity of the amygdala in the context of stressful life experiences and/or deficient cortical regulatory input.

Subsequent investigations were focused on the modifying impact of the limbic cortex in the context of 5-HTTLPR's role in depression risk (Figure 11.6). Patients with depression display a decreased volume in the subgenual division of the ACC, and together with altered activity of the limbic circuit components involving ACC and amygdala, an enduring disagreement remained whether these abnormalities predispose for the development of depression and comorbid conditions, or are a consequence of the depressed state. To address this question, Pezawas *et al.* (2005) used a complementary fMRI approach to confirm that the low-expressing s variant of the 5-HTTLPR is associated with depression-typical structural and functional alterations. Carriers of the s variant showed reduced gray matter volume of both the perigenual ACC and the amygdala. In addition, the findings revealed *5-HTT* genotype-dependent correlation of amygdala activity with the the activity of the rostral and caudal segment of the ACC, indicating a genetically regulated dynamic coupling which renders the amygdala more responsive to emotional stimuli. Heinz and colleagues (2005) also observed

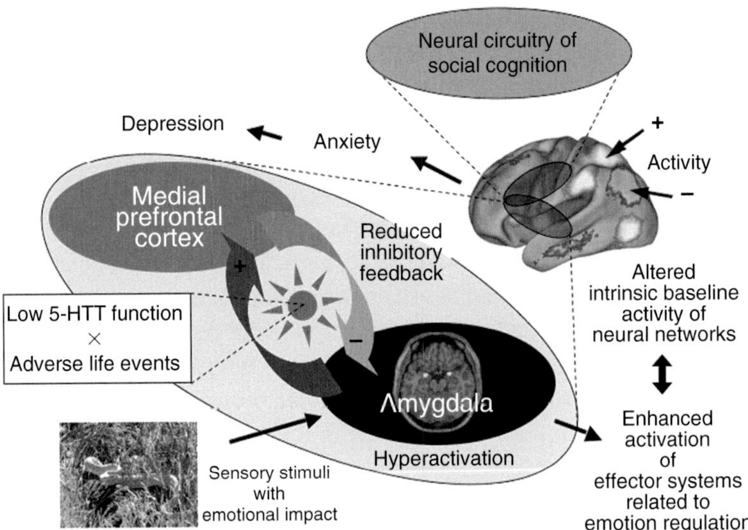

Figure 11.6 Influence of *5-HTT* × life stress interaction on neural networks of emotion regulation. Allelic variation of 5-HTT function is likely to represent a classic susceptibility factor for affective spectrum disorders by biasing the functional reactivity of the amygdala in the context of stressful life experiences and/or deficient cortical regulatory input.

increased amygdala activation in carriers of the 5-HTTLPR s variant, which was paralleled by enhanced functional coupling with the ventromedial prefrontal cortex. Moreover, it was shown that positively valenced emotional scenes also evoked amygdala activation, consistent with the general task for the amygdala in both positive and negative emotion regulation, but only the response to negative stimuli was associated with the *5-HTT* genotype.

Despite its obvious relevance beyond traits of emotionality and affective spectrum disorders, the assumption that the neutral baseline as the control condition does not itself produce changes in activation as a function of *5-HTT* genotype was not investigated in these studies. Recently, Canli *et al.* (2005) showed that allelic variation in 5-HTT function is associated with differential activation to negative, positive, *and* neutral stimuli in limbic, striatal, and cortical regions using the Stroop, an attentional interference task. This task is sensitive to individual differences in personality and mood, and activates both the cognitive division and affective division of the ACC and amygdala, depending on whether the stimuli are neutral or affectively valenced. While increased amygdala activation to negative, relative to neutral, stimuli in *5-HTTLPR* s variant carriers was confirmed, the differences were determined by decreased activation to neutral stimuli, rather than increased activation to negative stimuli. High-resolution structural images and automated processes also revealed *5-HTT* genotype-related volumetric and gray matter density differences in frontal cortical regions, anterior cingulate, and cerebellum. These findings are consistent with the notion that the ACC plays an integral role in both emotional (and non-emotional) cognitive processes, and is heavily interconnected with a number of cortical and subcortical regions and therefore implicate 5-HT transport efficiency in a wide-ranging spectrum of brain processes that affect neural systems controlling affective, cognitive, and motor processes (Figure 11.6).

The database of functional 5-HTT imaging was further extended, and its relevance was supported by several flanking investigations. Bertolino and coworkers (2005) studied two groups of volunteers categorized by contrasting cognitive/personality styles characteristic of variable salience to fearful stimuli, in phobic-prone versus eating disorders-prone subjects. The fMRI results showed that phobic-prone individuals selectively recruited the amygdala to a larger extent than eating disorders-prone subjects. Interestingly, amygdala activation was independently predicted by cognitive style and *5-HTT* genotype, suggesting that responsivity of the amygdala may represent an emergent property which is based on the association between genetic and psychological factors. It was concluded that certain aspects of cognitive/personality style are rooted in physiological responses of the fear circuitry which interact with processing of environmental stimuli. Furmark *et al.* (2004) scanned social phobic patients using positron emission tomography (PET) of cerebral blood flow to report greater amygdala activation during a public, compared to a private, speaking task as a function of *5-HTT* genotype. Finally, as the field is progressing toward exploration of epistatic mechanisms, both the 5-HTTLPR and variation in the gene coding for tryptophan hydroxylase 2 (*TPH2*), which specifically synthesizes 5-HT in the brain, additively modulate the sensory encoding of emotional stimuli during early steps of visual processing indicative of gene $\times$ gene interaction within a single neurotransmitter system (Canli *et al.*, 2008; Gutknecht *et al.*, 2007; Herrmann *et al.*, 2007; Strobel *et al.*, 2007).

All together, these lines of evidence support the notion that allelic variation of 5-HTT function and consequently 5-HT signaling contributes to the response of brain regions underlying human emotionality and resulting behavior impressively. They also indicate that differential excitability of limbic circuits to emotional stimuli contributes to exaggerated anxiety-related responses as well as increased risk for affective spectrum disorders. The combination of elaborate genetic, imaging, and behavioral analyses is certainly predestined to generate even more exciting insight into the role of the 5-HTT and other candidate genes in modulating neural function and behavior. It is concluded that the identification of *5-HTT* as a susceptibility gene for depression is a first step to an explanation of the molecular dimension of personality and behavior at risk, and holds the potential to predict response to antidepressant therapy and other treatments. The future, then, would hold improved premorbid risk assessment, preventive strategies, and treatment individualization.

NEURAL MECHANISMS OF EPIGENETIC PROCESSES: ARE SOCIAL COGNITION AND COMMUNICATION SKILLS MODERATED BY THE SEROTONIN TRANSPORTER?

As already outlined, clinical evaluation and self-report of life events revealed that the effect of psychosocial stress on depression and suicidal behavior is modifed by allelic variation of 5-HTT function, which renders carriers of the 5-HTTLPR s variant more vulnerable to depression, the neural mechanisms underlying this moderator effect are poorly understood. As a first approximation toward identification of neurocircuits in control of these epigenetic processes, individuals with self-reported life stress but no history of psychopathology were investigated with multimodal MRI-based imaging (functional, perfusion, and structural). Based on fMRI and perfusion data, support was found for a model by which life stress interacts with the effect of 5-HTTLPR genotype on amygdala and hippocampal resting activation, which may provoke a chronic state of vigilance, threat, or rumination (Canli *et al.*, 2006). Life events also affected differentially, as a function of 5-HTTLPR genotype, the functional connectivity of the amygdala and hippocampus in response to emotional stimuli with a wide network of other regions, as well as gray matter structural features. These interactions may constitute a neural mechanism for epigenetic vulnerability towards, or protection against, depression.

Intriguingly, whole-brain analyses of activation, functional connectivity, and gray matter density and volume revealed additional regions that were moderated by the interaction of 5-HTTLPR genotype

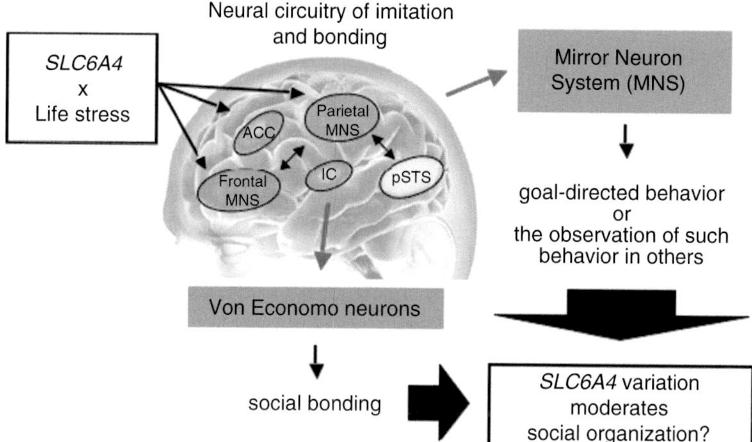

Figure 11.7 Beyond negative emotionality: *5-HTT* variation and neural correlates of social cognition. *5-HTT* × environment interaction may influence neural networks of social cognition and emotion regulation. These interactions are documented in brain regions that comprise the frontal and parietal Mirror Neuron System (MNS) or that contain Von Economo neurons, both of which play a role in social cognition and bonding. ACC, anterior cingulate cortex; IC, insular cortex, pSTS, posterior superior temporal sulcus (visual input to MNS).

and life stress. The remarkable fact about these regions is that they belong to circuits that integrate imitation-related behavior, from which social cognition and the behavior in a social world has evolved (Iacoboni, 2005). Social cognition is a construct comprising representations of internal somatic states, interpersonal knowledge and motivations as well as procedures used to decode and encode the self relative to other people. This complex set of processes, which is carefully orchestrated to support skilled social functioning and communication-facilitated networking, has recently been associated with activity in distinct neurocircuits of brain. Regions involved in imitation, imitative learning, social cognition, and communication skills (Amodio and Frith, 2006; Carr *et al.*, 2003), and affected by *5-HTT* × life stress, include the superior parietal lobule, superior temporal gyrus, inferior frontal gyrus, precentral gyrus, insula, anterior cingulate, and amygdala. Some of these regions contain mirror neurons (Rizzolatti and Craighero, 2004; Uddin *et al.*, 2005), which are activated during goal-directed behavior or the observation of such behavior in others, and Von Economo neurons, which are believed to play a role in social bonding (Figure 11.7). Dysfunction of both neural units are thought to cause social and communication disabilities associated with autistic syndromes (Allman *et al.*, 2005; Dapretto *et al.*, 2006). These findings suggest that social competence and behavior may be subject to an interaction between psychosocial stress and 5-HTTLPR genotype, while mirror or Von Economo neurons are neural targets of epigenetic moderation (Canli and Lesch, 2007). Future electrophysiological and imaging studies will have to address the question whether an interaction of 5-HTTLPR and life stress moderates neural activation during imitation or social processing tasks. As investigations have begun to refine the methodologies for capturing epigenetic effects on the brain, we may better understand the mechanisms that render some individuals susceptible and others resilient to depression and other affective spectrum disorders.

SEROTONIN TRANSPORTER DEFICIENT MOUSE: MODEL FOR MOLECULAR AND NEURAL MECHANISMS OF EPIGENETICS?

Rodents have become an indispensable tool for studying the biological function of genes that are involved in the pathogenesis of human diseases. Mice have almost the same genome size and gene number as humans, and with the introduction of gene targeting techniques the mouse is the only mammal uniting the top-down and bottom-up genetic approach, from phenotype to gene and from gene to phenotype, respectively. Mouse models make it possible to control and to manipulate the environment which will facilitate elucidation of gene × gene and gene × environment interactions. Inactivation of the murine 5-HTT and the resulting disturbance of brain 5-HT system homeostasis has considerably advanced our understanding of the neurobiological basis of anxiety- and depression-related behavior in mice (Figure 11.8) (Bengel *et al.*, 1998; Holmes *et al.*, 2003; Lesch, 2005; Murphy and Lesch, 2008; Murphy *et al.*, 2001). In addition, 5-HTT knock-out mice provide practical models to study the impact of genetic mechanisms on development and plasticity of the brain including regionalization and connectivity of the cortex, as well as subcortical structures (Altamura *et al.*, 2006; Di Pino *et al.*, 2004; Persico *et al.*, 2001, 2003; Salichon *et al.*, 2001). Despite growing evidence for a critical role of the 5-HTT in the integration of synaptic connections in the mouse brain during critical periods of development and adult life, knowledge of the machinery involved in these fine-tuning processes remains fragmentary. Investigations in rodents have shown that maternal behavior has long-lasting consequences on anxiety-like behavior of the offspring and that

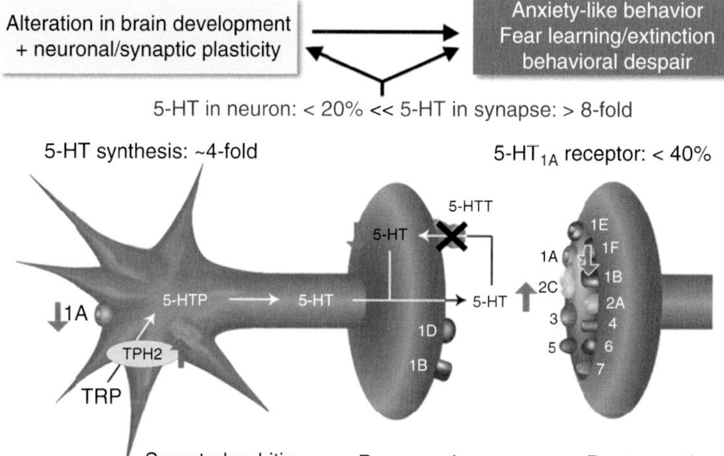

Figure 11.8 Altered brain 5-HT homeostasis in 5-HTT deficient mice: resolving the conundrum of the serotonin hypothesis of depression.

intra- and extra-uterine maternal signals can induce long-term plastic changes in anxiety- and depression-related neurocircuits synergistically (Gross and Hen, 2004; Gross *et al.*, 2002).

The molecular mechanisms by which early stress increases risk for disorder of emotion regulation in adulthood is not known, but is presumed to include epigenetic programming of gene expression (Weaver *et al.*, 2004, 2006). A gene × environment interaction screening paradigm was developed in the mouse to facilitate the study of the molecular mechanisms underlying epigenetic programming by early adverse environment in an animal model amenable to genetic manipulation (Figure 11.9). Using this gene × environment screen, it was shown that the effects of adverse rearing environment on anxiety-related behavior are modulated by mutations in 5-HTT in a way that mimics the interaction between early stress and 5-HTT seen in humans (Carola *et al.*, 2008). Mice experiencing low maternal care showed deficient GABA-A receptor binding in the amygdala and 5-HTT heterozygous knock-out mice showed increased anxiety and depression-like behavior and decreased 5-HT turnover in hippocampus and striatum. Strikingly, levels of brain-derived neurotrophic factor (BDNF) mRNA in hippocampus were elevated exclusively in 5-HTT heterozygous knock-out mice experiencing poor maternal care, suggesting that developmental programming of hippocampal circuits may underlie the *5-HTT* × environment risk factor. These findings demonstrate that 5-HT plays a similar role

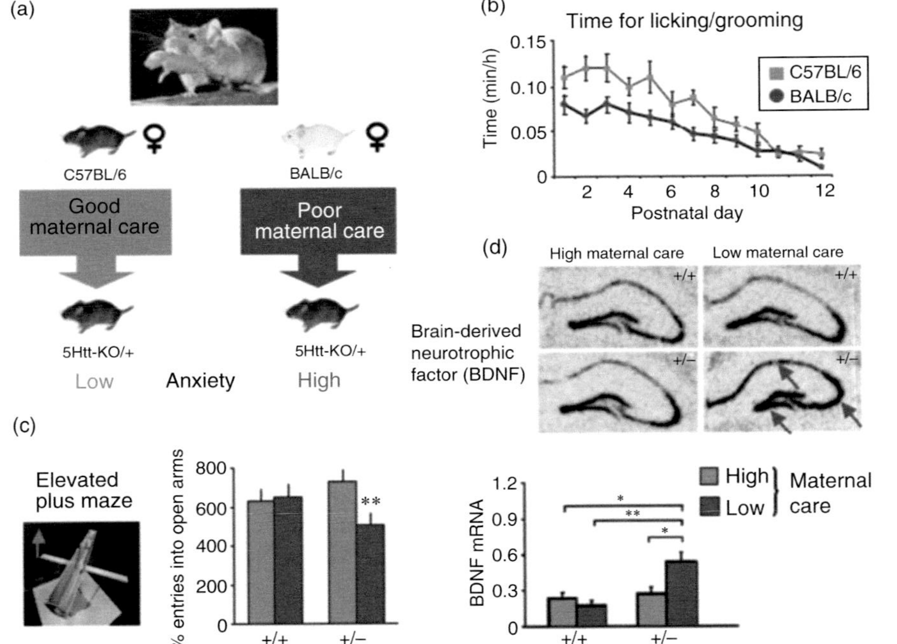

Figure 11.9 A–D Interaction between rearing environment and 5-HTT function: BDNF as a molecular substrate of both *5-HTT* genotype and maternal care (Carola *et al.*, 2008). (a) and (b) To study the molecular mechanisms underlying epigenetic programming by early adverse environment in an animal model amenable to genetic manipulation, an innovative gene × environment interaction screening paradigm (G×E screen) in the mouse was developed. Using this G×E screen it was shown that the effects of adverse rearing environment on anxiety-related behavior is modulated by mutations in 5-HTT in a way that mimics the interaction between early stress and 5-HTT seen in humans. (c) 5-HTT heterozygous null mice experiencing low maternal care showed increased anxiety-like behavior. (d) BDNF mRNA concentrations in hippocampus were elevated exclusively in 5-HTT heterozygous knock-out mice experiencing poor maternal care, suggesting that developmental programming of hippocampal circuits may underlie the *5-HTT* × E risk factor.

in modifying the long-term behavioral effects of rearing environment in diverse mammalian species and identifies BDNF as a molecular substrate of this risk factor. It is therefore predicted that the molecular mechanisms involved in the animal model are relevant to the etiology of anxiety disorders in humans.

To identify changes in mRNA expression of novel candidate genes associated with altered rearing environment and/or 5-HTT genotype, microarray-based expression profiling of mRNA extracted from brain region-specific tissue and laser-dissected single neurons will have to be performed in mice from the gene × environment screen (Ichikawa *et al.*, 2008). Whole-genome expression screening methods combined with high-throughput methylation and histone acetylation profiling microarray techniques both genome-wide and of selected genes in mice from the gene × environment screen promise to identify genes that are epigenetically regulated by rearing environment and *5-Htt* in the mouse (Figure 11.10). These genes are likely novel candidate susceptibility genes for disorders of emotion regulation and will serve as potential diagnostic and therapeutic targets. The evidence for epigenetic inheritance of anxiety-like behavior underscores the view that environmental influences can exert to persistently remodel circuits in the brain during early development. 5-HTT-deficient mice will therefore be essential for the dissection of the molecular and neural mechanisms of epigenetic processes and of the neurodevelopmental–behavioral interface (Lesch and Mössner, 2006).

FUTURE CHALLENGES

Although 5-HT system dysfunction is central to the pathophysiology of emotion regulation disorder including depression, etiological mechanisms continue to be understood inadequately at the neuronal and molecular level. A complementary approach to genetic studies of these disorders involves investigation of genes and their protein products (i.e. construction of transcriptome and proteome maps) implicated in the brain neurocircuitries of cognition, emotionality, and behavioral despair in humans and animal models (Kovas and Plomin, 2006). Based on converging lines of evidence that genetically driven variability of expression and function of proteins that regulate the function of neurotransmitter systems is associated with behavioral traits, research is now giving emphasis to the molecular basis of anxiety- and depression-related behaviors in rodents and, increasingly, non-human primates, as well as cognitive and emotional endophenotypes in healthy individuals and patient populations.

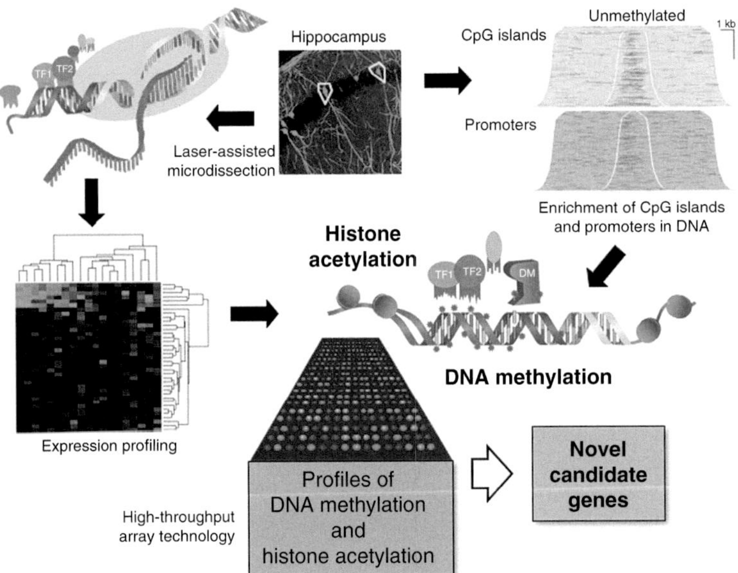

Figure 11.10 Changes in mRNA expression of novel candidate genes associated with altered rearing environment and/or 5-HTT genotype may be identified by microarray-based expression profiling of mRNA extracted from brain region-specific tissue and laser-dissected single neurons in mice from the G×E screen. Whole-genome expression screening methods combined with high-throughput methylation and histone acetylation profiling microarray techniques both genome-wide and of selected genes in mice from the G×E screen promise to identify genes that are epigenetically regulated by rearing environment and *5-HTT* in the mouse. These genes are likely novel candidate susceptibility genes for disorders of emotion regulation and will serve as potential diagnostic and therapeutic targets.

More functionally relevant polymorphisms in genes within a single neurotransmitter system, or in genes which comprise a functional unit in their concerted actions, need to be identified and assessed in both large population- and family-based association studies that carefully minimize stratification artifacts, and to elucidate complex interactions of multiple loci. It is now generally accepted that even pivotal regulatory proteins of neurotransmission will have only a modest impact, which may vary considerably among different patient populations, while noise from epigenetic mechanisms likely obstructs identification of relevant genes. Although current methods for the detection of environmental stressors in behavioral genetics are largely indirect and incomplete, the most relevant consequence of gene identification for behavioral traits related to depression may be that it will provide the tools required to systematically clarify the effects of both gene × gene and gene × environment interaction, and to apply this advanced knowledge to the design of preventive therapeutic strategies as well as manifest disease.

Faced with the new wealth of genomic data and the potential for manipulating genes, what are the challenges and limitations for determining the genetic influence on behavior? While it is obvious that certain genes play a pre-eminent role in the encoding of particular behaviors, and that the individual's current environment and past life events have a major impact on expression patterns and epigenetic programming, neither genes nor environment act alone in determining development and patterns of behavior. An as yet little-explored level of complexity comes from the interactions between genetic and epigenetic mechanisms involving DNA methylation and histone acetylation in determining gene expression. The future challenge for behavioral genetics applied to the elucidation of neurocircuitries of cognition, emotionality, and related brain pathology associated with depression will be the shift from the analysis of gene sequence and protein structure to gene and protein function as well as to the understanding of disease mechanisms. In order to achieve this goal, the application of biological knowledge in the elucidation of functional information will be essential. The sequel to the gene knowledge spiral will therefore be extraction and integration of experimental data, construction of gene and protein networks, and the creation of functional information by feedback from simulation to empirical approaches.

We are clearly a long way from completely understanding the neural mechanisms of social cognitive phenomena and effective social functioning (Amodio and Frith, 2006). Yet, the potential impact of *5-HTT* variation on social cognition is currently transcending the borders of behavioral genetics to embrace biosocial science, thus resulting in a new microcosm of "social neurogenetics of behavior" (Lesch, 2007). Biosocial science has been conceptualized to transform our understanding of problems ranging from gender-specific behavior, marriage and the family as a social institution, to "freedom of will" and legal responsibility, as well as to the natural history of moral obligation (Butz and Torrey, 2006). As analyses of genomes of humans, non-human primates, and other species has contributed fundamentally to understanding how humans have evolved and how they (mal)function, biosocially focused genomics is about to provide insight into phenomena such as prehistoric migrations of human populations. It has matured to explore the nature of genetic variation among humans and its influence on inter-individual differences, as well as the relative impact of genetic and environmental determinants on non-human primate and human cognition and behavior. Neurosocial science increasingly uses imaging to study the neural basis of economic, social, and political behavior, examining such phenomena as social conformity, decision-making, empathy, and time preference. For example, there is evidence for a neurobiological link entrenched deeply in multidimensional cognitive and emotional processes of decision-making, between the experienced displeasure of dread and subsequent decisions about unpleasant outcomes (Berns *et al.*, 2006). The integration of biosocial paradigms in behavioral genetics to test species generality of hypotheses contributes more and more observations that will eventually tear down some long-standing myths about the uniqueness of human behavior. Although the increasing impact of genetics on social sciences has long been anticipated and represents an inevitable, although preferred, development, the transition from complicated correlations to useful prediction is now the basic challenge.

ACKNOWLEDGMENTS

The writing of this chapter and the author's related research were supported by the European Commission (NEWMOOD LSHM-CT-2003-503474), Bundesministerium für Bildung und Forschung (IZKF 01 KS 9603) and the Deutsche Forschungsgemeinschaft (SFB 581, SFB TRR 58, KFO 125).

REFERENCES

Abkevich V, Camp N J, Hensel C H, *et al.* (2003). Predisposition locus for major depression at chromosome 12q22–12q23.2. *Am J Hum Genet* **73**: 1271–81.

Allman J M, Watson K K, Tetreault N A, Hakeem A Y (2005). Intuition and autism: a possible role for Von Economo neurons. *Trends Cogn Sci* **9**: 367–73.

Altamura C, Dell'Acqua M L, Moessner R, Murphy D L, Lesch K P, Persico A M (2006). Altered neocortical cell density and layer thickness in serotonin transporter knockout mice: a quantitation study. *Cereb Cortex* **17**: 1394–401.

Amodio D M, Frith C D (2006). Meeting of minds: the medial frontal cortex and social cognition. *Nat Rev Neurosci* **7**: 268–77.

Azmitia E C, Whitaker-Azmitia P M (1997). Development and adult plasticity of serotonergic neurons and their target cells. In Baumgarten H G, Göthert M, editors. *Serotonergic neurons and 5-HT receptors in the CNS.* Berlin: Springer, pp. 1–39.

Bachner-Melman R, Dina C, Zohar A H, *et al.* (2005). AVPR1a and SLC6A4 gene polymorphisms are associated with creative dance performance. *PLoS Genet* **1**: e42.

Ball D, Hill L, Freeman B, *et al.* (1997). The serotonin transporter gene and peer-rated neuroticism. *Neuroreport* **8**: 1301–04.

Barr C S, Newman T K, Becker M L, *et al.* (2003). The utility of the non-human primate; model for studying gene by environment interactions in behavioral research. *Genes Brain Behav* **2**: 336–40.

Barr C S, Newman T K, Lindell S, *et al.* (2004a). Interaction between serotonin transporter gene variation and rearing condition in alcohol preference and consumption in female primates. *Arch Gen Psychiatry* **61**: 1146–52.

Barr C S, Newman T K, Schwandt M, *et al.* (2004b). Sexual dichotomy of an interaction between early adversity and the serotonin transporter gene promoter variant in rhesus macaques. *Proc Natl Acad Sci USA* **101**: 12 358–63.

Baumeister R F, Tice D M (1990). Anxiety and social exclusion. *J Social Clin Psychol* **9**: 165–95.

Bengel D, Greenberg B, Cora-Locatelli G, *et al.* (1999). Association of the serotonin transporter promoter regulatory region polymorphism and obsessive–compulsive disorder. *Mol Psychiatry* **4**: 463–6.

Bengel D, Heils A, Petri S, *et al.* (1997). Gene structure and 5′-flanking regulatory region of the murine serotonin transporter. *Brain Res Mol Brain Res* **44**: 286–92.

Bengel D, Murphy D L, Andrews A M, *et al.* (1998). Altered brain serotonin homeostasis and locomotor insensitivity to 3,4-methylenedioxymethamphetamine ("Ecstasy") in serotonin transporter-deficient mice. *Mol Pharmacol* **53**: 649–55.

Bennett A J, Lesch K P, Heils A, *et al.* (2002). Early experience and serotonin transporter gene variation interact to influence primate CNS function. *Mol Psychiatry* **7**: 118–22.

Berns G S, Chappelow J, Cekic M, Zink CF, Pagnoni G, Martin-Skurski M E (2006). Neurobiological substrates of dread. *Science* **312**: 754–8.

Bertolino A, Arciero G, Rubino V, *et al.* (2005). Variation of human amygdala response during threatening stimuli as a function of 5′HTTLPR genotype and personality style. *Biol Psychiatry* **57**: 1517–25.

Blakely R D, Berson H E, Fremeau R T, Jr., *et al.* (1991). Cloning and expression of a functional serotonin transporter from rat brain. *Nature* **354**: 66–70.

Bloch M H, Landeros-Weisenberger A, Sen S, *et al.* (2008). Association of the serotonin transporter polymorphism and obsessive–compulsive disorder: systematic review. *Am J Med Genet B Neuropsychiatr Genet* **147B**: 850–8.

Bouchard T J (1994). Genes, environment and personality. *Science* **264**: 1700–01.

Brown G W, Harris T O (2008). Depression and the serotonin transporter 5-HTTLPR polymorphism: a review and a hypothesis concerning gene-environment interaction. *J Affect Disord.*

Buss D M (1991). Evolutionary personality psychology. *Annu Rev Psychol* **42**: 459–91.

Butz W P, Torrey B B (2006). Some frontiers in social science. *Science* **312**: 1898–900.

Canli T, Congdon E, Todd Constable R, Lesch K P (2008). Additive effects of serotonin transporter and tryptophan hydroxylase-2 gene variation on neural correlates of affective processing. *Biol Psychol* **79**: 118–25.

Canli T, Lesch K P (2007). Long story short: the serotonin transporter in emotion regulation and social cognition. *Nat Neurosci* **10**: 1103–09.

Canli T, Omura K, Haas B W, Fallgatter A, Constable R T, Lesch K P (2005). Beyond affect: a role for genetic variation of the serotonin transporter in neural activation during a cognitive attention task. *Proc Natl Acad Sci USA* **102**: 12 224–9.

Canli T, Qiu M, Omura K, *et al.* (2006). Neural correlates of epigenesis. *Proc Natl Acad Sci U S A* **103**: 16 033–8.

Carola V, Frazzetto G, Pascucci T, *et al.* (2008). Identifying molecular substrates in a mouse model of the serotonin transporter × environment risk factor for anxiety and depression. *Biol Psychiatry* **63**: 840–6.

Carr L, Iacoboni M, Dubeau M C, Mazziotta J C, Lenzi G L (2003). Neural mechanisms of empathy in humans: a relay from neural systems for imitation to limbic areas. *Proc Natl Acad Sci USA* **100**: 5497–502.

Caspi A, McClay J, Moffitt T E, *et al.* (2002). Role of genotype in the cycle of violence in maltreated children. *Science* **297**: 851–4.

Caspi A, Sugden K, Moffitt T E, *et al.* (2003). Influence of life stress on depression: moderation by a polymorphism in the 5-HTT gene. *Science* **301**: 386–9.

Champoux M, Bennett A, Shannon C, Higley J D, Lesch K P, Suomi S J (2002). Serotonin transporter gene polymorphism, differential early rearing, and behavior in rhesus monkey neonates. *Mol Psychiatry* **7**: 1058–63.

Cho H J, Meira-Lima I, Cordeiro Q, *et al.* (2005). Population-based and family-based studies on the serotonin transporter gene polymorphisms and bipolar disorder: a systematic review and meta-analysis. *Mol Psychiatry* **10**: 771–81.

Collier D A, Stober G, Li T, *et al.* (1996). A novel functional polymorphism within the promoter of the serotonin transporter gene: possible role in susceptibility to affective disorders. *Mol Psychiatry* **1**: 453–60.

Costa P, Jr, McCrae R R (1992). Revised NEO Personality Inventory (NEO PI-R) and NEO Five-Factor Inventory (NEO-FFI). Psychological Assessment Resources, Florida.

Dapretto M, Davies M S, Pfeifer J H, *et al.* (2006). Understanding emotions in others: mirror neuron dysfunction in children with autism spectrum disorders. *Nat Neurosci* **9**: 28–30.

David S P, Murthy N V, Rabiner E A, *et al.* (2005). A functional genetic variation of the serotonin (5-HT) transporter affects 5-HT1A receptor binding in humans. *J Neurosci* **25**: 2586–90.

de Waal F B M, Luttrell L M (1989). Toward a comparative socioecology of the genus *Macaca:* different dominance styles in rhesus and stumptailed macaques. *Am J Primatol* **19**: 83–109.

Di Bella D, Catalano M, Balling U, Smeraldi E, Lesch K P (1996). Systematic screening for mutations in the coding region of the human serotonin transporter (5-HTT) gene using PCR and DGGE. *Am J Med Genet* **67**: 541–5.

Di Pino G, Mössner R, Lesch K P, Lauder J M, Persico A M (2004). Serotonin roles in neurodevelopment: more than just neural transmission. *Curr Neuropharmacol* **2**: 403–17.

Dreary I J, Battersby S, Whiteman M C, Connor J M, Fowkes F G, Harmar A (1999). Neuroticism and polymorphisms in the serotonin transporter gene. *Psychol Med* **29**: 735–9.

Fallgatter A, Jatzke S, Bartsch A, Hamelbeck B, Lesch K (1999). Serotonin transporter promoter polymorphism influences topography of inhibitory motor control. *Int J Neuropsychopharmacol* **2**: 115–20.

Fallgatter A J, Herrmann M J, Roemmler J, *et al.* (2004). Allelic variation of serotonin transporter function modulates the brain electrical response for error processing. *Neuropsychopharmacology* **29**: 1506–11.

Felitti V J, Anda R F, Nordenberg D, *et al.* (1998). Relationship of childhood abuse and household dysfunction to many of the leading causes of death in adults. The Adverse Childhood Experiences (ACE) Study. *Am J Prev Med* **14**: 245–58.

Furmark T, Tillfors M, Garpenstrand H, *et al.* (2004). Serotonin transporter polymorphism related to amygdala excitability and symptom severity in patients with social phobia. *Neurosci Lett* **362**: 189–92.

Gaspar P, Cases O, Maroteaux L (2003). The developmental role of serotonin: news from mouse molecular genetics. *Nat Rev Neurosci* **4**: 1002–12.

Gelernter J, Kranzler H, Cubells J F (1997). Serotonin transporter protein (SLC6A4) allele and haplotype frequencies and linkage disequilibria in African- and European-American and Japanese populations and in alcohol-dependent subjects. *Hum Genet* **101**: 243–6.

Glatt C E, DeYoung J A, Delgado S, *et al.* (2001). Screening a large reference sample to identify very low frequency sequence variants: comparisons between two genes. *Nat Genet* **27**: 435–8.

Gould E (1999). Serotonin hippocampal neurogenesis. *Neuropsychopharmacology* **21**: 46S–51S.

Greenberg B D, Li Q, Lucas F R, *et al.* (2000). Association between the serotonin transporter promoter polymorphism and personality traits in a primarily female population sample. *Am J Med Genetics* **96**: 202–16.

Greenberg B D, Tolliver T J, Huang S J, Li Q, Bengel D, Murphy D L (1999). Genetic variation in the serotonin transporter promoter region affects serotonin uptake in human blood platelets. *Am J Med Genet* **88**: 83–7.

Gross C, Hen R (2004). The developmental origins of anxiety. *Nat Rev Neurosci* **5**: 545–52.

Gross C, Zhuang X, Stark K, *et al.* (2002). Serotonin1A receptor acts during development to establish normal anxiety-like behavior in the adult. *Nature* **416**: 396–400.

Gutknecht L, Jacob C, Strobel A, *et al.* (2007). Tryptophan hydroxylase-2 gene variation influences personality traits and disorders related to emotional dysregulation. *Int J Neuropsychopharmacol* **10**: 309–20.

Hammock E A, Young L J (2005). Microsatellite instability generates diversity in brain and sociobehavioral traits. *Science* **308**: 1630–4.

Hanna G L, Himle J A, Curtis G C, *et al.* (1998). Serotonin transporter and seasonal variation in blood serotonin in families with obsessive–compulsive disorder. *Neuropsychopharmacology* **18**: 102–11.

Hariri A R, Mattay V S, Tessitore A, *et al.* (2002). Serotonin transporter genetic variation and the response of the human amygdala. *Science* **297**: 400–03.

Heils A, Teufel A, Petri S, *et al.* (1995). Functional promoter and polyadenylation site mapping of the human serotonin (5-HT) transporter gene. *J Neural Transm Gen Sect* **102**: 247–54.

Heils A, Wichems C, Mossner R, *et al.* (1998). Functional characterization of the murine serotonin transporter gene promoter in serotonergic raphe neurons. *J Neurochem* **70**: 932–9.

Heinz A, Braus D F, Smolka M N, *et al.* (2005). Amygdala–prefrontal coupling depends on a genetic variation of the serotonin transporter. *Nat Neurosci* **8**: 20–1.

Heinz A, Jones D W, Mazzanti C, *et al.* (1999). A relationship between serotonin transporter genotype and in vivo protein expression and alcohol neurotoxicity. *Biol Psychiatry* **47**: 643–9.

Herman A I, Kaiss K M, Ma R, *et al.* (2005). Serotonin transporter promoter polymorphism and monoamine oxidase type A VNTR allelic variants together influence alcohol binge drinking risk in young women. *Am J Med Genet B Neuropsychiatr Genet* **133**: 74–8.

Herrmann M J, Huter T, Muller F, *et al.* (2007). Additive effects of serotonin transporter and tryptophan hydroxylase-2 gene variation on emotional processing. *Cereb Cortex* **17**: 1160–3.

Hertting G, Axelrod J (1961). Fate of tritiated noradrenaline at the sympathetic nerve-endings. *Nature* **192**: 172–3.

Higley J D, Linnoila M (1997). A nonhuman primate model of excessive alcohol intake. Personality and neurobiological parallels of type I- and type II-like alcoholism. *Recent Dev Alcohol* **13**: 191–219.

Higley J D, Suomi S J, Linnoila M (1991). CSF monoamine metabolite concentrations vary according to age, rearing, and sex, and are influenced by the stressor of social separation in rhesus monkeys. *Psychopharmacology* **103**: 551–6.

Higley J D, Suomi S J, Linnoila M (1992). A longitudinal assessment of CSF monoamine metabolite and plasma cortisol concentrations in young rhesus monkeys. *Biol Psychiatry* **32**: 127–45.

Holmans P, Zubenko G S, Crowe R R, *et al.* (2004). Genomewide significant linkage to recurrent, early-onset major depressive disorder on chromosome 15q. *Am J Hum Genet* **74**: 1154–67.

Holmes A, Lit Q, Murphy D L, Gold E, Crawley J N (2003). Abnormal anxiety-related behavior in serotonin transporter null mutant mice: the influence of genetic background. *Genes Brain Behav* **2**: 365–80.

Iacoboni M (2005). Neural mechanisms of imitation. *Curr Opin Neurobiol* **15**: 632–7.

Ichikawa M, Okamura-Oho Y, Shimokawa K, *et al.* (2008). Expression analysis for inverted effects of serotonin transporter inactivation. *Biochem Biophys Res Commun* **368**: 43–9.

Ishiguro H, Arinami T, Yamada K, Otsuka Y, Toru M, Shibuya H (1997). An association study between a transcriptional polymorphism in the serotonin transporter gene and panic disorder in a Japanese population. *Psychiatry Clin Neurosci* **51**: 333–5.

Jacob C P, Muller J, Schmidt M, *et al.* (2005). Cluster B personality disorders are associated with allelic variation of monoamine oxidase A activity. *Neuropsychopharmacology* **30**: 1711–8.

Jorm A F, Henderson A S, Jacomb P A, *et al.* (1998). An association study of a functional polymorphism of the serotonin transporter gene with personality and psychiatric symptoms. *Mol Psychiatry* **3**: 449–51.

Katsuragi S, Kunugi H, Sano A, *et al.* (1999). Association between serotonin transporter gene polymorphism and anxiety-related traits. *Biol Psychiatry* **45**: 368–70.

Kendler K S (1996). Major depression and generalised anxiety disorder. Same genes, (partly) different environments – revisited. *Br J Psychiatry* Suppl: 68–75.

Kendler K S (1998). Major depression and the environment: a psychiatric genetic perspective. *Pharmacopsychiatry* **31**: 5–9.

Kendler K S, Karkowski L M, Prescott C A (1999). Causal relationship between stressful life events and the onset of major depression. *Am J Psychiatry* **156**: 837–41.

Kendler K S, Walters E E, Neale M C, Kessler R C, Heath A C, Eaves L J (1995). The structure of the genetic and environmental risk factors for six major psychiatric disorders in women. Phobia, generalized anxiety disorder, panic disorder, bulimia, major depression, and alcoholism. *Arch Gen Psychiatry* **52**: 374–83.

Klauck S M, Poustka F, Benner A, Lesch K P, Poustka A (1997). Serotonin transporter (5-HTT) gene variants associated with autism? *Hum Mol Genet* **6**: 2233–8.

Knutson B, Wolkowitz O M, Cole S W, *et al.* (1998). Selective alteration of personality and social behavior by serotonergic intervention. *Am J Psychiatry* **155**: 373–9.

Kovacs M, Devlin B, Pollock M, Richards C, Mukerji P (1997). A controlled family history study of childhood-onset depressive disorder. *Arch Gen Psychiatry* **54**: 613–23.

Kovas Y, Plomin R (2006). Generalist genes: implications for the cognitive sciences. *Trends Cogn Sci* **10**: 198–203.

Kraemer G W, Ebert M H, Schmidt D E, McKinney W T (1989). A longitudinal study of the effect of different social rearing conditions on cerebrospinal fluid norepinephrine and biogenic amine metabolites in rhesus monkeys. *Neuropsychopharmacology* **2**: 175–89.

Kunugi H, Hattori M, Kato T, *et al.* (1997). Serotonin transporter gene polymorphisms: ethnic difference and possible association with bipolar affective disorder. *Mol Psychiatry* **2**: 457–62.

Langer S Z, Zarifian E, Briley M, Raisman R, Sechter D (1981). High-affinity binding of 3H-imipramine in brain and platelets and its relevance to the biochemistry of affective disorders. *Life Sci* **29**: 211–20.

Lauder J M (1990). Ontogeny of the serotonergic system in the rat: serotonin as a developmental signal. *Ann NY Acad Scie* **600**: 297–314.

Lesch K P (2005). Genetic alterations of the murine serotonergic gene pathway: the neurodevelopmental basis of anxiety. *Handb Exp Pharmacol* **169**: 71–112.

Lesch K P (2007). Linking emotion to the social brain. The role of the serotonin transporter in human social behavior. *EMBO Rep 8 Spec No* S24–9.

Lesch K P, Balling U, Gross J, *et al.* (1994). Organization of the human serotonin transporter gene. *J Neural Transm Gen Sect* **95**: 157–62.

Lesch K P, Bengel D, Heils A, *et al.* (1996). Association of anxiety-related traits with a polymorphism in the serotonin transporter gene regulatory region. *Science* **274**: 1527–31.

Lesch K P, Gutknecht L (2004). Focus on The 5-HT1A receptor: emerging role of a gene regulatory variant in psychopathology and pharmacogenetics. *Int J Neuropsychopharmacol* **7**: 381–5.

Lesch K P, Gutknecht L (2005). Pharmacogenetics of the serotonin transporter. *Prog Neuropsychopharmacol Biol Psychiatry* **29**: 1062–73.

Lesch K P, Meyer J, Glatz K, *et al.* (1997). The 5-HT transporter gene-linked polymorphic region (5-HTTLPR) in evolutionary perspective: alternative biallelic variation in rhesus monkeys. Rapid communication. *J Neural Transm* **104**: 1259–66.

Lesch K P, Mossner R (1998). Genetically driven variation in serotonin uptake: is there a link to affective spectrum, neurodevelopmental, and neurodegenerative disorders? *Biol Psychiatry* **44**: 179–92.

Lesch K P, Mössner R (2006). Inactivation of 5HT transport in mice: modeling altered 5HT homeostasis implicated in emotional dysfunction, affective disorders, and somatic syndromes. *Handb Exp Pharmacol* **175**: 417–56.

Lesch K P, Wolozin B L, Estler H C, Murphy D L, Riederer P (1993). Isolation of a cDNA encoding the human brain serotonin transporter. *J Neural Transm Gen Sect* **91**: 67–72.

Levinson D (2006). The genetics of depression: a review. *Biol Psychiatry* **60**: 84–92.

Little K Y, McLaughlin D P, Zhang L, *et al.* (1998). Cocaine, ethanol, and genotype effects on human midbrain serotonin transporter binding sites and mRNA levels. *Am J Psychiatry* **155**: 207–13.

Loehlin J C (1992). *Genes and environment in personality development*. Newburg Park, CA: Sage.

Lotrich F E, Pollock B G (2004). Meta-analysis of serotonin transporter polymorphisms and affective disorders. *Psychiatr Genet* **14**: 121–9.

Lowry C, Johnson P, Hay-Schmidt A, Mikkelsen J, Shekhar A (2005). Modulation of anxiety circuits by serotonergic systems. *Stress* **8**: 233–46.

Lyons M J, Eisen S A, Goldberg J, *et al.* (1998). A registry-based twin study of depression in men. *Arch Gen Psychiatry* **55**: 468–72.

Malhi G S, Moore J, McGuffin P (2000). The genetics of major depressive disorder. *Curr Psychiat Rept* **2**: 165–9.

Matsumura S (1999). The evolution of "egalitarian" and "despotic" social systems among macaques. *Primates* **40**: 23–31.

Mazzanti C M, Lappalainen J, Long J C, *et al.* (1998). Role of the serotonin transporter promoter polymorphism in anxiety-related traits. *Arch Gen Psychiatry* **55**: 936–40.

McDougle C J, Epperson C N, Price L H, Gelernter J (1998). Evidence for linkage disequilibrium between serotonin transporter protein gene (SLC6A4) and obsessive compulsive disorder. *Mol Psychiatry* **3**: 270–3.

McGue M, Bouchard T J (1998). Genetic and environmental influences on human behavioral differences. *Annu Rev Neurosci* **21**: 1–24.

McGuffin P, Katz R, Watkins S, Rutherford J (1996). A hospital-based twin register of the heritability of DSM-IV unipolar depression. *Arch Gen Psychiatry* **53**: 129–36.

McGuffin P, Knight J, Breen G, *et al.* (2005). Whole genome linkage scan of recurrent depressive disorder from the depression network study. *Hum Mol Genet* **14**: 3337–45.

Meyer-Lindenberg A, Buckholtz J W, Kolachana B, *et al.* (2006). Neural mechanisms of genetic risk for impulsivity and violence in humans. *Proc Natl Acad Sci USA* **103**: 6269–74.

Morales J C, Melnick D J (1998). Phylogenetic relationships of the macaques (Cercopithecidae: Macaca), as revealed by high resolution restriction site mapping of mitochondrial ribosomal genes. *J Hum Evo* **34**: 1–12.

Mortensen O V, Thomassen M, Larsen M B, Whittemore S R, Wiborg O (1999). Functional analysis of a novel human serotonin transporter gene promoter in immortalized raphe cells. *Mol Brain Res* **68**: 141–8.

Murphy D L, Lerner A, Rudnick G, Lesch K P (2004). Serotonin transporter: gene, genetic disorders, and pharmacogenetics. *Mol Interv* **4**: 109–23.

Murphy D L, Lesch K P (2008). Targeting the murine serotonin transporter: insights into human neurobiology. *Nat Rev Neurosci* **9**: 85–96.

Murphy D L, Li Q, Engel S, *et al.* (2001). Genetic perspectives on the serotonin transporter. *Brain Res Bull* **56**: 487–94.

Nakamura T, Muramatsu T, Ono Y, *et al.* (1997). Serotonin transporter gene regulatory region polymorphism and anxiety-related traits in the Japanese. *Am J Med Genet* **74**: 544–5.

Newman T K, Syagailo Y V, Barr C S, *et al.* (2005). Monoamine oxidase A gene promoter variation and rearing experience influences aggressive behavior in rhesus monkeys. *Biol Psychiatry* **57**: 167–72.

Nobile M, Begni B, Giorda R, *et al.* (1999). Effects of serotonin transporter promoter genotype on platelet serotonin transporter functionality in depressed children and adolescents. *J Am Acad Child Adolesc Psychiatry* **38**: 1396–402.

Ogilvie A D, Battersby S, Bubb V J, *et al.* (1996). Polymorphism in serotonin transporter gene associated with susceptibility to major depression. *Lancet* **347**: 731–3.

Ono Y, Yoshimura K, Sueoka R, *et al.* (1996). Avoidant personality disorder and taijin kyoufu: sociocultural implications of the WHO/ADAMHA international study of personality disorders in Japan. *Acta Psychiatr Scand* **93**: 172–6.

Ozaki N, Goldman D, Kaye W H, *et al.* (2003). Serotonin transporter missense mutation associated with a complex neuropsychiatric phenotype. *Mol Psychiatry* **8**: 895.

Ozsarac N, Santha E, Hoffman B J (2002). Alternative non-coding exons support serotonin transporter mRNA expression in the brain and gut. *J Neurochem* **82**: 336–44.

Persico A M, Baldi A, Dell'Acqua M L, *et al.* (2003). Reduced programmed cell death in brains of serotonin transporter knockout mice. *Neuroreport* **14**: 341–4.

Persico A M, Mengual E, Moessner R, *et al.* (2001). Barrel pattern formation requires serotonin uptake by thalamocortical afferents, and not vesicular monoamine release. *J Neurosci* **21**: 6862–73.

Pezawas L, Meyer-Lindenberg A, Drabant E M, *et al.* (2005). 5-HTTLPR polymorphism impacts human cingulate–amygdala interactions: a genetic susceptibility mechanism for depression. *Nat Neurosci* **8**: 828–34.

Phelps E A (2006). Emotion and cognition: insights from studies of the human amygdala. *Annu Rev Psychol* **57**: 27–53.

Plomin R, Owen M J, McGuffin P (1994). The genetic basis of complex human behaviors. *Science* **264**: 1733–9.

Raisman R, Briley M, Langer S Z (1979). Specific tricyclic antidepressant binding sites in rat brain. *Nature* **281**: 148–50.

Reif A, Lesch K P (2003). Toward a molecular architecture of personality. *Behav Brain Res* **139**: 1–20.

Reif A, Rosler M, Freitag C M, *et al.* (2007). Nature and nurture predispose to violent behavior: serotonergic genes and adverse childhood environment. *Neuropsychopharmacology* **32**: 2375–83.

Rizzolatti G, Craighero L (2004). The mirror-neuron system. *Annu Rev Neurosci* **27**: 169–92.

Rogers J, Kaplan J, Garcia R, Shelledy W, Nair S, Cameron J (2006). Mapping of the serotonin transporter locus (SLC6A4) to rhesus chromosome 16 using genetic linkage. *Cytogenet Genome Res* **112**: 341A.

Salichon N, Gaspar P, Upton A L, *et al.* (2001). Excessive activation of serotonin (5-HT) 1B receptors disrupts the formation of sensory maps in monoamine oxidase A and 5-HT transporter knock-out mice. *J Neurosci* **21**: 884–96.

Samochowiec J, Lesch K P, Rottmann M, *et al.* (1999). Association of a regulatory polymorphism in the promoter region of the monoamine oxidase A gene with antisocial alcoholism. *Psychiatry Res* **86**: 67–72.

Schinka J A, Busch R M, Robichaux-Keene N (2004). A meta-analysis of the association between the serotonin transporter gene polymorphism (5-HTTLPR) and trait anxiety. *Mol Psychiatry* **9**: 197–202.

Schmidt L G, Sander T, Kuhn S, *et al.* (2000). Different allele distribution of a regulatory MAOA gene promoter polymorphism in antisocial and anxious-depressive alcoholics. *J Neural Transm* **107**: 681–9.

Sen S, Burmeister M, Ghosh D (2004). Meta-analysis of the association between a serotonin transporter promoter polymorphism (5-HTTLPR) and anxiety-related personality traits. *Am J Med Genet B Neuropsychiatr Genet* **127**: 85–9.

Serretti A, Benedetti F, Zanardi R, Smeraldi E (2005). The influence of serotonin transporter promoter polymorphism (SERTPR) and other polymorphisms of the serotonin pathway on the efficacy of antidepressant treatments. *Prog Neuropsychopharmacol Biol Psychiatry* **29**: 1074–84.

Silberg J, Pickles A, Rutter M, *et al.* (1999). The influence of genetic factors and life stress on depression among adolescent girls. *Arch Gen Psychiatry* **56**: 225–32.

Sirota L A, Greenberg B D, Murphy D L, Hamer D H (1999). Non-linear association between the serotonin transporter promoter polymorphism and neuroticism: a caution against using extreme samples to identify quantitative trait loci. *Psychiatric Genet* **9**: 35–8.

Strobel A, Dreisbach G, Muller J, Goschke T, Brocke B, Lesch K P (2007). Genetic variation of serotonin function and cognitive control. *J Cogn Neurosci* **19**: 1923–31.

Sullivan P F, Neale M C, Kendler K S (2000). Genetic epidemiology of major depression: review and meta-analysis. *Am J Psychiatry* **157**: 1552–62.

Sutcliffe J S, Delahanty R J, Prasad H C, *et al.* (2005). Allelic heterogeneity at the serotonin transporter locus (SLC6A4) confers susceptibility to autism and rigid-compulsive behaviors. *Am J Hum Genet* **77**: 265–79.

Thapar A, McGuffin P (1997). Anxiety and depressive symptoms in childhood – a genetic study of comorbidity. *J Child Psychol Psychiatry* **38**: 651–6.

Thierry B (1990). Feedback loop between kinship and dominance: the macaque model. *J Theor Biol* **145**: 511–21.

Thierry B (2000). Covariation of conflict management patterns across macaque species. In Aureli F, de Waal FBM, editors. *Natural conflict resolution*. Berkeley, CA: University of California Press, pp. 106–28.

Thierry B, Iwaniuk A N, Pellis S M (2000). The influence of phylogeny on the social behavior of macaques (Primates: Cercopithecidae, genus *Macaca*). *Ethology* **106**: 713–28.

Uddin L Q, Kaplan J T, Molnar-Szakacs I, Zaidel E, Iacoboni M (2005). Self-face recognition activates a frontoparietal "mirror" network in the right hemisphere: an event-related fMRI study. *Neuroimage* **25**: 926–35.

Uher R, McGuffin P (2008). The moderation by the serotonin transporter gene of environmental adversity in the aetiology of mental illness: review and methodological analysis. *Mol Psychiatry* **13**: 131–46.

Weaver I C, Cervoni N, Champagne F A, *et al.* (2004). Epigenetic programming by maternal behavior. *Nat Neurosci* **7**: 847–54.

Weaver I C, Meaney M J, Szyf M (2006). Maternal care effects on the hippocampal transcriptome and anxiety-mediated behaviors in the offspring that are reversible in adulthood. *Proc Natl Acad Sci USA* **103**: 3480–5.

Wendland J R, Lesch K P, Newman T K, *et al.* (2006a). Differential functional variability of serotonin transporter and monoamine oxidase a genes in macaque species displaying contrasting levels of aggression-related behavior. *Behav Genet* **36**: 163–72.

Wendland J R, Martin B J, Kruse M R, Lesch K P, Murphy D L (2006b). Simultaneous genotyping of four functional loci of human SLC6A4, with a reappraisal of 5-HTTLPR and rs25531. *Mol Psychiatry* **11**: 224–6.

Wilson E O (1975). *Sociobiology: the new synthesis*. Cambridge, MA: Harvard University Press.

Wilson E O (1978). *On human nature*. Cambridge, MA: Harvard University Press.

Zubenko G S, Maher B, Hughes H B, 3rd, *et al.* (2003). Genome-wide linkage survey for genetic loci that influence the development of depressive disorders in families with recurrent, early-onset, major depression. *Am J Med Genet* **123B**: 1–18.

Index

Locators in *italic* refer to figures/tables
Locators in **bold** refer to especially significant coverage of the topic
Locators for headings with subheadings refer to general aspects of that topic